Butterworths International Medical Reviews

Clinical Endocrinology 2

Calcium Disorders

Butterworths International Medical Reviews

Clinical Endocrinology 2

Editorial Board
D. C. Anderson
C. G. Beardwell
C. G. D. Brook
C. R. W. Edwards
D. A. Heath
S. J. Marx
G. L. Robertson
D. M. Styne
J. Winter

Published in this Series

Volume 1 The Pituitary
Edited by Colin Beardwell *and* Gary L. Robertson

Next Volume

Endocrine Effects of Dopamine

Butterworths
International
Medical
Reviews

Clinical
Endocrinology 2

Calcium Disorders

Edited by
David Heath, MB ChB, MRCP
Reader in Medicine
Queen Elizabeth Hospital
Birmingham, UK

and

Stephen J. Marx, MD
Senior Investigator
Metabolic Diseases Branch
National Institute of Arthritis, Diabetes, Digestive and
Kidney Diseases
National Institutes of Health
Bethesda
Maryland, USA

Butterworth Scientific
London Boston
Sydney Wellington Durban Toronto

First published 1982

© Butterworth & Co (Publishers) Ltd. 1982

British Library Cataloguing in Publication Data

Clinical endocrinology.–2.–(Butterworths
    international medical reviews)
    1. Endocrinology–Periodicals
    616.4′05   RC648

    ISBN 0-407-02273-2
    ISSN 0260-0072

Photoset by Butterworths Litho Preparation Department
Printed and bound in England by Hartnoll Print Ltd., Bodmin,
Cornwall.

Preface

In the past decade, major discoveries have been made in the field of mineral metabolism and its endocrine controls. Many of these discoveries have resulted in rapid changes in clinical practice. The physician must now select judiciously among an array of sophisticated and often expensive diagnostic tests. He or she should make decisions that are justified by basic principles of mineral homeostasis. This volume contains material reviewing many of the topics in which knowledge has accumulated most rapidly.

We have tried to select topics of interest to a wide variety of endocrinologists as well as clinicians working in other branches of medicine. It was not our intention that contributors should write an exhaustive and complete review of their subject but to concentrate where possible on the recent literature and where alternative managements are available to outline their own personal policy.

Authors were encouraged to limit the number of references using wherever possible recent reports which themselves can be used as sources of the previous literature.

We would like to thank our contributors for making the effort to produce what we hope will be an important book. Finally, we wish to record our gratitude to the staff of Butterworths for their patience and persistence throughout the evolution of this volume.

David Heath
Stephen Marx

List of Contributors

J. M. Aitken, MD, FRCP
Consultant Physician, Essex County Hospital, Colchester, Essex, UK

Jack W. Coburn, MD
Medical and Research Services, VA Wadsworth Medical Center and Department of Medicine, UCLA School of Medicine, Los Angeles, Calif., USA

M. G. Dunnigan, MD, FRCP
Consultant Physician, Department of Medicine, Stobhill General Hospital, Glasgow, UK

J. A. Ford, MRCP
Consultant Paediatrician, Paediatrics Unit, Rutherglen Maternity Hospital, Rutherglen, UK

D. Fraser, MD, PhD
Professor of Pediatrics and Physiology, Departments of Pediatrics and Physiology, University of Toronto; and Research Institute, The Hospital for Sick Children, Toronto, Ont., Canada

John G. Haddad, MD
Professor of Medicine and Director, Endocrine Section, University of Pennsylvania Medical School, Philadelphia, Penn., USA

David A. Heath, MB ChB, MRCP
Reader in Medicine, University of Birmingham, Queen Elizabeth Hospital, Birmingham, UK

Hunter Heath III, MD
Consultant in Endocrine Research, Mayo Clinic; and Associate Professor of Medicine, Mayo Medical School, Rochester, Minn., USA

Laura S. Hillman, MD
Associate Professor of Pediatrics, Department of Neonatology, St Louis Children's
Hospital, St Louis, Mo., USA

S. W. Kooh, MD, PhD
Assistant Professor of Paediatrics and Physiology, University of Toronto; and
Research Institute, The Hospital for Sick Children, Toronto, Ont., Canada

Burt A. Liebross, MD
Medical and Research Services, VA Wadsworth Medical Center and Department
of Medicine, UCLA School of Medicine, Los Angeles, Calif., USA

P. A. Lucas, MB, MRCP
Lecturer in Medicine, Department of Renal Medicine, Welsh National School of
Medicine, Cardiff, UK

Stephen J. Marx, MD
Senior Investigator, Metabolic Diseases Branch, National Institute of Arthritis,
Diabetes, Digestive and Kidney Diseases, National Institutes of Health, Bethesda,
Md., USA

W. B. McIntosh, FIMLS
Senior Chief Medical Laboratory Officer, Department of Biochemistry, Stobhill
General Hospital, Glasgow, UK

Don C. Purnell, MD
Consultant in Endocrinology and Internal Medicine, Mayo Clinic; and Associate
Professor of Medicine, Mayo Medical School, Rochester, Minn., USA

B. Lawrence Riggs, MD
Professor of Medicine, Mayo Medical School; and Chairman, Division of
Endocrinology, Metabolism and Internal Medicine, Mayo Clinic, Rochester,
Minn., USA

Iris Robertson, BSc, DipStat
Lecturer, Department of Mathematics, University of Strathclyde, Glasgow, UK

R. G. G. Russell, PhD, DM, FRCP, MRCPath
Professor of Human Metabolism and Clinical Biochemistry, University of Sheffield
Medical School, Sheffield, UK

C. R. Scriver, MD
Professor of Pediatrics, Biology and Human Genetics, Department of Biology and
Center for Human Genetics, McGill University, Montreal, PQ, Canada

Ego Seeman, MD
Research Fellow in Endocrinology, Mayo Graduate School of Medicine,
Rochester, Minn., USA

J. S. Woodhead, PhD
Senior Lecturer, Department of Medical Biochemistry, Welsh National School of
Medicine, Cardiff, UK

Contents

1
Hereditary rickets

C. R. Scriver, D. Fraser and S. W. Kooh

INTRODUCTION

Since the first description of 'vitamin D-resistant osteomalacia' by Albright *et al.*[1], in 1937, it has become obvious that there exists an increasingly large and diversified list of heritable rachitic conditions. The early classifications[33, 50] of the various syndromes were descriptive. However, as more discrete conditions are added to the list, and as more information is acquired about the pathogenetic mechanisms of the human diseases and their animal analogues, it becomes clear that the individual conditions represent paradigms of genetic phenomena.

Our approach in this paper will be to look first at the evolutionary steps through which phosphate has become central to the energetics of all cell processes and calcium has become a key mediator of cellular function. In the evolutionary scheme, genes determine enzymes and hormones which in turn establish homeostatic mechanisms. Accordingly, we will examine mechanisms of phosphate and calcium homeostasis, and consider how they can be targets for mutation leading to various rachitic syndromes. With this background, we will describe specific forms of rickets and osteomalacia,* examine how they fit in with the present knowledge of cell control and function, and finally indicate how the understanding of pathogenetic mechanisms can be used to design logical therapies.

The heritability† of rickets has, in general, been increasing in modern man because environmental causes have abated. Accordingly, our emphasis on intrinsic causes of rickets is appropriate. Our goal is to encourage the physician to anticipate and prevent the consequences of rickets by the application of genetic principles to the patient.

---

* The term *rickets* in this article refers to a disorder of mineral deposition in preosseous cartilage of growth plates and matrix of growing bone; *osteomalacia* refers to a similar disorder of endosteal remodeling in bone matrix.

† Heritability (h^2) is a population statistic parameter that expresses the genetic contribution to the observed trait[152]. In the broad sense, h^2 is defined by the relationship V_G/V_P where V_G and V_P refer to the total genotypic and phenotypic variance respectively. Since V_G is relatively constant over short intervals of time in human populations, increase in h^2 reflects a decrease in the environmental variance (V_P).

THE COMPONENTS OF MINERAL METABOLISM: THE EVOLUTIONARY PERSPECTIVE

Earth cooled and solidified during her first billion years of geochemical evolution, and phosphate was trapped in igneous rocks of the lithosphere[67]. Since molecular oxygen was also present in the lithosphere, phosphorus occurred as phosphate. The anion became available to biological evolution when leaching by oceans produced sedimentary deposits of inorganic phosphates. Phosphate became sufficiently abundant to support evolution of prokaryotes at least 1.5 billion years ago and probably as long ago as 3 billion years. When cellular energy metabolism became irrevocably coupled with phosphate and oxygen in solution, evolution of eukaryotes and multicellular organisms could be sustained[119].

Vertebrate evolution began about 400 million years ago. The skeleton of later vertebrate evolution is bone, a tissue with adaptive advantages over cartilage. Attainment of a stable internal phosphate pool was necessary for the evolution of mineralization. Thus, cells and organisms became dependent on phosphate long ago, and those that possessed mechanisms to capture the anion from the environments to compartmentalize it and to control its cellular content were more fit in the Darwinian sense. Phosphate transport systems in membranes were the phenotype, and genes to control them were the genotype that conferred advantage. Mutant phenotypes with disturbed phosphate transport are found throughout evolution, from prokaryotes to man, and are the price paid for the selective advantage attached to the normal genes at the relevant loci.

The case for calcium is somewhat similar. Biologists consider calcium to be so important 'that evolution simply could not help bestowing upon it one role after another'[88]. Calcium was available in primeval oceans but whereas phosphate was first selected for the energetics of biological systems, calcium seems to have been selected initially for its role in excitation–response coupling in cells. Later, during vertebrate evolution, it was readily stored in chemical union with phosphate, as hydroxyapatite $(Ca_{10}(PO_4)_6(OH_2))$, in the skeleton from whence it could be recalled to maintain calcium pools in biological fluids and be controlled within narrow limits by hormones.

Parathyroid hormone and vitamin D are the principal hormone products of vertebrate evolution that regulate extracellular phosphorus and calcium homeostasis. Calmodulin[156] and vitamin D-dependent calcium-binding protein[155] are the principal intracellular gene products controlling calcium activity. The role of calcitonin is less well understood and some consider it a vestigial hormone in man[5]. Parathyroid hormone and vitamin D both expose mineral pools in bone. The former also acts on kidney to conserve calcium and reject the attendant phosphate anion in glomerular filtrate; the latter also acts on the intestine to enhance absorption of both calcium and phosphate.

Parathyroid hormone is synthesized, processed, and secreted by the parathyroid chief cell; the signal for control of hormone release is the activity of calcium ion on the parathyroid cell. The hormone acts on target cells by binding to a specific plasma membrane receptor. Its signal is translated by a membrane coupling protein to activate adenylcyclase; the product is a cyclic nucleotide that acts to modulate a cellular component and its function. Mendelian disorders of biosynthesis and release (such as familial hyperparathyroidism), and target cell response (such as pseudohypoparathyroidism) are known.

Vitamin D is produced by skin (in stratum spinosum, and stratum basale) through a complex mechanism[76]. 7-Dehydrocholesterol is photoisomerized to previtamin D_3 by ultraviolet radiation (290–320 nm); previtamin D_3 can be photoisomerized to inert isomers (lumisterol₃ and tachysterol₃) that are in slow reversible chemical equilibrium with previtamin D_3 or thermally isomerized to vitamin D_3. The vitamin is released from skin to blood and bound to an α-globulin (vitamin D binding protein) for transport to liver.

Two factors have a major influence on biosynthesis of vitamin D^{76}. First, the amount of previtamin D_3 formed is dependent on u.v. dosage; at higher latitudes, where dosage is less per unit time than at the equator, exposure to sunlight must be lengthened to obtain the amount of product equivalent to that formed at lower latitudes. Second, melanin competes with 7-dehydrocholecalciferol for u.v. photons; photoproduction of previtamin D_3 and lumisterol₃ is greater per unit time in hypopigmented skin. It follows that conversion to lumisterol₃ and tachysterol₃ is an adaptive mechanism to avert vitamin D_3 intoxication from excessive exposure to sunlight; and hypopigmentation is an adaptive response to enhance vitamin D_3 synthesis in temperate zones. The occurrence of endemic rickets in Asian populations that have migrated to European countries in recent times highlights this relation.

Among the intrinsic factors controlling transport of the vitamins is the plasma vitamin D binding protein (DBP – also known as group-specific substance); though polymorphic in man, to our knowledge this polymorphism is without influence on mineral homeostasis[13]. Hydroxylation to 25-hydroxyvitamin D_3 (25-OHD₃) follows delivery of vitamin D_3 to liver[30]; this step is susceptible to the influence of drugs and hepatobilitary disease. Upon release from liver, the polar metabolite is bound to the vitamin D binding protein in plasma where it constitutes the major circulating form of vitamin D^{53}. The active form of the hormone is attained after intramitochondrial hydroxylation in kidney to form $1,25(OH)_2D_3^{54}$; this step is susceptible to metabolic regulation and it is also the target of at least one Mendelian disorder of vitamin D metabolism, autosomal recessive vitamin D dependency Type I (ARVDD Type I). $1,25(OH)_2D_3$ binds to specific 3.2–3.5s high-affinity intracellular receptors in many target tissues and elicits its spectrum of responses by regulating gene expression; a mutation affecting receptor function in various tissues (intestine, skin, bone, kidney, etc.) is now known (vitamin D dependency Type II–ARVDD Type II).

Organisms do not exist in a vacuum. Interaction with the environment is a constant and obligatory aspect of life. Change, either in the environment or in a gene, can be disadaptive. The organism can respond and maintain homeostasis or decompensate and express disease. Rickets is such a disease.

Human history reveals a constant burden of rickets. Neanderthal man experienced the disease[79], presumably as a consequence of reduced exposure to sunlight during the Ice Age and reduced access to dietary sources of vitamin D. Modern man also experienced rickets as an endemic problem of industrialized societies in northern latitudes[89], again as the consequence of environmental events involving lifestyle and atmospheric pollution. When the antirachitic substance, now known as vitamin D, was discovered[93, 96] and the role of irradiation in its formation recognized[78, 135], preventive measures could be prescribed. The result was a public health enterprise that soon achieved a dramatic decline in the prevalence of endemic rickets. But rickets did not disappear from twentieth-century human society; there have been persistent cases that were 'resistant' to optimization of the environment[87].

The 'new' forms of resistant rickets illuminate the nature: nurture paradigm[23, 122]; rickets in the era of vitamin D fortification has high heritability*. The modern 'cause' of rickets is not so much in the nurture as it is in the nature (genes) of the patient. Mendelian rickets is the laboratory wherein we can discover how evolution committed genes to cellular homeostasis of phosphate and calcium.

CLASSIFICATION OF RICKETS

The process of decompensation during exogenous deficiency of vitamin D occurs in stages in man[48] wherein is the germ of our classification (*Table 1.1*). Hypocalcemia characterizes the initial stage of vitamin D deficiency; blood phosphate is normal. The compensatory response to hypocalcemia involving parathyroid hormone is blunted for reasons yet to be determined. There is no evidence of rickets although subtle changes in the X-ray image of the skull indicate perturbation of mineralization. It may be possible to define the extent of demineralization in the first stage of human vitamin D deficiency by bone histomorphometry but the data have yet to be obtained (Marie, P.J., personal communication, 1981).

The second stage is characterized by normalization of blood calcium. On the other hand, hypophosphatemia emerges as parathyroid hormone is secreted and exerts its renal effect. At this stage, signs of rickets become apparent.

As vitamin D deficiency increases, calcium and phosphate homeostasis are further compromised. The third stage is characterized by severe hypophosphatemia, a return of hypocalcemia, and florid rickets. The tubulopathy of late-stage vitamin D deficiency impairs net reabsorption of many solutes including phosphate. Apparently, both intracellular depletion of calcium activity and the action of parathyroid hormone are necessary to generate the tubulopathy[94].

The appearance of rickets with increasing vitamin D deficiency depends on the occurrence of hypophosphatemia. This observation is the key to our classification[51, 121]. We propose that rachitogenic events are disturbing signals to homeostasis; they are either primarily *calcipenic* or *phosphopenic*. In the concept of homeostasis, a disturbing signal provokes a controlled response to which a controlling response replies. In calcipenic rickets, it is the controlling response (parathyroid hormone secretion) that causes hypophosphatemia. In phosphopenic rickets, the controlled/controlling response loop involves phosphate directly and is inadequate to restore phosphate homeostasis. The concept recognizes extrinsic

*See footnote, p. 1.

Table 1.1 Classification of rickets according to the primary event and heritability (h^2) of the condition

h^2	Calcipenic event	Phosphopenic event
High*	Vitamin D dependency (Type I) (AR)† Vitamin D dependency (Type II) (AR)	Hypophosphatemia [XLH] (XLD) Hypophosphatemia [HBD] (AD¹)§ Hypophosphatemia [ADHR] (AD²)§ Fanconi syndromes (Mendelian forms) (AD, AR)
Intermediate	Idiosyncratic response to anticonvulsant medication; malabsorption syndromes; hepatobiliary disease; renal osteodystrophy	
Low	Vitamin D deficiency** Calcium deficiency	Fanconi syndromes (acquired) Oncogenic rickets Phosphate deficiency

* Only diseases in this category are discussed in detail in the text.
† Abbreviations: AR, autosomal recessive; AD, autosomal dominant; XLD, X-linked dominant; XLH, X-linked hypophosphatemia; HBD, hypophosphatemic bone disease.
§ AD¹ means hypophosphatemic bone disease (HBD); AD² is an autosomal form of hypophosphatemic rickets. (ADHR) distinguished from XLH by inheritance, from HBD by severity of phenotype (see text and *Table 1.4*).
** Vitamin D deficiency has a deviant sex ratio (M:F, 2:1)[25, 52]; therefore it has heritability.

(environmental) and intrinsic (hereditary) disturbing signals (*see Table 1.1*). It also directs treatment. Primary repair of calcium homeostasis with vitamin D or calcium is indicated in calcipenic rickets; primary repair of phosphate homeostasis by anion replacement is indicated in phosphopenic rickets. Since the latter may perturb calcium homeostasis[110] the use of supplemental vitamin D is often indicated in treatment of phosphopenia.

MECHANISMS OF HOMEOSTASIS

In this section we examine homeostasis of the principal determinants of rachitic disease: phosphate, calcium and vitamin D. Phosphopenic rickets is the consequence of primary disruptions of phosphate homeostasis. Calcipenic rickets follows impairment of vitamin D homeostasis which in turn will perturb phosphate metabolism. Accordingly, to understand the mechanism of Mendelian rickets, we must understand the homeostasis of phosphate and the metabolism of vitamin D.

Phosphate homeostasis

Free phosphate anion is absorbed from intestine, distributed throughout extracellular and intracellular fluids, lost from the body in the glomerular filtrate, and largely retrieved by tubular reabsorption. Free anion enters additional pools both as organic derivatives in cells (primarily phosphorylated compounds) and as inorganic derivatives in bone (primarily hydroxyapatite). All endogenous pools of phosphate

Table 1.2 Components of phosphate* homeostasis in the average human adult

Distribution in body pools (mg)		
extracellular	400	
intracellular	900	
bone	40 000	
Renal handling (mg/day)		
filtered†	6500	
reabsorbed	5500	
excreted§		1000
Net absorption from diet (mg/day)		1000
Net balance		0

* Expressed as phosphorus.
† Assuming a Donnan equilibrium across membranes of 1.09, and approximately 20% binding of phosphorus to plasma proteins, the filtered fraction is $0.95 \times GFR \times [P]$ plasma (see Goldberg *et al.*[64] and Dennis *et al.*[32])
§ In this example fractional excretion of phosphate anion

$$FE_P = 1 - \frac{reabsorbed_P}{filtered_P}$$

is 0.153. When phosphorus balance is zero (net intestinal absorption = renal loss) in the steady-state, it follows that any change in FE_P will rapidly influence the extracellular pool.

are ultimately at steady state, usually far from equilibrium, with extracellular phosphate. Within the physiological range, mammals are primarily dependent on diet for supply and on kidney for homeostasis of phosphate (*Table 1.2*).

We consider here the mechanisms that supply and maintain the extracellular concentration of phosphate anion within the narrow limits characteristic of the normal (healthy) phenotype*. Our interest is to show that mutation, impeding membrane transport, will affect phosphate homeostasis and, thus, skeletal mineralization. The nature of the membrane and its carriers is described first. We then address the important and complex issue of vectorial transcellular transport of phosphate and its implications for the epithelia involved in phosphate homeostasis. Lastly we discuss topological aspects of transport along the intestine and nephron.

Membrane transport of phosphate anion

Membranes are an organizing principle in biology[141]. Cellular evolution is characterized by the partitioning of compartments to achieve differentiation of content and function. The earliest cells partitioned extracellular environment from intracellular aqueous phase by a hydrophobic lipid bilayer membrane; subcellular compartments were further defined by internal boundary membranes.

* The serum phosphate concentration (measured as phosphorus) is age and sex dependent (*see Figure 1.3*). Phosphate anion is partitioned as $H_2PO_4^-/HPO_4^=$; at pH 7.4 the ratio of anion species is 19:81.

Lipids in contact with aqueous phases have an organizing force exerted on them; that force is the hydrophobic effect and it determines assembly and structure of lipid bilayers[141]. Assembly of lipids is under thermodynamic control and they aggregate in water as micelles, vesicles, or bilayers according to their chemical nature and the prevailing physical conditions. In the absence of strong attractive forces between constituent molecules, lipid membranes are fluid and deformable. Their plastic nature permits mobility of cells, insertion of components such as proteins, packing for functional organization and resealing after injury. These properties allow the study of phosphate transport in isolated membranes.

Biological membranes play many roles. For example, they have receptor and binding activities, an ability to maintain electrochemical gradients, and the capacity to transfer substances in selective vectorial fashion across their domain. These functions all have specificity. Only proteins can confer specificity to biological functions and it is not surprising that membranes contain proteins as well as lipids. The specificity of a protein is determined by the gene that directs its synthesis. It follows that membrane proteins committed to phosphate transport could be modified by mutation and further, that mutations which impair phosphate homeostasis can be 'markers' of specific phosphate transport processes.

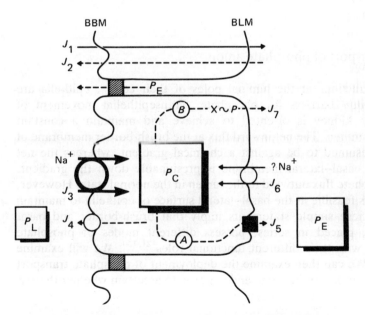

Figure 1.1 A model of transepithelial transport of phosphate applicable to nephron and small intestine. Abbreviations: BBM, brush-border membrane; BLM, basal–lateral membrane; Na^+, sodium ion; P_L, luminal phosphate; P_C, cellular phosphate; P_E, extracellular (antiluminal) phosphate (size of boxes indicates relative concentrations); J, flux; J_1, transcellular absorptive flux; J_2, transcellular outward flux; J_3, absorptive flux at BBM; J_4, backflux at BBM; J_5, outward flux at BLM; J_6, uptake flux at BLM; J_7, metabolic runout flux; A, permeability runout of P_C at steady-state; B, metabolic runout of P_C at steady-state; ◀---P_E, diffusional flux of phosphate from intercellular space at lumen via tight junction; ○, ■, carrier-mediated transport of P

Permeation of living cells by phosphate deviates from its oil–water partition coefficient. Since passive diffusion across the boundary (plasma) membrane does not explain phosphate accumulation, mediation of the process must be considered. Substrate-specific facilitated or exchange diffusion is one possibility; saturable, active, or secondary-active transport is another*. Facilitated diffusion is apparent in erythrocyte membranes[144]; active transport coupled with a Na^+ gradient is found in brush-border membranes of intestine[9] and kidney[75] (*Figure 1.1*), and in the plasma membrane of some somatic cells[84].

Specificity allows the process to differentiate the functional groups of phosphate anion, strip the anion of the water of hydration, and position it correctly for vectorial translocation through the membrane. Little is known about the molecular mechanisms of phosphate transport specificity and the physical nature of anion migration through the membrane but we presume they are analagous to transport on the anion carrier in erythrocyte membrane[114]. Moreover, one presumes the phosphate transport protein – or proteins – span(s) the membrane; if so, the parathyroid hormone-sensitive phosphate carrier in kidney brush-border membranes[42] is accessible to intracellular phosphorylation by protein kinases when activated by cyclic nucleotide.

Transepithelial transport of phosphate anion

By virtue of tight junctions at the luminal poles of their cells[36], epithelia are continuous permeability barriers for phosphate. Transepithelial movement of phosphate in gut or kidney is oriented to achieve and maintain a constant extracellular internal milieu. The net inward flux at the brush-border membrane of epithelial cells is presumed to be against a chemical gradient, whereas the net outward flux at the basal–lateral membrane is presumably down the gradient. There is no net phosphate flux outward to the lumen in the normal state. However, net uptake of anion is feasible at the basal–lateral surface of epithelia to maintain cellular nutrition. These simple statements imply that brush-border and basal –lateral membranes, placed in series, possess different modes of phosphate transport in keeping with their different functional roles[121, 130]. We will examine this possibility first. We can then examine the deployment of phosphate transport along the epithelial cylinders of intestine and nephron to ascertain whether there is further evidence for functional heterogeneity of phosphate transport by epithelia.

---

* Movement of phosphate anion is down its chemical gradient during simple facilitated diffusion; the flux is accelerated when exchange of the 'carrier' is achieved by counter-flux with anion of the same or related species. Active transport implies movement against a chemical gradient and requires energy. Secondary active transport[4] implies that energy is expended to maintain a gradient of another anion which is then co-transported to drive the flux of the primary anion.

NET ABSORPTIVE FLUX (ASYMMETRY OF FLUX)

For net absorption of phosphate to occur in the intestine or nephron, transepithelial inward flux (J_1) must exceed the transepithelial outward flux (J_2) (*see Figure 1.1*). Each flux observes the general relationship:

$$J = K \cdot Pi^* \tag{1}$$

where K is the rate coefficient and Pi^* is the activity of the anion. For net absorption from lumen to occur, only flux J_3 (that influx component of J_1 which is located at brush-border membrane) need exceed efflux J_4 (that component of J_2 which is located at the brush-border membrane). If we assume that the paracellular flux component is a passive diffusion, it follows that net absorption (that is, fractional delivery of phosphate along the cylinder is less than input at the origin) is achieved by events at the brush-border membrane.

Phosphate transport at brush-border membranes of intestinal and renal epithelia is saturable, carrier-mediated, and coupled with the Na^+ gradient[9,75]. Moreover, growth hormone and parathyroid hormone exert their modulating effects (enhancement and inhibition respectively) on phosphate transport *in vivo* by their effect on brush-border membrane transport specifically[42,69]. The absorptive flux can be described by the appropriately combined Michaelis and diffusional equation:

$$J_3 = J_{in} = \frac{J_{max_{in}} \cdot [Pi]_\ell}{Km_{in} + [Pi]_\ell} + Kd \cdot Pi^*_\ell \tag{2}$$

where subscripts 'in' and 'ℓ' refer to influx and lumen respectively. The corresponding equation for backflux is:

$$J_4 = J_{eff} = \frac{J_{max_{eff}} \cdot [Pi]_c}{Km_{eff} + [Pi]_c} + Kd \cdot Pi^*_c \tag{3}$$

where subscripts 'eff' and 'c' refer to efflux and cell, respectively.

The Na^+-coupled, secondary-active transport of phosphate inward at the brush-border membrane uses the potential energy in the Na^+ electrochemical potential gradient ($\Delta\mu_{Na}$). This gradient[117] is described by the equation:

$$\Delta\mu_{Na} = \frac{-RT_{\ell n} [Na^+]_e}{[Na^+]_\ell} = -F - V_{BBM} \tag{4}$$

where R is the gas constant, T absolute temperature, F the Faraday constant, V_{BBM} the brush-border membrane potential (cytoplasm relative to lumen).

Measurements of intracellular phosphate in kidney imply that net uptake from lumen occurs against a chemical gradient; a similar situation apparently exists in the small intestine. However, it is important to know whether free phosphate anion is uniformly distributed in cytoplasm and, specifically, whether the concentration adjacent to the cytoplasmic surface of the brush-border membrane is uniform with phosphate elsewhere in cytoplasm. There is no reason to believe that cytosolic binding proteins exist for phosphate that are analogous to those controlling the intracellular movement and distribution of calcium (CaBP)*. Nevertheless, essential knowledge about partitioning of cellular phosphate will remain unattainable until methods such as nuclear magnetic resonance analysis[17] show how phosphate anion is distributed in epithelial cells and at what concentrations.

Given the asymmetry of phosphate flux at the brush-border membrane and the ability to concentrate phosphate in the cell, we must consider how flux is achieved in the steady-state. Two possibilities deserve consideration: either the effective $[Pi]_c$ is kept below that which is at equilibrium with $[Pi]_{ej}$, or Km_{eff} exceeds Km_{in} for flux kinetics. Little is known about the latter possibility. However, mechanisms to accomplish the former can be identified. They are:

(1) *metabolic runout* of phosphate into other pools (for example, organified phosphates [$\sim P$ in *Figure 1.1, see page 7*] and the mitochondrial pool), with net flux away from apical cytosolic region;

(2) *membrane (permeability) runout*, in which J_5 exceeds J_6 (*see Figure 1.1*) at the basal–lateral membrane. Phosphate permeation outward at the basal–lateral membrane is carrier-mediated but it is not dependent on a Na^+ gradient[74].

Thus, there is evidence that the respective characteristics of phosphate transport at brush-border and basal–lateral membranes are different. The implications are clear: first, net transepithelial flux essential to net absorption can be accounted for by the transporting characteristics of membranes in series; second, mutation could impair net flux of phosphate by modifying carriers in either the brush-border or the basal–lateral membrane.

Phosphate transport along the intestine and nephron

Primitive kidney (metanephros) is derived from primitive hindgut. Accordingly, a similarity in the functional orientation of phosphate transport across luminal and antiluminal membranes of intestinal and renal epithelium is not surprising. Nonetheless, interorgan heterogeneity of phosphate transport is apparent. First, only renal transport is clearly modulated by parathyroid hormone[30]; second, whereas the effect of vitamin D on intestinal transport of phosphate is unequivocal[30], its physiological significance for renal transport of phosphate is not clear[32, 159]. We examine two aspects of phosphate transport in this section: axial heterogeneity of transport activity and hormonal influences on transporting segments.

INTESTINE

Phosphate absorption is achieved along the whole length of small intestine[30, 153]. In rat and mouse, where measurement of *in vitro* transport is feasible, it is apparent

---

* Should there be an intracellular phosphate-binding protein, we would need to postulate a new class of phosphate transport disorders and our present view of phosphate transport would require careful revision.

that steady-state uptake by the everted gut-sac or enterocyte preparation is maximal in midgut segments of rat and in the more distal segments of mouse small intestine[143]. Phosphate transport is calcium-dependent in the proximal portion and calcium-independent in the distal part of rodent small intestine[20, 153]. Comparable data for man are not available.

Intestine lacks binding sites for parathyroid hormone[30] and intestinal transport of phosphate is unresponsive to this hormone. On the other hand, intestinal phosphate transport is stimulated by vitamin D hormone, 1,25-dihydroxyvitamin D_3 $(1,25(OH)_2D_3)$[20, 153]. The response is mediated by two mechanisms. In the first, phosphate is the attendant anion for the vitamin D-stimulated calcium transport process in proximal small intestine. In the second, vitamin D stimulates trans-epithelial transport of phosphate by a mechanism independent of calcium transport; the latter is Na^+-dependent, concentrative, and located in the brush-border membrane.

NEPHRON

Under normal day-to-day conditions, there is a small variation in the normal interindividual distribution of plasma phosphate both in the normal adult (at values

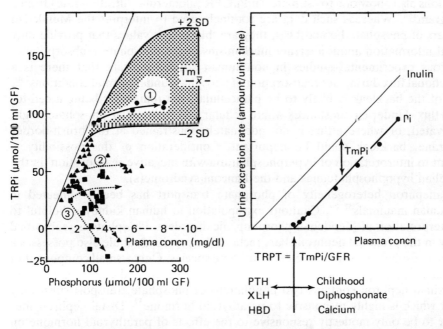

Figure 1.2 Left: TRPi at endogenous levels of filtered phosphate (left of dotted sloping lines) and during phosphate infusion in normal subjects, ①, ● and patients with HBD ②,▲ and XLH ③,■; range of TmPi values is indicated for each phenotype; negative reabsorption is also indicated. *Right*: generalized diagram showing phosphate-dependent TmPi, TmPi/GFR (or TRPT) value and various physiological and pathological events that shift TmPi/GFR

below 4 mg/dl or less than 1.29 mAtom/l)* and in the child (at values above 4 mg/dl). Within individuals, there is also a small circadian variation in plasma phosphate[64]. Such variation in plasma phosphate is, in part, a reflection of variation in net tubular reabsorption of phosphate. Kidney is the key organ of phosphate homeostasis (*see Table 1.2*). We will consider the general aspects of renal phosphate handling before addressing the specific phenomenon of intra-nephron and internephron heterogeneity.

Plasma phosphate is virtually ultrafilterable at pH 7.4 (*see Table 1.2*). Fractional phosphate excretion in human bladder urine is less than 20% of filtered phosphate under normal conditions. Under conditions of phosphate deprivation, fractional excretion approaches zero, implying adaptation of net tubular reabsorption (TRPi). On the other hand, elevation of plasma phosphate leads to saturation of reabsorption and attainment of a maximum rate of reabsorption (TmPi) (normal value: 130 ± 20 μmol/100 ml glomerular filtrate, mean ± SD); the latter implies a finite capacity for net phosphate transport along the nephron (*Figure 1.2*).

Three parameters of renal phosphate reabsorption have been investigated in man by means of standardized infusion methods and normal values have been defined for TRPi, TmPi and TmPi/GFR (theoretical renal phosphate threshold) (*Figure 1.2*). Single measurements of phosphate in plasma and in short-term urine collections also allow one to estimate TmPi/GFR (glomerular filtration rate) from a nomogram[154]. Whereas such data are routinely used to interpret the Mendelian disorders of phosphate homeostasis, they are 'black-box' values that provide only general information about aberrant mechanisms of net phosphate reabsorption.

Various experimental studies in non-human species indicate that there is a bidirectional flux during net reabsorption of phosphate under normal conditions[130]. Some of the backleak is likely to be paracellular, the remainder being a cell-to-lumen flux. Under circumstances where cellular and peritubular phosphate might be elevated, or where efflux is not adequately constrained at the brush-border membrane, backleak could be important. Consideration of this possibility is relevant to interpretation of hyperphosphaturia with 'negative reabsorption' in the Mendelian hypophosphatemias and the Fanconi syndrome(s).

Intranephron heterogeneity of phosphate transport has been delineated in non-human mammals[32, 64]. Cautious extrapolation to human kidney is helpful to the interpretation of Mendelian phosphopenic disorders. Phosphate is reabsorbed largely in the proximal nephron. Pars recta of the proximal tubule also possesses a specific phosphate transport capability in some species. Only a small component of phosphate reabsorption occurs in distal convoluted tubule and collecting tubules.

Proximal nephron contains two populations of phosphate transport sites, only one of which is highly responsive to parathyroid hormone[32]. Distal nephron sites appear to be only modestly responsive to the effects of parathyroid hormone on phosphate reabsorption. The distribution of growth hormone effects on phosphate transport in the nephron[70] has not received comparable attention. Parathyroid hormone-dependent cyclic AMP (cAMP) formation occurs at several sites in the

---

* Since at pH 7.4, the anion exists as two species, its concentration cannot be expressed as a single molar equivalent; the convention milliAtom recognizes that phosphate anion is measured as phosphorus (atomic weight 30.975).

nephron[98], not only in proximal nephron but also in distal nephron segments and collecting tubules. The proximal sites clearly pertain to phosphate transport; the distal sites probably modulate calcium reabsorption primarily. The physiological significance of these findings for the fine tuning of net phosphate reabsorption by the nephron is of great interest. For an understanding of X-linked and autosomal disorders of phosphate homeostasis, we are most interested in the heterogeneity of proximal tubule sites and their response to parathyroid hormone.

Internephron heterogeneity must also be considered. Deep and superficial nephrons in mammalian kidney appear to be similar in their handling of phosphate in proximal segments[95]. Deep and superficial nephrons differ at the level of distal segments in their responsiveness to parathyroid hormone and its effect on phosphate transport; superficial nephrons are insensitive, whereas deep nephrons appear to be sensitive[32]. These conclusions, derived from *in vivo*, *in situ* observations in non-human mammals, are compatible with the distribution of adenylate cyclase responsiveness to parathyroid hormone; only deep nephrons possess such responsiveness[98].

Two other facets of intranephron heterogeneity merit comment. They concern the sites of calcitonin and vitamin D interaction with the nephron. While both may bear on the interpretation of X-linked hypophosphatemia, we see no clear resolution of the difficulties raised by these observations. Calcitonin stimulates adenylate cyclase only in the distal nephron[98]. The importance of calcitonin in the pathophysiology of phosphate homeostasis is still not clear[5], but there is evidence that *in situ* renal sensitivity to the hormone is increased in the murine form of X-linked hypophosphatemia[15]. Furthermore, the precise role of vitamin D in renal phosphate transport is also not clear[32, 159]. However, the nephron is endowed with two forms of vitamin D interaction; 25-OH-D$_3$ is converted to 1,25(OH)$_2$D$_3$ by the proximal nephron[16]. On the assumption that parathyroid hormone and phosphate anion are regulators of 1α-hydroxylase activity, it is appropriate that the principal sites for uptake of phosphate and binding of parathyroid hormone are found together in proximal segments. The cellular effect of 1,25(OH)$_2$D$_3$ hormone is intimately dependent on its receptor; the fact that there are not large numbers of the latter in proximal segments[140] suggests that the hormone is not intimately coupled with the principal modes of phosphate transport in kidney and their contribution to whole-body phosphate homeostasis. The distal nephron is well endowed with 1,25(OH)$_2$D$_3$ receptors where they may play a role in calcium reabsorption[140]. Why and how 1,25(OH)$_2$D$_3$ enhances net phosphate reabsorption in the autosomal form of hypophosphatemic bone disease (HBD) and not in the X-linked form (XLH) is not revealed by the physiological data.

Vitamin D metabolism

In this section we summarize some recent advances in vitamin D metabolism pertinent to an understanding of vitamin D dependency and treatment of the phosphopenic conditions. Vitamin D is essential for calcium homeostasis (for review, see references[30, 53, 83]). The human being acquires vitamin D in two forms:

vitamin D_3 (cholecalciferol) synthesized in skin and vitamin D_2 (ergocalciferol of plant origin) ingested in fortified foods and medications. Both forms are transported in plasma by the vitamin D binding protein (DBP).

Vitamin D_2 and D_3 as such are biologically inactive and must undergo two enzymatic hydroxylations before either can exert physiological action at target sites. Vitamins D_2 and D_3 appear to be metabolized in the same manner and, in man, are believed to have equal potency. Of the metabolites identified to date, the dihydroxylated derivative $1,25(OH)_2D$ has the most potent effect on calcium transport.

The first hydroxylation to yield 25-hydroxyvitamin D (25-OHD) occurs in the liver. The conversion is catalyzed by a specific microsomal enzyme, vitamin D-25-hydroxylase. Recent findings indicate that homogenates of chick small intestine and kidney are also able to hydroxylate vitamin D. It is not known whether such extrahepatic 25-hydroxylation takes place in man. Early experiments[10] suggested that synthesis of hepatic 25-OHD is regulated by product-feedbacks but other findings[150] place this concept in question. Plasma 25-OHD levels are greatly elevated in patients treated with large doses of vitamin D.

Studies in countries where vitamin D_2 is the form commonly used to fortify foods show that $25\text{-}OHD_3$ rather than $25\text{-}OHD_2$ is the major circulating form in most individuals[69, 80, 133]. This finding indicates that endogenous biosynthesis is the principal source of vitamin D in man.

Development of rickets in anticonvulsant-treated patients is well established[35]. Anticonvulsants induce hepatic microsomal enzymes that inactivate vitamin D and metabolites. In addition, they disturb calcium homeostasis independent of vitamin D[73].

Although 25-OHD is about three times more active than vitamin D in preventing or curing rickets[82], it requires further hydroxylation to express its full biological potency. Further hydroxylation of 25-OHD occurs in kidney mitochondria, and is catalyzed by the enzyme 25-hydroxyvitamin D-1α-hydroxylase (1α-hydroxylase), yielding the active metabolite, $1\alpha,25(OH)_2D$. Placenta[65] and bone[151] also possess very modest capabilities to convert 25-hydroxyvitamin D to $1,25(OH)_2D$. The metabolism of vitamin D responds to the physiological state of the individuals. Thus, in times of need (for example, hypocalcemia, vitamin D deficiency, secondary hyperparathyroidism and probably hypophosphatemia), 1α-hydroxylase activity is stimulated and synthesis of $1,25(OH)_2D$ takes place. On the other hand, when $1,25(OH)_2D$ is not required (for example, normocalcemia or hypercalcemia, normophosphatemia or hyperphosphatemia), 1α-hydroxylation is inhibited, and 25-OH-D is converted to $24,25(OH)_2D$ by another enzyme (24-hydroxylase) or to other metabolites. Other hormones, such as estrogens, testosterone, prolactin, glucocorticoid, and insulin also influence 1α-hydroxylase activity, but their physiological importance is yet to be determined.

Vitamin D hormone stimulates intestinal absorption of calcium and phosphate and, in conjunction with parathyroid hormone, stimulates mineral resorption from bone. It also enhances renal tubular reabsorption of calcium[77]. $1,25(OH)_2D_3$ receptors are found in parathyroid gland but their role in the control of hormone synthesis and release is not clear.

With a sufficient supply of $1,25(OH)_2D$, 1α-hydroxylase activity is inhibited and 25-OHD is converted by another hydroxylating activity (25-hydroxyvitamin D-24-hydroxylase (24-hydroxylase) to 24,25-dihydroxyvitamin D $(24,25(OH)_2D)$. This vitamin D metabolite is a substance of uncertain physiological action, but several studies suggest that it may play an essential role in normal mineral metabolism[11, 55, 81].

Vitamin D deficiency impairs intestinal absorption of calcium and mobilization of calcium from bone, resulting in hypocalcemia. Hypocalcemia stimulates parathyroid hormone secretion, but vitamin D depletion renders the organism relatively insensitive to the calcium-mobilizing effects of parathyroid hormone. A high concentration of parathyroid hormone is therefore required to offset hypocalcemia. At the same time the hyperparathyroidism results in hyperphosphaturia and hyperaminoaciduria[48], and enhances $1,25(OH)_2D$ synthesis. It is of interest that whereas 25-OHD is depressed in advanced vitamin D deficiency serum $1,25(OH)_2D$ is sometimes normal[38].

Toxic doses of vitamin D cause increased synthesis of 25-OHD but plasma levels of $1,25(OH)_2D$ remain within the normal range. The hypercalcemia that accompanies this situation implies that very high concentrations of 25-OHD *per se* increase absorption of calcium from the intestinal tract and skeleton. The resultant hypercalcemia suppresses parathyroid hormone secretion. Eventually, hypercalcemia may impair renal function. These untoward effects explain the toxicity of vitamin D and are of major clinical concern in the management of the 'vitamin D-resistant' forms of rickets. Protein binding assays and immunoassays are now available to measure 25-OHD and $1,25(OH)_2D$ in plasma. These methods are of great clinical value for diagnosis and management of the Mendelian forms of rickets.

MENDELIAN RICKETS/OSTEOMALACIA

Normal mineralization of the skeleton requires an adequate supply of calcium and inorganic phosphate in the appropriate ratio at nucleation sites in osteoid. Normal matrix and epiphyseal growth cartilage are also essential and there must be no excess of inhibitors of the calcification process. Any interruption in the process results in osteomalacia and rickets. Mendelian disorders of phosphate conservation and of vitamin D hormone biosynthesis and action are discussed here. Hereditary disorders of matrix (for example, hypophophatasia) are omitted simply because their pathogenesis is so poorly understood.

The term 'osteomalacia' is applied to conditions of the skeleton in which there is a failure of bone mineral to be deposited promptly in the recently formed protein matrix of endosteal remodeling sites in bone. In rickets, the pediatric counterpart of osteomalacia, the defect in mineralization occurs also in preosseous cartilage and at the zones of provisional calcification of growth plates.

Osteomalacia and rickets connote morphological changes. Thus, the diagnosis of osteomalacia and rickets can be made by radiography. Course trabeculation, deformation, and pseudofractures are characteristic radiographic features of osteomalacia. In rickets, linear growth is impaired and deformities of the long bones occur – genu varum if rickets occurs before 3 years of age, and genu valgum if onset is after that age. Findings can be quantified by histological examination of undecalcified material from a full thickness iliac crest trephine biopsy[12]. Excessive osteoid and a reduced calcification front are the generally accepted histological criteria of ostomalacia[18].

Phosphopenic rickets/osteomalacia

Four Mendelian disorders (or phenotypes) are described. *X-linked hypophosphatemia* (XLH)[107] is characterized by persistent postnatal hypophosphatemia with essentially normal serum calcium and parathyroid hormone levels; it is associated with early onset of rickets and growth retardation and is more uniform and severe in males than females. The phenotype is variable from one heterozygous X-linked hypophosphatemic female to another because of lyonization (random inactivation of one X_q chromosome). *Autosomal dominant hypophosphatemic bone disease* (HBD)[127] has the equivalent degree of postnatal-onset hypophosphatemia, without hypocalcemia, but, unlike X-linked hypophosphatemia, the bone disease is primarily osteomalacic, rarely rachitic, and not accompanied by significant growth failure. Genu varum in mid-infancy is the usual presenting sign and male and female phenotypes are comparable. *Autosomal dominant hypophosphatemic rickets* (ADHR)[73] resembles the X-linked hypophosphatemia phenotype in severity of bone disease, but critical pedigrees with male-to-male transmission exclude X-linkage. Only the X-linked hypophosphatemia and autosomal hypophosphatemic bone disease forms have been sufficiently characterized to indicate that different renal mechanisms are involved in the origins of hypophosphatemia. The *Fanconi syndrome*[99, 118] is a set of diseases that is distinguished from the conditions mentioned above, because it exhibits a generalized disturbance of tubular functions including phosphate reabsorption. The phenotype of each form of the Fanconi syndrome is a combination of the particular primary Mendelian disease and the impact it has on tubular function.

An analysis of the phosphopenic mechanisms in these four phenotype groups follows.

X-linked hypophosphatemia (XLH)

This disease is the prototype of Mendelian phosphopenic rickets, formally refined as 'familial vitamin D-resistant rickets'[123]. Described initially by Albright *et al.*[1] and Christensen[24], it was first interpreted as a heritable disorder of mineralization resulting from target organ resistance to vitamin D. However, key evidence was missing to support a calcipenic mode of rickets and an alternative hypothesis involving a phosphopenic mode of rickets was soon advanced[33, 112]. X-linked dominant inheritance of the hypophosphatemic component of the phenotype was not recognized until many years later[160] when evidence confirmed that X-linked hypophosphatemia is an inborn error of phosphate homeostasis. Another decade passed before data could be gathered implicating the disease as a selective disorder of renal phosphate transport[60]. The important findings for this interpretation of X-linked hypophosphatemia, both quantitative and qualitative[125] are as follows:

(1) Serum parathyroid hormone levels are not significantly elevated in XLH[2]; thus, a key component of the calcipenic hypothesis is missing.

(2) TRPi and TmPi values are intermediate in obligate heterozygotes relative to normal and mutant hemizygous subjects[60]; this finding indicates a gene dosage effect and implies that the mutant gene product is a component of renal phosphate transport or closely related to it.

(3) Negative TRPi values are occasionally encountered in X-linked hypophosphatemia males, particularly after phosphate loading. This finding indicates backflux of phosphate from tubular epithelium and implies that the defect in phosphate transport is likely to be found at the brush-border membrane[124].

(4) Phosphate transport by the erythrocyte, a model for facilitated diffusional transport of phosphate in a plasma membrane, is normal in X-linked hypophosphatemia[144] and implies selective expression of the X-linked hypophosphatemia mutation among membrane gene products serving phosphate transport.

(5) About one-third to one-half of normal phosphate reabsorption is retained in mutant hemizygotes. This residual component of phosphate transport is hyposensitive to inhibition by parathyroid hormone in mutant hemizygotes under endogenous conditions despite an adequate urinary cyclic nucleotide response to the hormone[61, 125]. Heterozygotes show intermediate degrees of phosphaturia after parathyroid hormone relative to normal and hemizygous subjects. Prolonged calcium infusion restores inhibition of phosphate reabsorption by parathyroid hormone[131], but calcium infusion itself, both short-term and long-term, enhances phosphate reabsorption in X linked hypophosphatemia[49, 61]. These findings must be interpreted in the context of a controversy about serum $1,25(OH)_2D_3$ levels in the disease. The levels are considered inappropriately low for the degree of hypophosphatemia[37] and appear to be depressed by phosphate and vitamin D treatment (*see below*). Accordingly, if vitamin D hormone plays a permissive role in the phosphaturic effect of parathyroid hormone[107], a secondary disorder of vitamin D metabolism may affect the tubular response to parathyroid hormone in X-linked hypophosphatemia.

(6) Phosphate replacement therapy[63], intended to restore phosphate homeostasis by an effect of mass action on intestinal absorption[132], raises serum phosphate, stimulates linear growth rate, and heals rickets in XLH. On the other hand, this difficult form of therapy does not completely heal the osteomalacia[26, 59] and apparently disturbs regulation of $1,25(OH)_2D_3$ biosynthesis[21, 31, 59, 128]. Combined therapy with phosphate and $1,25(OH)_2D_3$ in children[26, 59], or with $1,25(OH)D_3$ alone in adults[42] improves phosphate homeostasis and bone mineralization, presumably through the effect of vitamin D hormone on intestinal transport of phosphate. There is no significant change in the renal phosphate transport defect with this form of treatment.

Table 1.3 Features of the common types of hereditary rickets

	X-linked hypophosphatemia (XLH)	Autosomal dominant hypophosphatemic bone disease (HBD)
Genetics	X-linked dominant	Autosomal dominant
Onset of physical signs	12–18 months (hypophosphatemia present shortly after birth)	12–24 months
Mode of presentation	Bow-legs when starting to walk, short stature, slight to severe deformities	Bow-legs when starting to walk
Additional signs and symptoms	Healthy, short and stocky, strong, females usually less severely affected than males, and may have no deformities or dwarfism. Sagittal craniosynostosis common. No enamel hypoplasia in permanent teeth, but interglobular dentin occurs and pulp spaces enlarged. No urinary symptoms	Healthy, deformities mild; males and females equally affected. No urinary symptoms
Radiographs	Mild to severe 'chronic' rickets; shafts usually wide, cortices thick, coarse trabecular pattern, total skeletal calcium increased. Some hypophosphatemic females have no physical or radiographic abnormalities	Osteomalacia with or without mild rickets – less severe than in XLH
Plasma		
Ca	Normal	Normal
Pi	Marked decrease	Marked decrease
alkaline phosphatase	Slight to moderate increase	Slight to moderate increase
electrolytes	Normal	Normal
acid/base	Normal	Normal
BUN, creatinine	Normal	Normal
aminoacids	Normal	Normal
iPTH	Normal	Normal
25-OHD	Normal	Normal
1,25(OH)$_2$D	Normal	
Urine		
protein	0	0
glucose	0	0
pH	Normal range	Normal range
concentration	Normal range	Normal range
aminoacids	Normal	Normal
Prognosis	Probably require lifelong therapy in most cases; normal life expectancy; remain hypophosphatemic; males and most females remain stunted and deformed	Probably require lifelong therapy in most cases; normal life expectancy; remain hypophosphatemic; deformities tend to be mild or absent in adult life
Therapy	Phosphate supplements and 1,25(OH)$_2$D$_3$	Phosphate supplements and 1,25(OH)$_2$D$_3$

Autosomal recessive vitamin D dependency Type I (ARVDD Type I)	Vitamin D dependency Type II (VDD Type II)	Fanconi syndrome
Autosomal recessive	Autosomal recessive or sporadic, female preponderance	Autosomal recessive usually (unless due to a toxic agent)
3–12 months (biochemical signs present shortly after birth)	Infancy, childhood	Infancy, childhood, adulthood
Irritability, tetany, convulsions, delayed walking, severe rickets, failure to thrive	Bow-legs, deformities, convulsions	Infancy: irritability, anorexia, failure to thrive, polydipsia, polyuria, dehydration
Severe, rapidly increasing deformities, short stature, muscle weakness, enamel hypoplasia, interglobular dentin in permanent teeth. No urinary symptoms	Alopecia, very common; oligodentia, and amelogenesis imperfecta, rare	Cystinosis: fair complexion; grey-blonde hair; cystine in leukocytes, cornea, conjunctiva; peripheral retinopathy
Severe rachitic changes in growth plates and shafts; bones have thin cortices and tend toward osteoporosis	Rickets, mild to severe	Mild to severe rickets; osteoporosis in most cases
Moderate to marked decrease	Decrease (variable)	Normal to moderate decrease
Decrease	Decrease (variable)	Early, marked decrease; late, normal or increased
Increased, usually markedly	Increased	Moderate increase
Normal	Normal	Serum K decreased
Normal	Normal	Mild acidosis
Normal	Normal	Early, normal; late, increased
Normal	Normal	Normal (except in hereditary tyrosinemia)
Increased	Increased	Normal to increased
Normal	Normal	Normal
Marked decrease	Marked increase	Normal
0	0	+ to +++ (tubular protein)
0 (occasionally +)	0	+ to +++
Normal (in some cases, mild proximal RTA)	Normal range	Tends to be alkaline
Normal range	Normal range	Dilute
Generalized aminoaciduria	Generalized aminoaciduria	Generalized aminoaciduria
Require lifelong therapy; normal life expectancy with vitamin D therapy; condition is compatible with normal mineral balance, bone mineralization and growth	Probably lifelong therapy required; deformities variable; alopecia permanent	Cystinosis: infant (Type I): severe uremia by end of 1st decade. Adolescent (Type II): shortened life expectancy. Other forms of Fanconi: variable
Large doses of vitamin D or small doses of 1,25(OH)$_2$D$_3$	Large doses of vitamin D or vitamin D analogue	Phosphate supplements, potassium supplements, sodium bicarbonate, vitamin D, 1,25(OH)$_2$D$_3$

This resumé omits many interesting but more peripheral findings (for more detail, see Rasmussen and Anast[107]). Nonetheless, it is clear that all is still not known about the basic defect in X-linked hypophosphatemia and that its treatment is not at the point where expression of the mutant gene can be completely offset. However, the interpretation of X-linked hypophosphatemia has been clarified by two independent lines of investigation: one, in the X-linked hypophosphatemic (*Hyp*) mouse; the other in the autosomal dominant form of human hypophosphatemic bone disease (HBD). The principal distinguishing features of both human diseases are summarized in *Table 1.3*.

MURINE X-LINKED HYPOPHOSPHATEMIA

The *Hyp* mouse represents a homologue of the disease process in human X-linked hypophosphatemia[39]. The *Hyp* gene is located at a distal locus on the mouse X chromosome. Affected male mice (*Hyp*/Y) are mutant hemizygotes; affected females (*Hyp*/+) are heterozygotes. Conservation of genes on the X chromosome characterizes mammalian evolution[101, 102] and equivalent X-linked genes code for gene products with equivalent function in different species. Homologous mutant phenotypes in mice and men bearing the X-linked mutation (*see Table 1.3*) imply that comparable gene products are indeed involved in the two species. Therefore, the *Hyp* mouse can be used to ascertain the nature of the phosphate transport defect in human XLH.

The following is a summary of findings in the *Hyp* mouse[142]:

(1) A defect in renal handling of phosphate is apparent *in vivo* and *in situ* in *Hyp* kidney[27, 57, 147]. Whole-kidney fractional excretion of phosphate is increased; negative reabsorption occurs after phosphate loading. Single-nephron studies reveal reduced fractional and absolute reabsorption in proximal nephron segments and probably in pars recta; distal nephron segments are not involved. Parathyroidectomy does not correct the transport defect.

(2) *Hyp* renal cortex slices expose basal–lateral membranes preferentially and transport phosphate normally; overall phosphate incorporation into organic pools is also normal[147]. These findings eliminate impaired metabolic runout or altered basal–lateral membrane permeability as the mechanisms of disturbed phosphate transport and homeostasis in *Hyp* kidney.

(3) Whereas the pools for total phosphorus and inorganic phosphorus in *Hyp* kidney appear to be normal, the distribution of nucleotide phosphate is abnormal with an increased AMP/ATP ratio[116].

(4) *Hyp* renal brush-border membranes have deficient Na^+/Pi cotransport activity[145, 153]; the Na^+-dependent, arsenate-inhibited component of saturable transport activity is about half-normal in mutant hemizygous mice. The residual transport activity adapts adequately to the signal of dietary phosphorus deprivation[136]. Renal brush-border membrane enzymes, including alkaline phosphatase, are normal in *Hyp* membranes[145, 148]. These findings indicate a specific and selective defect in secondary-active phosphate transport in *Hyp* kidney.

(5) Intestinal transport of phosphate does not appear to be abnormal in the *Hyp* phenotype[143] despite earlier evidence to the contrary.

(6) Treatment with phosphate enhances mineralization of *Hyp* growth plates[90]. Treatment with $1,25(OH)_2D_3$ does not correct the renal defect in phosphate transport but improves homeostasis by enhancing intestinal transport of phosphate[146]. These findings are the equivalent of those described above for human X-linked hypophosphatemia.

(7) *Hyp* nephrons have a blunted adenylcyclase response to parathyroid hormone in defined proximal segments[15, 142]. The abnormality is apparently related to change in sensitivity of the basal–lateral membrane receptor to the hormone and not to change in cyclase itself or in the coupling protein. The same nephrons have enhanced sensitivity to calcitonin in distal segments. The meaning of these observations is not clear.

(8) There is a paradoxical relation between serum $1,25(OH)_2D_3$ and phosphate in *Hyp* mice[96]. Under endogenous conditions, vitamin D hormone levels are slightly elevated; with phosphate deprivation *Hyp* animals have decreased serum $1,25(OH)_2D_3$. Findings in +/Y mice are the reverse. Extrapolation from these findings in *Hyp* mice to the X-linked hypophosphatemia phenotype is awkward and perhaps ill-advised because phosphate homeostasis is set at different levels in man and mouse and the relative importance of phosphate anion in regulation of $1,25(OH)_2D_3$ in the two species is unknown.

With the exceptions indicated, the foregoing observations illustrate the similarity of disturbed phosphate homeostasis in *Hyp* and X-linked hypophosphatemia phenotypes and, by homology, imply that human X-linked hypophosphatemia is the result of a selective defect in secondary-active transport of phosphate in the brush-border membrane of proximal nephron; the defect is not modified by $1,25(OH)_2D_3$[25, 37, 59, 146].

Autosomal dominant hypophosphatemic bone disease (HBD)

This disease is autosomal dominant, not X-linked. All the subjects we have studied have a similar phenotype; one key pedigree shows male-to-male transmission of the hypophosphatemic phenotype[123, 127]. Accordingly, both hypophosphatemic bone disease and X-linked hypophosphatemia are the result of different mutations. Therefore, the mechanisms of the hypophosphatemia in the two diseases must be different.

The following is a summary of findings in the hypophosphatemic bone disease phenotype[123, 127].

(1) The degree of hypophosphatemia is similar in both diseases (*see Figure 1.2*).

(2) Renal handling of phosphate is different in the two conditions (*see Figure 1.2*). Fractional TRPi is normal under endogenous conditions in hypophosphatemic bone disease but clearly decreased in all X-linked hypophosphatemic males and many females. TmPi is decreased and negative reabsorption can occur in both conditions.

(3) Under endogenous conditions decreased fractional TRPi follows parathyroid hormone infusion in hypophosphatemic bone disease (but not in X-linked hypophosphatemia). However, the onset of the phosphaturic response after parathyroid hormone infusion is delayed in the former compared to normal; the urinary cyclic nucleotide response is normal.

(4) TRPi, TmPi/GFR, and serum phosphate rise when childhood hypophosphatemic bone disease is treated with $1,25(OH)_2D_3$; it is probable that the renal response contributes to the serum response in hypophosphatemic bone disease, which is clearly not the case in childhood X-linked hypophosphatemia treated with $1,25(OH)_2D_3$[26, 59].

(5) The major distinguishing clinical feature concerns the bone disease. It is less severe in hypophosphatemic bone disease than in X-linked hypophosphatemia at the equivalent serum phosphate concentration. Osteomalacia occurs in metaphyseal and diaphyseal cortical bone, but rachitic changes at the epiphyseal plate and growth impairment are mild or absent in hypophosphatemic bone disease.

(6) Phosphate transport by the erythrocyte membrane is normal in hypophosphatemic bone disease[144].

These findings, in conjunction with our knowledge of X-linked hypophosphatemia (and *Hyp*), suggest that different forms of phosphate transport are involved in both conditions. The renal sites (presumably in proximal nephron) controlled by the X-linked gene are apparently more sensitive to inhibition by parathyroid hormone than those controlled by the autosomal locus. Fractional TRPi and parathyroid hormone-response data suggest the possibility that X-linked carriers are 'downstream' from autosomal carriers in the proximal nephron. While this is only a speculation, it is not incompatible with the findings of Dennis *et al.*[32] on the distribution of parathyroid hormone-sensitive and insensitive phosphate transport sites along the proximal (rabbit) nephron.

Whereas different selective disorders of renal phosphate transport produce a common effect on phosphate homeostasis in both hypophosphatemic bone disease and X-linked hypophosphatemia, the impact on bone mineralization is quite different in the two conditions. This important observation implies that extracellular phosphate is not the sole determinant of homeostasis in the bone compartment[123], as it is, for example, in the erythrocyte[149]. The fact that bone disease is more severe in X-linked hypophosphatemia suggests either that the X-linked gene is expressed also in bone and affects transport in that compartment or that a specific and secondary manifestation of the X-linked phenotype accounts for the bone disease. Regarding the latter, there are no significant differences in steady-state serum levels of parathyroid hormone or $1,25(OH)_2D_3$ in untreated patients with both conditions. Regarding the former, a functional endosteal membrane has been proposed at the interface between bone and extracellular fluid[91]. Moreover, Na^+-dependent, saturable transport of nutrients on carriers, perhaps at the putative membrane, is a feature of bone metabolism[43]. Mutation affecting an X-linked secondary-active type of phosphate transport in the bone compartment may be a feature of X-linked hypophosphatemia that would not be expressed in hypophosphatemic bone disease. Such a hypothesis is of interest primarily for the experiments it suggests in the *Hyp* mouse and as a source of insight regarding the mechanisms of rickets in phosphopenic states.

Autosomal dominant hypophosphatemic rickets (ADHR)

Harrison and Harrison[73] described a phenotype strongly resembling X-linked hypophosphatemia in its severity that was dominantly inherited yet clearly autosomal in linkage. Insufficient experimental data are offered[73] to discern how this condition might differ from both X-linked hypophosphatemia and hypophosphatemic bone disease in renal handling of the phosphate. Nevertheless, the findings are important because they imply further heterogeneity in renal transport of the phosphate beyond that described above; they are a further challenge to the clinician who tries to interpret the heterogeneity of phosphopenic rickets and osteomalacia and the problems of its treatment.

Fanconi syndrome(s)

The Fanconi syndrome[48] has two components of interest for this chapter: a complex disorder of net tubular reabsorptive processes that is distinguishable from the selective phosphaturic disorders already described, and a metabolic bone disease generally similar to the other phosphopenic forms of bone disease (rickets/osteomalacia) (*see Table 1.3*). The syndrome has many causes that are both inherited and acquired (*Table 1.4*). The bone disease is a consequence of the renal dysfunction and is essentially dependent on the renal loss of phosphate, although

Table 1.4 Mendelian forms of the Fanconi syndrome

Primary diagnosis	Primary disorder (deficiency of)	Inheritance
Idiopathic form(s)	?	AR
Idiopathic forms(s)	?	AD (or sporadic)
Cystinosis		
infantile nephropathic	?	AR
adolescent nephropathic	?	AR
Hereditary fructose intolerance	F-1-P aldolase B	AR
Hereditary tyrosinemia	Furasyl acetoacetase?	AR
Galactosemia	Gal-1-P-uridyl-transferase	AR
Wilson's disease	Ceruloplasmin?	AR
Oculocerebrorenal syndrome	?	XLR
Vitamin D dependency Type I (ARVDD Type I)	25-OHD-1-α-hydroxylase	AR
Vitamin D dependency Type II (VDD Type II)	Nuclear uptake of 1,25(OH)$_2$D	AR?

AR, autosomal recessive; AD, autosomal dominant; XLR, X-linked recessive.

renal tubular acidosis may be a complicating factor. Therefore, the mechanism of the bone disease is primarily phosphopenic. We will consider the renal problem primarily. Treatment of the bone disease involves management of the primary disease, administration of vitamin D, and replacement of phosphate if necessary.

CLINICAL ASPECTS

All aspects of the *syndrome* (which is to be distinguished from the primary *disease*), reflect impaired tubular transport (*see Table 1.3*). They comprise all or several of the following: generalized renal hyperaminoaciduria, hyperphosphaturia and hypophosphatemia, low-Tm glucosuria, type-2 (proximal) renal tubular acidosis with impaired bicarbonate reabsorption, hyperkaluria with hypokalemia, high free-water clearance with dehydration, and hyperuricosuria with hypouricemia.

The metabolic bone disease is coupled with hypophosphatemia resulting from impaired phosphate reabsorption. Vitamin D metabolism is specifically impaired in the syndrome associated with autosomal recessive vitamin D dependency Type I (ARVDD Type I), but synthesis of $1,25(OH)_2D$ may also be non-specifically impaired in other forms of Fanconi syndrome[22]. Under these circumstances, homeostasis of phosphate is both primarily and secondarily impaired and the bone disease is both phosphopenic and calcipenic in origin.

THE RENAL LESION

The causes of the tubular dysfunction are manifold in the syndrome (*see Table 1.4*). Whatever the primary cause, a final, perhaps common, cellular lesion results that disturbs net transepithelial transport of phosphate and other solutes.

Two lines of investigation suggest what the nature of the cellular lesion might be:

(1) Studies in hereditary fructose intolerance[99] implicate disturbed intracellular renal phosphate homeostasis. Fructose-induced experimental renal dysfunction suggests the following sequence: fructose-1-phosphate→ ↓ cellular phosphate → ↓ cellular (adenosine 5′-triphosphate) (ATP). These events may further perturb oxidative phosphorylation in renal mitochondria. However, depletion of cellular ATP is not enough to provoke the syndrome, as evidenced in the *Hyp* form of X-linked hypophosphatemia in which renal steady-state cellular ATP is decreased significantly yet there is no Fanconi syndrome[116].
(2) Maleic acid has long been used to produce an experimental form of Fanconi syndrome. Micropuncture studies[68] in the maleic acid-treated rat indicate generalized impairment of mediated transport in the proximal nephron. Stop–flow studies[8] show that permeability in the distal nephron is also affected, permitting exaggerated cell-to-lumen flux of solutes. Both studies imply that net reabsorptive transport is depressed in the nephron. Studies with isolated brush-border membranes prepared from the rat[41] show that maleate binds to such membranes but does not impair Na^+-gradient-dependent transport by brush-border membrane vesicles. These findings imply that the maleate-induced Fanconi syndrome is an intracellular event of metabolic nature that compromises net transcellular flux *in situ*.

As models for the Fanconi syndrome, fructose intolerance and maleate toxicity represent quite different 'causes' but they have a 'common' effect in perturbing cellular events that sustain absorptive transport. If those events determine permeability of renal membranes along the nephron, and in particular permeability related to secondary-active transport in the proximal nephron, a general mechanism for the syndrome and for its phosphaturic component can be envisaged.

Calcipenic rickets/osteomalacia

Autosomal recessive vitamin D dependency Type I (ARVDD Type I)

Fraser and Salter[50] recognized that vitamin D dependency rickets was a condition separate from other vitamin D-resistant rickets in 1958; they called the condition hypophosphatemic vitamin D refractory rickets with aminoaciduria. In 1961, Prader *et al.*[106] described the disease further under the name of pseudovitamin D deficiency rickets. Others have also discussed the problem[3, 34, 115, 120, 139].

This condition has all the features of advanced vitamin D deficiency, but it occurs in spite of adequate prophylactic vitamin D intake (*see Table 1.3*). Onset is before 2 years of age and often during the first 6 months of life. Irritability, hypotonia and convulsions are common presenting complaints. Hypocalcemia, hypophosphatemia and elevated alkaline phosphatase activity are consistently present. The plasma iPTH concentration is increased and there is generalized hyperaminoaciduria. Occasionally a defect in urine acidification is also present. Radiographically, there are features of severe vitamin D deficiency rickets, including epiphyseal lesions, coarse trabeculation, hypomineralization, varying degrees of deformity and fractures. The permanent teeth show marked hypoplasia of the enamel[100, 120], a feature never observed in X-linked hypophosphatemia. Treatment with high doses of vitamin D reverses all the biochemical and clinical features of the disease; if it is started early, there is no residual deformity and stature is normal. The condition is autosomal recessive in inheritance.

In recent years the pathogenesis of autosomal recessive vitamin D dependency Type I has become clear[47]. The speculation that the bone lacked the ability to mineralize and that the intestine was unable to absorb calcium and phosphorus due to some primary abnormality of the gut has been ruled out. The possibility of abnormal vitamin D metabolism was suggested by the fact that clinical manifestations completely mimic vitamin D deficiency and the finding that pharmacological doses of vitamin D or 'physiological' doses of $1,25(OH)_2D_3$ reverse all the clinical and biochemical abnormalities.

Three mechanisms have been suggested to explain vitamin D dependency: (a) poor absorption of vitamin D; (b) inadequate conversion of vitamin D to $1,25(OH)_2D$; and (c) inability of target tissues to respond satisfactorily to physiological concentrations of the active metabolites. Specific malabsorption of vitamin D is ruled out because normal levels of the vitamin have been found in the serum of untreated patients. Furthermore, assays of vitamin D and 25-OHD show high concentrations when patients are given large doses of vitamin D. Of the two remaining possibilities, evidence excludes the possibility that target tissues are refractory to the action of active metabolites of vitamin D in autosomal recessive vitamin D dependency Type I.

There is now sufficient information to assign the cause of vitamin D dependency to an inborn error in conversion of 25-OHD to $1,25(OH)_2D$ due presumably to recessively inherited deficiency of 25-hydroxyvitamin D-1α-hydroxylase in the kidney[47]. Initial evidence for a block in vitamin D metabolism was obtained indirectly by observing the relative doses of vitamin D, 25-OHD_3 and $1,25(OH)_2D_3$ required to heal the biochemical and radiographic lesions. Massive doses of vitamin D_2 and D_3 (1000–3000 μg/day, 100–300 times the normal requirement) are required to maintain biochemical and radiographic healing in autosomal recessive vitamin D dependency Type I. The maintenance requirement of 25-OH-D_3 is also very high (200–900 μg/day) in the same patients[6]. By contrast, a dose of only 1 μg/day $1,25(OH)_2D_3$ or less is required to correct hypocalcemia, increase intestinal calcium absorption, establish positive calcium balance and initiate radiographic healing in hereditary vitamin D dependency. A similar response is achieved with very small doses of synthetic analogue 1-α-hydroxyvitamin D_3 ($1α\text{-OHD}_3$)[108].

Development of a sensitive method to measure the product of the enzyme in question has provided support for the suggestion that autosomal recessive vitamin D dependency Type I is the result of deficient 1α-hydroxylase activity. Using the competitive binding assay of Eisman *et al.*[41] to measure the levels of $1,25(OH)_2D$ in the serum of patients with autosomal recessive vitamin D dependency Type I, Scriver *et al.*[128] and DeLuca[22, 29] have shown that conversion of 25-OHD to $1,25(OH)_2D$ is indeed greatly impaired in the condition. In the first-mentioned study the serum $1,25(OH)_2D$ level in five vitamin D_2-treated children was 9.5 ± 2.9 pg/ml (means ± SD), as compared to 37.1 ± 11.1 pg/ml in age-matched normal children[125]. The difference in the means was significant ($P < 0.01$). In the other study[22], patients were investigated under four different conditions. Eight determinations of serum $1,25(OH)_2D$ in untreated patients with active rickets averaged 22 pg/ml, significantly less than measurements in a series of normal children whose mean serum value averaged 92 pg/ml. Treatment of patients with vitamin D or 25-OHD_3 caused no significant change in the serum 1,25-OHD concentration. In contrast, two patients controlled with $1,25(OH)_2D$ had levels comparable to those of normal children.

These investigations imply that the metabolism of vitamin D is seriously impaired at the 1α-hydroxylation step in autosomal recessive vitamin D dependency Type I. The observed low values may signify a small residual conversion to the active metabolite or may represent a spurious value due to methodological problems at such low concentrations of sterol. Further, the studies indicate that pharmacological doses of vitamin D and 25-OHD_3 correct the metabolic disturbances by a mechanism other than through generation of physiological amounts of $1,25(OH)_2D$ by a hypothetical 'leaky' 1α-hydroxylase. To account for the efficacy of high-dosage vitamin D therapy in autosomal recessive vitamin D dependency Type I, one must conclude that appropriately high concentrations of 25-OHD have the capacity to subserve the action of physiological concentrations of $1,25(OH)_2D$ at the end-organs. Direct proof that defective vitamin D metabolism is due to a defective kidney 1α-hydroxylase enzyme is still not available.

PORCINE AUTOSOMAL RECESSIVE VITAMIN D DEPENDENCY RICKETS

Soon after the first reports of autosomal recessive vitamin D dependency Type I in humans, a similar syndrome in a mutant strain of domestic pigs was reported from Hanover, West Germany[71, 72, 105, 158]. The model has been propagated and studied intensively at the School of Veterinary Medicine in Hanover. In almost all respects reported to date, the human and porcine conditions are similar. The porcine condition is inherited as an autosomal recessive trait. The homozygote develops hypocalcemia, hypophosphatemia, hyperparathyroidism, generalized aminoacidur-ia and severe rickets within 6 weeks of birth, and the animal dies between 3 and 4 months of age if it is not treated. Physical, radiographic and biochemical lesions revert to normal with high doses of vitamin D. The serum 25-OHD concentrations are approximately four times normal in the porcine model. This finding differs from that in human autosomal recessive vitamin D dependency Type I. The difference is unexplained.

As indicated above, proof that human autosomal recessive vitamin D depend-ency Type I is caused by a defect in the 1α-hydroxylase enzyme awaits direct measurement of enzyme activity in renal tissue from an affected individual. Although, as in the human, 1α-hydroxylase activity has not yet been assayed in the porcine model, there are no ethical restraints against making this measurement in the pig. It should be pointed out, however, that data regarding the porcine disease cannot be transposed with certainty to the human, because phenotypical similarity between recessively inherited conditions does not necessarily imply genetic homol-ogy. Nevertheless, additional information on the metabolic defect in the mutant vitamin D-dependent pig could give valuable insight into the cause and treatment of the human disease.

Vitamin D dependency rickets Type II (VDD Type II)

Vitamin D dependency rickets Type II is the designation of a recently reported rachitic syndrome believed to be due to target-organ resistance to $1,25(OH)_2D$. Since 1978, some 14 patients have been described[6, 7, 14, 85, 91, 113, 149, 161], and a reasonably accurate general description of the condition can now be made.

Rickets usually appears by 1 year of age, and tends to be severe. Plasma calcium and phosphate concentrations are decreased, plasma parathyroid hormone is elevated, and there is generalized aminoaciduria – features comparable to those in advanced vitamin D deficiency (Stage III rickets) and autosomal recessive vitamin D dependency Type I. The condition is distinguished from the latter two diseases by higher than normal concentrations of $1,25(OH)_2D$ in plasma or by lack of response to physiological doses of $1,25(OH)_2D_3$. Calcium and phosphate homeo-stasis and the rachitic bone lesions are usually but not necessarily improved by very large doses of vitamin D or $1,25(OH)_2D_3$. Cultured skin fibroblasts show deficient nuclear uptake of $[^3H]$-$1,25(OH)_2D_3$[40]. Vitamin D dependency rickets Type II joins the list of endocrine deficiency syndromes attributable not to a defect in hormone synthesis or secretion, but to deficient end-organ responsiveness. (Pseudohypoparathyroidism, nephrogenic diabetes insipidus, and Laron-type dwarfism are other examples of endocrine disorders attributable to defective target organ responsiveness.)

Vitamin D dependency rickets Type II is a rare condition. However, since the metabolic disturbance cannot be readily differentiated from autosomal recessive vitamin D dependency Type I except by measuring the level of $1,25(OH)_2D_3$, the disease may have been missed in the past, and may possibly prove to be of more frequent occurrence when the above diagnostic tests are applied.

A strong hereditary tendency is evident from the published reports. Two or more sibs were affected in four of the eight reported kindreds[7, 85, 91, 113]. Absence of stigmata of the condition in parents or other relatives and the high prevalence of first and second cousin marriages in the parents of affected children[7, 85, 113, 149] are consistent with autosomal recessive inheritance. Accordingly, this hereditary condition could perhaps be designated autosomal recessive vitamin D dependency Type II. However, there is a marked female sex preponderance that remains unexplained. Of the 11 patients in whom the sex was mentioned, 10 were females; the only male patient was one of the sibs reported by Marx *et al.*[91]. There is also a marked tendency to alopecia totalis (10:14 patients) usually before 1 year of age[6, 7, 85, 149].

At first glance the literature suggests the existence of two different phenotypes – a group of patients with alopecia and a strong family history, and a less frequent, possibly sporadic group without alopecia. However, an attempt to differentiate the disease into two forms breaks down when all the reported findings are considered.

Vitamin D dependency Type II is evidently a lifelong affliction since some patients with rickets in infancy were still affected in adult life[14, 91, 161]. In infancy, the biochemical and skeletal manifestations may be very incapacitating. Convulsions are reported and four infants have died[7, 85]. Children have usually had typical rachitic deformities with stunted stature. Only in one child did signs of rickets first appear during school age[14]. This child, like several others, required orthopedic surgery to correct deformities.

All patients had received high-dosage vitamin D treatment for various periods in various doses and with varying degrees of success before diagnosis of end-organ refractoriness to $1,25(OH)_2D$ was established. Some were young adults when the definitive tests were carried out[14, 91, 161]. With one exception, referred to below, these young adult individuals had the same biochemical abnormalities as did affected children and they had radiographic and histological signs of osteomalacia, their growth plates having fused. In general, their deformities were less than during infancy, though most patients were stunted in stature at the time of study. Evidently, phenotypical expression of the abnormal gene becomes less conspicuous with time.

In treating this newly identified condition, the first approach has been to use high doses of vitamin D or vitamin D analogues. Although data on response are still somewhat scant, one gains the general impression that these agents usually had beneficial effects on calcium and phosphate homeostasis and on the skeletal lesions if given in sufficient dosage[7, 14, 91, 149, 161]; alopecia was not altered, however. Some patients on the other hand failed to show any biochemical or radiographic response to extremely high doses of vitamin D or metabolites given for periods that one would have expected to be effective[6, 85, 113]. One adult patient showed dramatic and lasting correction of calcium and phosphate homeostasis following a brief combined course of $24,25(OH)_2D_3$ and $1\alpha\text{-OHD}_3$ treatment[85]. Interestingly, plasma $24,25(OH)_2D$ was undetectable before treatment in this patient, but increased to normal concentrations during $24,25(OH)_2D_3$ therapy. Two children who were unresponsive to moderate doses of vitamin D showed radiographic healing on oral phosphate supplementation alone[110], but were subsequently treated with high-dose $1,25(OH)_2D_3$ alone[40].

The hypothesis that end-organ resistance to $1,25(OH)_2D$ is the pathophysiological mechanism underlying vitamin D dependency Type II is based on the following considerations. The constellation of rickets associated with hypocalcemia, hypophosphatemia, elevated plasma iPTH, generalized aminoaciduria and deficient intestinal absorption of calcium[90, 113, 149] categorizes the disease as a calcipenic condition. Since there is no evidence that dietary calcium intake or intestinal fat absorption are abnormal[113], it follows that an intrinsic defect in calcium transport exists, and that there must be a perturbation of either parathyroid or vitamin D physiology. Hypoparathyroidism is ruled out as the cause of hypocalcemia by the demonstration of high plasma levels of iPTH in all patients. Pseudohypoparathyroidism (which hypothetically could cause both hypocalcemia and elevated plasma, $1,25(OH)_2D$) was ruled out by significantly elevated rates of urinary cyclic AMP excretion[6, 14, 91, 113, 149, 161], and a by a rise in plasma calcium concentration and further increase in urinary cyclic AMP excretion in response to exogenous parathyroid extract[84, 110].

Plasma 25-OHD levels in untreated patients were normal[6, 7, 14, 91, 113, 161], from which it can be deduced that vitamin D nutrition was satisfactory and hepatic 25-hydroxylation was normal. Plasma levels of $24,25(OH)_2D$ are also normal or slightly elevated[6, 7, 91, 149], except for the seemingly atypical patient of Liberman *et al.*[85] in whom $24,25(OH)_2D$ could not be detected prior to vitamin D treatment.

Elevated plasma levels of $1,25(OH)_2D$ – at least three times normal – are a salient feature of the condition. The mean value for eight untreated patients was 350 pg/ml and ranged from 137 to 916 pg/ml[6, 14, 85, 91, 113, 161]. This finding, which distinguishes autosomal recessive vitamin D dependency Type II from Type I, led to the suggestion that end-organ refractoriness was the basis for the disease. Two additional observations lend strong support to this hypothesis: (a) there is lack of response to treatment with vitamin D_2, vitamin D_3, 25-OHD$_3$ and $1,25(OH)D_2D_3$ in moderately high, sometimes extremely high doses; and (b) cultured skin fibroblasts from members of two kindreds showed markedly deficient nuclear uptake of $[^3H]\text{-}1,25(OH)_2D_3$[40]. Whether the latter abnormality is due to an impairment in cytoplasmic or nuclear component(s) is not yet established (Marx, S.J. personal communication, 1981).

The elevated levels of $1,25(OH)_2D$ in the plasma of untreated patients have been attributed to stimulation of renal 1α-hydroxylase activity by hypocalcemia, hypophosphatemia and secondary hyperparathyroidism. This reasoning does not explain, however, the observation that plasma $1,25(OH)_2D$ levels remained elevated[161], or in some instances appeared actually to increase[7, 14, 91] during treatment with large doses of vitamin D or 25-OHD$_3$ sufficient to cause normocalcemia and normophosphatemia, and to reduce plasma iPTH to physiological levels[14, 91, 161].

Although the clinical features and some of the underlying pathogenetic mechanisms of vitamin D dependency Type II seem now to be falling into place, there are many questions that still cannot be answered. Alopecia totalis commencing early in life is a striking and frequent feature of vitamin D dependency Type II. It is possible that 1,25(OH)$_2$D plays some role in maintenance of normal skin function. Several authors have demonstrated 1,25(OH)$_2$D$_3$ effector systems in skin[40], but their physiological significance is unknown. The marked preponderance of affected females over males suggests that the X-chromosome may in some way contribute to the expression of 1,25(OH)$_2$D unresponsiveness, but a plausible explanation for this effect has not been presented.

Mention should also be made of the perplexing history and findings in the surviving female sib reported by Liberman *et al.*[85]. This patient was hypocalcemic, normophosphatemic and rachitic in infancy. However, the bone lesions had disappeared by 6 years of age, although hypocalcemia and elevated alkaline phosphatase persisted. When this individual was studied between the ages of 13 and 15 years, she was not rachitic, she suffered from cataracts, oligodentia and amelogenesis imperfecta, and though she was still hypocalcemic she had hyperphosphatemia at this time. The plasma iPTH level was slightly elevated and plasma 1,25(OH)$_2$D was approximately 700 pg/ml. Interestingly, the plasma 24,25(OH)$_2$D level was undetectable; on the other hand, this metabolite was present in normal concentrations in the other five patients tested. Some of the biochemical features suggested hypoparathyroidism, others pseudohypoparathyroidism, but the various observations failed to meet all the criteria for either diagnosis. Hypocalcemia and hyperphosphatemia did not respond to 1α-OHD$_3$, dihydrotachysterol, or 1,25(OH)$_2$D$_3$. However, plasma calcium, phosphate and alkaline phosphatase became normal during a short combined course of 24,25(OH)$_2$D$_3$ and 1α-OHD$_3$, and unaccountably remained normal 9 months after withdrawing these medications. Nonetheless, the plasma 1,25(OH)$_2$D level remained markedly raised (339 pg/ml). Unfortunately, the plasma iPTH level was not stated at this phase of treatment.

Implications of the pathophysiological findings for treatment of the rachitic syndromes

We are far from understanding any of the rachitic syndromes at the gene level. However, the knowledge we already have points to logical therapeutic approaches to the management of the various rachitic syndromes we have discussed.

Treatment of X-linked hypophosphatemia (XLH)

At present, it is not possible to correct the defect in transepithelial transport of inorganic phosphate. Consequently treatment is aimed at neutralizing the effects of the transport defect. The objectives therefore, are (a) to control hypophosphatemia, (b) to prevent deformities, (c) to achieve normal growth, and (d) to reduce bone lesions. Treatment with vitamin D or its metabolites and oral phosphate supplementation have been used with varying success.

Vitamin D is known to reduce rachitic lesions; however, only in near-toxic doses does it have any beneficial effect on the skeleton. Vitamin D treatment increases plasma phosphate slightly although not to the physiological range; it decreases plasma alkaline phosphatase activity but rarely to the normal value, it 'heals' rachitic lesions in the growth plates as judged radiographically[50], and it improves skeletal deformities such as genu varum. However, the characteristic coarse trabecular pattern rarely disappears, osteoid seams persist on microscopic examination, and the bone lesions probably never heal completely[26, 59, 62]. Vitamin D therapy alone rarely corrects dwarfism[104], and even if started in early infancy may fail to prevent its development[45, 134, 137]. As is necessary in any treatment with large doses of vitamin D, care must be taken to avoid vitamin D intoxication. The plasma calcium level must be measured accurately at least every 3 months. Even with diligence on the part of the physician and vigilance by the patient, occasional episodes of hypercalcemia are very difficult to prevent, and in consequence functional and histological abnormalities of the kidney occur in a significant number of patients after long-term vitamin D therapy[28].

Treatment with 25-hydroxyvitamin D offers no advantage over vitamin D treatment. Short-term treatment with $1,25(OH)_2D_3$ has proved to be ineffective in correcting the renal transport defect, restoring plasma phosphate concentrations to normal, and healing rachitic lesions[58, 62, 125]. Results of long-term treatment with $1,25(OH)_2D_3$ are more promising[26, 37, 59]. $1,25(OH)_2D_3$ therapy increases the intestinal absorption of phosphate and raises TmPi/GFR somewhat, resulting in increased plasma Pi concentrations and positive balance for phosphate and calcium. Moreover, striking improvement is noted in bone histology; $1,25(OH)_2D_3$ treatment almost completely normalizes the mineralization defect[26, 37], a feature that remains abnormal with vitamin D and oral phosphate treatment[58]. Radiographically, the rachitic lesions at the growth plates disappear and coarse trabeculation improves with $1,25(OH)_2D_3$ treatment. Some postulate[37, 128] that there may be altered vitamin D homeostasis in X-linked hyphosphatemia. This proposition is based on the observations that X-linked hyphosphatemic patients have normal concentrations of plasma $1,25(OH)_2D$ in the presence of severe hypophosphatemia and that several biochemical and histological abnormalities resolve after long-term $1,25(OH)_2D_3$ therapy. The question whether the abnormalities in vitamin D metabolism are primary or secondary requires further investigation. However, there is consensus that $1,25(OH)_2D_3$ is more effective than vitamin D as an adjunct to oral phosphate therapy and its rapid action and quick correction of hypercalcemia when discontinued are additional advantages. Whether these advantages reduce renal complications over many years of treatment is unknown.

When the skeletal lesions of X-linked hypophosphatemia were found to be caused by defective renal phosphate conservation, oral phosphate therapy became the cornerstone of treatment[63]. It has been known for over 100 years that dietary phosphate heals rachitic lesions in animals[86]. Intravenous infusion of phosphate has been found to promote rapid healing of rickets in human hypophosphatemic states without the aid of high doses of vitamin D[45, 46, 126, 136]. Various investigators[56] observed radiographic improvement in rachitic lesions and found positive external balances for phosphorus and calcium in X-linked hypophosphatemia after oral supplementation with phosphate salts. However, the healing effect was evident only during the first 1–2 months of treatment after which rachitic lesions reappeared despite phosphate supplementation (Fraser, D. and Kooh, S. W., unpublished data, 1981). Others have also reported failure of oral phosphate treatment[44, 138]. However, poor results from oral phosphate therapy are caused more often by lack of patient compliance than by failure of bone to respond. Photodensitometry of standard X-ray images of the middle phalanx has shown satisfactory bone density in treated patients when compared with age-matched control subjects[52]. Of greater clinical importance is the striking increase in linear growth velocity after initiation of treatment with supplemental phosphate. Glorieux *et al.*[63] observed that the average linear growth velocity in untreated X-linked hypophosphatemia was only 63% of normal; when treated with vitamin D alone in the traditional manner, the growth rate was not greatly increased. However, in patients receiving phosphate treatment and vitamin D, the average growth rate was approximately twice the pretreatment rate. Others have also shown that phosphate therapy permits true catch-up growth in X-linked hypophosphatemia, thus reducing the likelihood of dwarfism[74, 157]. Phosphate loading decreases the level of ionized calcium and thus causes an increase in the plasma concentration of parathyroid hormone[63, 109]. It is not obvious why X-linked hypophosphatemia patients receiving oral phosphate therapy develop secondary hyperparathyroidism. Such patients are not hyperphosphatemic even when receiving large doses of phosphate, and hypocalcemia, the presumed stimulus of parathyroid hormone hypersecretion, is difficult to document. At any rate, through its action on the residual PTH-sensitive component of tubular phosphate reabsorption, the elevated PTH level causes an even greater impairment in renal phosphate reclamation, thereby reducing the therapeutic efficacy of oral phosphate therapy.

The major complication of phosphate therapy is the development of secondary hyperparathyroidism. This can be avoided by using vitamin D or metabolites as an adjunct to phosphate therapy. Recent reports[19, 26, 59] indicate that the combination of oral phosphate and $1,25(OH)_2D_3$ produces better results than are achieved with either drug by itself or by conventional phosphate and vitamin D therapy. With the oral phosphate – $1,25(OH)_2D_3$ combination, higher concentrations of plasma phosphate are maintained, rachitic lesions are satisfactorily controlled, the mineralization front is almost normalized, and secondary hyperparathyroidism is prevented. However, to date there are only a few patients in whom increased stature has been reported[19, 59].

The objective in children is to attain plasma phosphate levels of approximately 4 mg/dl. The response of the plasma inorganic phosphate to single phosphate load is shortlived. For this reason phosphate supplements must be given every 4 hours and the child should receive a dose five times daily[25, 63]. Initially, phosphate supplementation may cause diarrhea, but tolerance to the regimen usually develops within 1 or 2 weeks. A dose of 1–5 g elemental phosphorus per day is needed to achieve the desired phosphate level.

The dose of $1,25(OH)_2D_3$ is 0.025–0.050 μg/kg bodyweight per day, preferably given in divided doses. Treatment should be monitored by measuring plasma calcium at least every 2 months, preferably monthly. Whether measurement of the ratio of calcium/creatinine in a fasting urine sample is preferable to monitoring plasma calcium is under investigation. At present a major deterrent to the use of $1,25(OH)_2D_3$ is its high cost compared to vitamin D therapy. The assessment regimen for long-term management is described in detail below.

COUNSELLING

Because the gene for hypophosphatemia is transmitted as an X-linked dominant trait, parents with one affected child have a 50% probability of having an affected child in each subsequent pregnancy. An affected mother transmits the condition to 50% of her children regardless of their sex, whereas if the father is affected, all his daughters and none of his sons will be affected. Hypophosphatemia cannot be detected by amniocentesis. However, in a pregnancy in which the father has X-linked hypophosphatemia, knowledge of the sex of the fetus will provide information whether the offspring is affected. Offspring of affected parents should be monitored for phosphate concentration monthly from birth, to allow early diagnosis. Since there is a normal decline in phosphate concentrations after birth, measurements should be checked against those for age-matched controls (*Figure 1.3*). The parent should also be informed of sex differences in severity of the

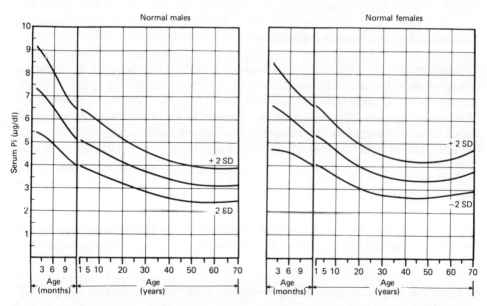

Figure 1.3 Age-related variation in normal serum inorganic phosphate concentrations in males and females. The curves depict the mean and 95% confidence limits. Data from infants aged 0–6 months are from Owen *et al.*[103]. Data for subjects 1 year of age and older are from Greenberg *et al.*[66]

disease. In general, males with X-linked hypophosphatemia are more severely affected, more likely to have short stature, and more likely to require corrective surgery than females. Some carrier females are asymptomatic and attain normal height, although they are hypophosphatemic and their bones are osteomalacic histologically.

Treatment of autosomal dominant hypophosphatemic bone disease (HBD)

Combination of $1,25(OH)_2D_3$ and oral phosphate provides the best control of biochemical and skeletal lesions of hypophosphatemic bone disease. In most patients the epiphyseal lesions are absent or less prominent than in patients with X-linked hypophosphatemia, but osteomalacic lesions, manifested by coarse trabeculation in the radiographs, are invariably present. The recommendations outlined for the treatment of X-linked hypophosphatemia apply also to treatment of hypophosphatemic bone disease. In one child, $1,25(OH)_2D_3$ treatment raised serum phosphate, improved tubular reabsorption of phosphate, and healed the bone deformities[129]. However, patients usually require oral phosphate supplementation.

COUNSELLING
An affected individual has a 50% probability of having affected children. The manifestations are equally express in males and females.

Treatment of the Fanconi syndromes

Treatment of the Fanconi syndromes is a two-fold process. One treatment component is aimed at offsetting the primary disease (eliminating or preventing the accumulation of toxic substances, for example, fructose, tyrosine, copper, drugs). The other component is to administer vitamin D and to replace phosphate and other solutes if necessary (for example, bicarbonate, potassium, etc.). Prevention or treatment of rickets/osteomalacia in the Fanconi syndrome is usually not a major clinical challenge.

COUNSELLING
The Fanconi syndrome(s) may be acquired or inherited. Depending on the specific form, inheritance may be autosomal dominant, X-linked recessive, or, for most syndromes, autosomal recessive (*see Table 1.4*).

Treatment of autosomal recessive vitamin D dependency Type I (ARVDD Type I)

As would be predicted from knowledge of the pathophysiology, a characteristic of autosomal recessive vitamin D dependency Type I is complete healing of the biochemical and skeletal lesions with appropriately large doses of vitamin D or with small presumably physiological doses of $1,25(OH)_2D_3$. In our experience, vitamin D_2 or D_3, 1000 iu/kg bodyweight per day (25 µg/kg bodyweight per day) or $1,25(OH)_2D_3$ (0.0075 µg/kg bodyweight per day) is an appropriate starting dose. Response is usually evaluated at weekly intervals initially and then at 4–6 weekly intervals until the maintenance requirement is ascertained. If no biochemical or radiographic improvement is evident, the dose of vitamin D or $1,25(OH)_2D_3$ is increased by 20% every 2 months until healing occurs. Once the maintenance dose is established, assessments of plasma calcium, Pi, alkaline phosphatase, blood urea nitrogen, and creatinine and urinary calcium/creatinine ratio are made regularly at 2-monthly intervals (monthly for $1,25(OH)_2D_3$). Radiographs of the knees and wrists are obtained less frequently. The maintenance dose of vitamin D is 1000–1600 iu/kg bodyweight per day (25–40 µg/kg bodyweight per day); the maintenance dose of $1,25(OH)_2D_3$ is 0.005–0.01 µg/kg bodyweight per day.

With appropriate therapy, all biochemical and radiographic abnormalities revert to normal, deformities disappear and normal growth returns. However, the defect in vitamin D metabolism is permanent and treatment must be continued into adulthood to prevent recurrence of osteomalacia.

COUNSELLING

At present there is no test to identify carriers of the mutant gene. Plasma $1,25(OH)_2D$ concentrations of parents of affected patients have not been reported. The risk of recurrence of this trait is 25% in each subsequent pregnancy. The diagnosis of an affected offspring can be made within weeks of birth and treatment started. Thus, phenotypic manifestations of the gene are completely preventable.

Treatment of vitamin D dependency Type II (VDD Type II)

In patients with this disease, the target tissues are insensitive to the actions of vitamin D hormone, but the defect appears to be relative since very large doses of vitamin D, $25\text{-}OHD_3$, $1\alpha\text{-}OHD_3$ or $1,25(OH)_2D_3$ corrected hypocalcemia and secondary hyperparathyroidism in most reported patients. Alopecia is not corrected. Lifelong therapy is presumably necessary since the biochemical and radiographic lesions have been reported in adults[14, 91, 161]. To date, there is little information on the long-term effects of treatment.

COUNSELLING

Vitamin D dependency Type II is probably an autosomal recessive condition. Most of the patients reported to date have been females, but a genetic mechanism has not been established to explain this observation. No physical or biochemical stigmata have been reported in obligate heterozygotes. The nuclear uptake of $1,25(OH)_2D_3$ in cultured skin fibroblasts of the heterozygote has not been reported.

References

1 ALBRIGHT, F., BUTLER, A. M. and BLOOMBERG, E. Rickets resistant to vitamin D therapy. *American Journal of Diseases of Children*, **54**, 529–547 (1937)

2 ARNAUD, C., GLORIEUX, F. and SCRIVER, C. Serum parathyroid hormone in X-linked hypophosphatemia. *Science*, **173**, 845–847 (1971)

3 ARNAUD, C., MAIJER, R., READE, T., SCRIVER, C. R. and WHELAN, D. T. Vitamin D dependency: an inherited postnatal syndrome with secondary hyperparathyroidism. *Pediatrics*, **46**, 871–880 (1970)

4 ARONSON, P. S. Identifying secondary active solute transport in epithelia. *American Journal of Physiology*, **240**, F1–F11 (1981)

5 AUSTIN, L. A. and HEATH, H. III. Calcitonin: physiology and pathophysiology. *New England Journal of Medicine*, **304**, 269–278 (1981)

6 BALSAN, S., GARABEDIAN, M., LIEBERHERR, M., GUERIS, J. and ULMANN, A. Serum 1,25-dihydroxyvitamin D concentrations in two different types of pseudo-deficiency rickets. In *Vitamin D, Basic Research and its Clinical Application*, edited by A. W. Norman, K. Schaefer, D. V. Herrath, H. G. Grigoleit, E. B. Mawer, T. Suda, H. F. DeLuca and J. W. Coburn, pp. 1143–1149. New York, de Gruyter (1979)

7 BEER, S., TIEDER, M., KOHELET, D., LIBERMAN, A. O., VURE, E., BAR-JOSEPH, G., GAVIZON, D., BOROCHOWITZ, Z. U., VARON, M. and MODAI, D. Vitamin D resistant rickets with alopecia: a form of end-organ resistance to 1,25-dihydroxyvitamin D. *Clinical Endocrinology*, **14**, 395–402 (1981)

8 BERGERON, M., DUBORD, L., HAUSSER, C. and SCHWAB, C. Membrane permeability as a cause of transport defects in experimental Fanconi syndrome: a new hypothesis. *Journal of Clinical Investigation*, **57**, 1181–1189 (1976)

9 BERNER, W., KINNE, R. and MURER, H. Phosphate transport into brush-border membrane vesicles isolated from rat small intestine. *Biochemical Journal*, **160**, 467–474 (1976)

10 BHATTACHARYYA, M. H. and DeLUCA, H. F. The regulation of rat liver calciferol-25-hydroxylase. *Journal of Biological Chemistry*, **248**, 2969–2973 (1973)

11 BORDIER, P., RASMUSSEN, H., MARIE, P., MIRAVET, L., GUERIS, J. and RYCKWAERT, A. Vitamin D metabolites and bone mineralization in man. *Journal of Clinical Endocrinology and Metabolism*, **46**, 284–294 (1978)

12 BORDIER, P. J. and TUN CHOT, S. Quantitative histology of metabolic bone disease. *Clinics in Endocrinology and Metabolism*, **1**, 197–215 (1972)

13 BRISSENDEN, J. E. and COX, D. W. Electrophoretic and quantitative assessment of vitamin D-binding protein (group-specific component) in inherited rickets. *Journal of Laboratory and Clinical Medicine*, **91**, 455–462, 1978

14 BROOKS, M. H., BELL, N. H., LOVE, L., STERN, P. H., ORFEI, E., QUEENER, S. F., HAMSTRA, A. J. and DeLUCA, H. F. Vitamin-D-dependent rickets Type II: resistance of target organs to 1,25-dihydroxyvitamin D. *New England Journal of Medicine*, **298**, 996–999 (1978)

15 BRUNETTE, M. G., CHABARDES, D., IMPERT-TEBOUL, M., CLIQUE, A., MONTÉGUT, M. and MOREL, F. Hormone-sensitive adenylate cyclase along the nephron of genetically hypophosphatemic mice. *Kidney International*, **15**, 357–369 (1979)

16 BRUNETTE, M. G., CHAN, M., FERRIERE, C. and ROBERTS, K. D. Site of 1,25(OH)$_2$ vitamin D$_3$ synthesis in the kidney. *Nature*, **276**, 287–288 (1978)

17 BURT, C. T., COHEN, S. M. and BARANY, M. Analysis of intact tissue with ^{31}P NMR. *Annual Review of Biophysics and Bioengineering*, **8**, 1–25 (1979)

18 BYERS, P. D. The diagnostic value of bone biopsies. In *Metabolic Bone Disease*, **1**, edited by L. V. Avioli and S. M. Krane, pp. 184–236. New York, Academic Press (1977)

19 CHAN, J. C. M. and BARTTER, F. C. Hypophosphatemic rickets: effects of 1α,25-dihydroxyvitamin D$_3$ on growth and mineral metabolism. *Pediatrics*, **64**, 488 –495 (1979)

20 CHEN, T. C., CASTILLO, L., KORYCKA-DAHL, M. and DeLUCA, H. F. Role of vitamin D metabolites in phosphate transport of rat intestine. *Journal of Nutrition*, **104**, 1056–1060 (1974)

21 CHESNEY, R. W., MAZESS, R. B., ROSE, P., HAMSTRA, A. J. and DeLUCA, H.F. Supranormal 25-hydroxyvitamin D and subnormal 1,25-dihydroxyvitamin D: their role in X-linked hypophosphatemic rickets. *American Journal of Diseases of Children*, **134**, 140–143 (1980)

22 CHESNEY, R. W., ROSEN, J. F., HAMSTRA, A. J. and DeLUCA, H. F. Serum 1,25-dihydroxyvitamin D levels in normal children and in vitamin D disorders. *American Journal of Diseases of Children*, **134**, 135–139 (1980)

23 CHILDS, B. Persistent echoes of the nature–nurture argument. *American Journal of Human Genetics*, **29**, 1–13 (1977)

24 CHRISTENSEN, J. F. Three familial cases of atypical late rickets. *Acta Paediatrica*, **28**, 247–270 (1941)

25 CLOW, C. L., READE, T. M. and SCRIVER, C. R. Management of hereditary metabolic disease: the role of allied health personnel. *New England Journal of Medicine*, **284**, 1292–1298 (1971)

26 COSTA, T., MARIE, P. J., SCRIVER, C. R., COLE, D. E. C., READE, T. M., NOGRADY, B., GLORIEUX, F. H. and DELVIN, E. E. X-linked hypophosphatemia: effect of calcitriol on renal handling of phosphate serum phosphate and bone mineralization. *Journal of Clinical Endocrinology and Metabolism*, **54**, 463–476 (1981)

27 COWGILL, L. D., GOLDFARB, S., LAU, K., SLATOPOLSKY, E. and AGUS, Z. S. Evidence for an intrinsic renal tubular defect in mice with genetic hypophophatemic rickets. *Journal of Clinical Investigation*, **63**, 1203–1210 (1979)

28 CURTIS, J., HSU, A. C., BAUMAL, R., RANCE, C. P., STEELE, B., KOOH, S. W. and FRASER, D. Risk of renal damage from large dose vitamin D therapy. *Pediatric Research*, **15**, 396 (1981) (Abstract)

29 DeLUCA, H. F. Vitamin D metabolism and function. *Archives of Internal Medicine*, **138**, 836–847 (1978)

30 DeLUCA, H. F. Some new concepts emanating from a study of the metabolism and function of vitamin D. *Nutrition Reviews*, **38**, 169–182 (1980)

31 DELVIN, E. E. and GLORIEUX, F. H. Serum 1,25-dihydroxyvitamin D concentration in hypophosphatemic vitamin D-resistant rickets. *Calcified Tissue International*, **33**, 173–175 (1981)

32 DENNIS, V. W., STEAD, W. W. and MYERS, J. L. Renal handling of phosphate and calcium. *Annual Review of Physiology*, **41**, 257–271 (1979)

33 DENT, C. E. Rickets and osteomalacia from renal tubule defects. *Journal of Bone and Joint Surgery*, **34B,** 266–274 (1952)

34 DENT, C. E., FRIEDMAN, M. and WATSON, L. Hereditary pseudo-vitamin D deficiency rickets ('hereditare pseudo-mangelrachitis'). *Journal of Bone and Joint Surgery*, **50B,** 708–719 (1968)

35 DENT, C. E., RICHENS, A., ROWE, D. J. F. and STAMP, T. C. B. Osteomalacia with long-term anticonvulsant therapy in epilepsy. *British Medical Journal*, **4,** 69–72 (1970)

36 DIAMOND, J. M. Tight and leaky junctions of epithelia: a perspective on kisses in the dark. *Federation Proceedings*, **33,** 2220–2224 (1974)

37 DREZNER, M. K., LYLES, K. W., HAUSSLER, M. R. and HARRELSON, J. M. Evaluation of a role for 1,25-dihydroxyvitamin D_3 in the pathogenesis and treatment of X-linked hypophosphatemic rickets and osteomalacia. *Journal of Clinical Investigation*, **66,** 1020–1032 (1980)

38 EASTWOOD, J. B., De WARDENER, H. E., GRAY, R. W. and LEMANN, J. L. Jr. Normal plasma-1,25-$(OH)_2$-vitamin D concentrations in nutritional osteomalacia. *Lancet*, **1,** 1377–1378 (1979)

39 EICHER, E. M., SOUTHARD, J. L., SCRIVER, C. R. and GLORIEUX, F. H. Hypophosphatemia: mouse model for human familial hypophosphatemic (vitamin D-resistant) rickets. *Proceedings of the National Academy of Sciences of the United States of America*, **73,** 4667–4671 (1976)

40 EIL, C., LIBERMAN, U. A., ROSEN, J. F. and MARX, S. J. A cellular defect in hereditary vitamin-D-dependent rickets Type II: defective nuclear uptake of 1,25-dihydroxyvitamin D in cultured skin fibroblasts. *New England Journal of Medicine*, **304,** 1588–1591 (1981)

41 EISMAN, J. A., JAMSTRA, A. J., KREAM, B. E. and DeLUCA, H. F. A sensitive, precise, and convenient method for determination of 1,25-dihydroxyvitamin D in human plasma. *Archives of Biochemistry and Biophysics*, **176,** 235–243 (1976)

42 EVERS, C., MURER, H. and KINNE, R. Effect of parathyrin on the transport properties of isolated renal brush-border vesicles. *Biochemical Journal*, **172,** 49–56 (1978)

43 FINERMAN, G. A. M. and ROSENBERG, L. E. Amino acid transport in bone: evidence for separate transport systems for neutral amino and imino acids. *Journal of Biological Chemistry*, **241,** 1487–1493 (1966)

44 FRAME, B., SMITH, R. W. Jr, FLEMING, J. L. and MANSON, G. Oral phosphates in vitamin-D-refractory rickets and osteomalacia. *American Journal of Diseases of Children*, **106,** 147–153 (1963)

45 FRASER, D., GEIGER, D. W., MUNN, J. D., SLATER, P. E., JAHN, R. and LIU, E. Calcification studies in clinical vitamin D deficiency and in hypophosphatemic vitamin D-refractory rickets: the induction of calcium deposition in rachitic cartilage without the administration of vitamin D. *American Journal of Diseases of Children*, **96,** 460–461 (1958) (Abstract)

46 FRASER, D., JACO, N. T., YENDT, E. R., MUNN, J. D. and LIN, E. The induction of *in vitro* and *in vivo* calcification in bones of children suffering from vitamin D-resistant rickets without recourse to large doses of vitamin D. *American Journal of Diseases of Children*, **93,** 84–84 (1957) (Abstract)

47 FRASER, D., KOOH, S. W., KIND, H. P., HOLICK, M. F., TANAKA, Y. and DeLUCA, H. F. Pathogenesis of hereditary vitamin-D-dependent rickets: An inborn error of

vitamin D metabolism involving defective conversion of 15-hydroxyvitamin D to 1α,25-dehydroxyvitamin D. *New England Journal of Medicine*, **289**, 817–822 (1973)

48 FRASER, D., KOOH, S. W. and SCRIVER, C. R. Hyperparathyroidism as the cause of hyperaminoaciduria and phosphaturia in human vitamin D deficiency. *Pediatric Research*, **1**, 425–435 (1967)

49 FRASER, D., LEEMING, J. M. and CERWENKA, E. A. Über die Handhabung von Phosphat durch die nieren bei hypophosphatämischer vitamin-D-resistenter Rachitis der einfachen Art und bei Cystinspeicherkrankheit: Reaktion auf verlängerte Calciuminfusion. *Helvetica Paediatrica Acta*, **14**, 497–404 (1959)

50 FRASER, D. and SALTER, R. B. The diagnosis and management of the various types of rickets. *Pediatric Clinics of North America*, **5**, 417–441 (1958)

51 FRASER, D. and SCRIVER, C. R. Familial forms of vitamin D-resistant rickets revisited. X-linked hypophosphatemia and autosomal recessive vitamin D dependency. *American Journal of Clinical Nutrition*, **29**, 1315–1329 (1976)

52 FRASER, D. and SCRIVER, C. R. Disorders associated with hereditary or acquired abnormalities in vitamin D function: hereditary disorders associated with vitamin D resistance or defective phosphate metabolism. In *Endocrinology*, **2**, edited by L. J. DeGroot, G. F. Cahill, Jr, L. Martini, D. H. Nelson, W. D. Odell, J. T. Potts, Jr., E. Steinberger and A. I. Winegrad, pp. 797–807. New York, Grune and Stratton (1979)

53 FRASER, D. R. Regulation of the metabolism of vitamin D. *Physiological Reviews*, **60**, 551–613 (1980)

54 FRASER, D. R. and KODICEK, E. Unique biosynthesis of a biologically active vitamin D metabolite. *Nature*, **228**, 764–766 (1970)

55 GALUS, K., SZYMENDERA, J., ZALESKI, A. and SCHREYER, K. Effects of 1α-hydroxyvitamin D_3 and 24R, 25-dihydroxyvitamin D_3 on bone remodelling. *Calcified Tissue International*, **31**, 209–213 (1980)

56 GERBEAUX-BALSAN, S. L'absorption intestinale du phosphore dans le rachitisme vitamino-résistant hypophosphatémique héréditaire. Effets de fortes surcharges de phosphore et des régimes très pauvres en calcium. *Revue Française d'Études Cliniques et Biologiques (Paris)*, **10**, 65–72 (1965)

57 GIASSON, S. D., BRUNETTE, M. G., DANAN, G., VIGNEAULT, N. and CARRIERE, S. Micropuncture study of renal phosphorus transport in hypophosphatemic vitamin D resistant rickets mice. *Pflügers Archiv, European Journal of Physiology*, **371**, 33–38 (1977)

58 GLORIEUX, F. H., BORDIER, P. J., MARIE, P., DELVIN, E. E. and TRAVERS, R. Inadequate bone response to phosphate and vitamin D in familial hypophosphatemic rickets (FHR). In *Homeostasis of Phosphate and Other Minerals*, edited by S. G. Massry, E. Rictz and A. Rapaso, pp. 227–232. New York, Plenum Publishing Corporation (1978)

59 GLORIEUX, F. H., MARIE, P. J., PETTIFOR, J. M. and DELVIN, E. E. Bone response to phosphate salts, ergocalciferol, and calcitriol in hypophosphatemic vitamin D-resistant rickets. *New England Journal of Medicine*, **303**, 1023–1131 (1980)

60 GLORIEUX, F. and SCRIVER, C. R. Loss of a parathyroid hormone-sensitive component of phosphate transport in X-linked hypophosphatemia. *Science*, **175**, 997–1000 (1972)

61 GLORIEUX, F. H. and SCRIVER, C. R. Transport metabolism and clinical use of inorganic phosphate in X-linked hypophosphatemia. In *Clinical Aspects of Metabolic Bone Disease*, edited by B. Frame, A. M. Parfitt and H. Duncan, pp. 421–426. Amsterdam, Excerpta Medica (1973)

62 GLORIEUX, F. H., SCRIVER, C. R., HOLICK, M. F. and DeLUCA, H. F. X-linked hypophosphataemic rickets: inadequate therapeutic response to 1-25-dihydroxycholecalciferol. *Lancet*, **2**, 287–289 (1973)

63 GLORIEUX, F. H., SCRIVER, C. R., READE, T. M., GOLDMAN, H. and ROSEBOROUGH, A. Use of phosphate and vitamin D to prevent dwarfism and rickets in X-linked hypophosphatemia. *New England Journal of Medicine*, **287**, 481–487 (1972)

64 GOLDBERG, M., AGUS, Z. S. and GOLDFARB, S. Renal handling of phosphate, calcium and magnesium. In *The Kidney*, **3**, edited by B. M. Brenner and F. C. Rector, Jr, pp. 344–390. Philadelphia, W. B. Saunders (1976)

65 GRAY, T. K., LESTER, G. E. and LORENC, R. S. Evidence for extra-renal 1α-hydroxylation of 25-hydroxyvitamin D_3 in pregnancy. *Science*, **204**, 1311–1313 (1979)

66 GREENBERG, B. R., WINTERS, R. W. and GRAHAM, J. B. The normal ranges of serum inorganic phosphorus and its utility as a discriminant in the diagnosis of congenital hypophosphatemia. *Journal of Clinical Endocrinology and Metabolism*, **20**, 364 (1960)

67 GRIFFITH, E. J., PONNAMPERUMA, C. and GABEL, N. W. Phosphorus, a key to life on the primitive earth. *Origins of Life*, **8**, 71–85 (1977)

68 GÜNTHER, R., SILBERNAGL, S. and DEETJEN, P. Maleic acid induced aminoaciduria, studied by free flow micropuncture and continuous microperfusion. *Pflügers Archiv, European Journal of Physiology*, **382**, 109–114 (1979)

69 HADDAD, J. G. Jr and HAHN, T. J. Natural and synthetic sources of circulating 25-hydroxyvitamin D in man. *Nature*, **244**, 515–517 (1973)

70 HAMMERMAN, M. R., KARL, I. E. and HRUSKA, K. A. Regulation of canine renal vesicle P_1 transport by growth hormone and parathyroid hormone. *Biochimica et Biophysica Acta*, **603**, 322–335 (1980)

71 HARMEYER, J., GRABE, C. V. and MARTENS, H. Effects of metabolites and analogues of vitamin D in hereditary pseudovitamin D deficiency of pigs. In *Vitamin D: Biochemical, Chemical and Clinical Aspects Related to Calcium Metabolism*, edited by A. W. Norman, K. Schaefer, J. W. Coburn, H. F. DeLuca, D. Fraser, H. G. Grigoleit and D. V. Herrath, pp. 785–788. Berlin, De Gruyter (1977)

72 HARMEYER, J. and PLONAIT, H. Generalisierte Hyperaminoacidurie mit erblicher Rachitis bei Schweinen. *Helvetica Paediatrica Acta*, **22**, 216–229 (1967)

73 HARRISON, H. E. and HARRISON, H. C. Disorders of calcium and phosphate metabolism in childhood and adolescence. *Major Problems in Clinical Pediatrics*, **20**, (1979)

74 HARRISON, H. E., HARRISON, H. C., LIFSHITZ, F. and JOHNSON, A. D. Growth disturbance in hereditary hypophosphatemia. *American Journal of Diseases of Children*, **112**, 290–297 (1966)

75 HOFFMAN, N., THEES, M. and KINNE, R. Phosphate transport by isolated renal brush border vesicles. *Pflügers Archiv, European Journal of Physiology*, **362**, 147–156 (1956)

76 HOLICK, M. F., MacLAUGHLIN, J. A. and DOPPELT, S. H. Regulation of cutaneous previtamin D_3 photosynthesis in man: skin pigment is not an essential regulator. *Science*, **211**, 590–593 (1981)

77 HUGI, K., BONJOUR, J. P. and FLEISCH, H. Renal handling of calcium: influence of parathyroid hormone and 1,25-dihydroxyvitamin D_3. *American Journal of Physiology*, **236**, F349–F356 (1979)

78 HULDSCHINSKY, K. Heilung von Rachitis durch Künstliche Höhensonne. *Deutsche Medizinische Wochenschrift*, **45**, 712–713 (1919)

79 IVANHOE, F. Was Virchow right about Neandertal? *Nature*, **277**, 577–579 (1970)

80 JONES, G. Assay of vitamins D_2 and D_3 and 25-hydroxyvitamins, D_2 and D_3 in human plasma by high-performance liquid chromatography. *Clinical Chemistry*, **24**, 287–298 (1978)

81 KANIS, J. A., CUNDY, T., BARTLETT, M., SMITH, R., HEYNEN, G., WARNER, G. T. and RUSSELL, R. G. G. Is 24,25-dihydroxycholecalciferol a calcium-regulating hormone in man? *British Medical Journal*, **1**, 1382–1386 (1978)

82 KOOH, S. W., FRASER, D., DeLUCA, H. F., HOLICK, M. F., BELSEY, R. E., CLARK, M. B. and MURRAY, T. K. Treatment of hypoparathyroidism and pseudohypoparathyroidism with metabolites of vitamin D: evidence for impaired conversion of 25-hydroxyvitamin D to 1α,25-dihydroxyvitamin D. *New England Journal of Medicine*, **293**, 840–844 (1975)

83 LAWSON, D. E. M. (editor). *Vitamin D*. London, Academic Press (1978)

84 LEVER, J. E. Phosphate ion transport in fibroblast plasma membrane vesicles. *Annals of the New York Academy of Sciences*, **341**, 37–47 (1980)

85 LIBERMAN, U. A., SAMUEL, R., HALABE, A., KAULI, R., EDELSTEIN, S., WEISMAN, Y, PAPA-POULOS, S. E., CLEMENS, T. L., FRAHER, L. J. and O'RIORDAN, J. L. H. End-organ resistance to 1,25-dihydroxycholecalciferol. *Lancet*, **1**, 504–507 (1980)

86 LILLY, C. A., PEIRCE, C. B. and GRANT, R. L. The effect of phosphates on the bones of rachitic rats. *Journal of Nutrition*, **9**, 25–35 (1935)

87 LITMAN, N. N., ULSTROM, R. A. and WESTIN, W. W. Vitamin D-resistant rickets. *California Medicine*, **86**, 248–253 (1953)

88 LOEWENSTEIN, W. R. and ROSE, B. Calcium in (junctional) intercellular communication and a thought on its behavior in intracellular communication. *Annals of the New York Academy of Sciences*, **307**, 285–307 (1978)

89 LOOMIS, W. F. Rickets. *Scientific American*, **223** (6), 77–91 (1970)

90 MARIE, P. J., TRAVERS, R. and GLORIEUX, F. H. Healing of rickets with phosphate supplementation in the hypophosphatemic male mouse. *Journal of Clinical Investigation*, **67**, 911–914 (1981)

91 MARX, S. J., SPIEGEL, A. M., BROWN, E. M., GARDNER, D. G., DOWNS, R. W., Jr, ATTIE, M., HAMSTRA, A. J. and DeLUCA, H. F. A familial syndrome of decrease in sensitivity to 1,25-dihydroxyvitamin D. *Journal of Clinical Endocrinology and Metabolism*, **47**, 1303–1310 (1978)

92 MATTHEWS, J. L., WIEL, C. V. and TALMAGE, R. V. Bone lining cells and the bone fluid compartment, an ultrastructural study. *Advances in Experimental Medicine and Biology*, **103**, 451–458 (1978)

93 McCOLLUM, E. V. and DAVIS, M. The necessity of certain lipids in the diet during growth. *Journal of Biological Chemistry*, **15**, 167–175 (1913)

94 McINNES, R. R. and SCRIVER, C. R. Effect of calciotropic hormones and cyclic nucleotides on aminoaciduria and phosphaturia. *Pediatric Research*, **14**, 218–223 (1980)

95 McKEOWN, J. W., BRAZY, P. C. and DENNIS, V. W. Intrarenal heterogeneity for fluid, phosphate and glucose absorption in the rabbit. *American Journal of Physiology*, **237**, F312–F318 (1979)

96 MELLANBY, E. *Experimental Rickets*. Medical Research Council, Special Report Series No. 61. London, HMSO (1921)

97 MEYER, R. A., Jr., GRAY, R. W. and MEYER, M. H. Abnormal vitamin D metabolism in the X-linked hypophosphatemic mouse. *Endocrinology*, **107**, 1577–1581 (1980)

98 MOREL, F. Sites of hormone action in the mammalian nephron. *American Journal of Physiology*, **241**, F159–F164 (1981)

99 MORRIS, R. C., Jr., McINNES, R. R., EPSTEIN, C. J., SEBASTIAN, A. and SCRIVER, C. R. Genetic and metabolic injury of the kidney. In *The Kidney*, **2**, edited by B. M. Brenner and F. C. Rector, Jr, pp. 1193–1256. Philadelphia, W. B. Saunders (1976)

100 NIKIFORUK, G. and FRASER, D. Etiology of enamel hypoplasia and interglobular dentin: the roles of hypocalcemia and hypophosphatemia. *Metabolic Bone Disease and Related Research*, **2**, 17–23 (1979)

101 OHNO, S. Sex chromosomes and sex-linked genes. In *Monographs on Endocrinology*, **1**, edited by A. Labhart, T. Mann, L. T. Samuels and J. Zanders, pp. 46–73. New York, Springer-Verlag, Chapter 4 (1967)

102 OHNO, S. Ancient linkage groups and frozen accidents. *Nature*, **244**, 259–262 (1973)

103 OWEN, G. H., GARRY, P. and FOMON, S. J. Concentrations of calcium and inorganic phosphorus in serum of normal infants receiving various feedings. *Pediatrics*, **31**, 495 (1963)

104 PARFITT, A. M. Hypophosphatemic vitamin D refractory rickets and osteomalacia. *Orthopedic Clinics of North America*, **3**, 653–680 (1972)

105 PLONAIT, H. Klinische Fragen der Calciumstoffwechselstörungen beim Schwein. *Deutsche Tieraerztliche Wochenschrift*, **69**, 198–202 (1962)

106 PRADER, A., ILLIG, R. and HEIERLI, E. Eine besondere Form der primären vitamin D-resistenten Rachitis mit Hypocälcämie und autosomal-dominantem Erbgang: die hereditare Pseudo-Mangelrachitis. *Helvetica Paediatrica Acta*, **16**, 452–468 (1961)

107 RASMUSSEN, H. and ANAST, C. Familial hypophosphatemic (vitamin D-resistant) rickets and vitamin D-dependent rickets. In *The Metabolic Basis of Inherited Disease*, *4th edition*, edited by J. B. Stanbury, J. B. Wyngaarden and D. S. Fredrickson, pp. 1537–1562. New York, McGraw-Hill (1978)

108 READE, T. , SCRIVER, C. R., GLORIEUX, F. H., NOGRADY, B., DELVIN, E., POIRIER, R., HOLICK, M. F. and DeLUCA, H. F. Response to crystalline 1α-hydroxyvitamin D_3 in vitamin D dependency. *Pediatric Research*, **9**, 593–599 (1975)

109 REISS, E. and CANTERBURY, J. M. The effect of phosphate on parathyroid hormone secretion. In *Calcium-Regulating Hormones* (Proceedings of the 5th Parathyroid Conference, Oxford, 1974), edited by R. V. Talmage, M. Owen and J. A. Parsons, pp. 66–71. Amsterdam, Excerpta Medica (1975)

110 REISS, E., CANTERBURY, J. M., BERCOVITZ, M. A. and KAPLAN, E. L. The role of phosphate in the secretion of parathyroid hormone in man. *Journal of Clinical Investigation*, **49**, 2146–2149 (1970)

111 REYNOLDS, R., McNAMARA, P. D. and SEGAL, S. On the maleic acid induced Fanconi syndrome: effects on transport by isolated rat kidney brush-border membrane vesicles. *Life Sciences*, **22**, 39–44 (1978)

112 ROBERTSON, B. R., HARRIS, R. C. and McCUNE, D. J. Refractory rickets: mechanism of therapeutic action of calciferol. *American Journal of Diseases of Children*, **64**, 948–949 (1942)

113 ROSEN, J. F., FLEISCHMAN, A. R., FINBERG, L., HAMSTRA, A. and DeLUCA, H. F. Rickets with alopecia: an inborn error of vitamin D metabolism. *Journal of Pediatrics*, **94**, 729–735 (1979)

114 ROTHSTEIN, A., CABANTCHIK, Z. I. and KNAUF, P. Mechanism of anion transport in red blood cells: role of membrane proteins. *Federation Proceedings*, **35**, 3–10 (1976)

115 ROYER, P., LESTRADET, H., FRÉDÉRICH, A. and DARTOIS, A. M. Les rachitismes vitaminorésistants hypophosphatémiques idiopathiques de l'enfant. *Archives Françaises de Pédiatrie*, **18**, 41–64 (1961)

116 SABINA, R. L., DREZNER, M. K. and MOLNER, E. W. Phosphate depletion: a derangement in nucleoside triphosphate metabolism. *Clinical Research*, **29**, 544A (1981)

117 SCHAFER, J. A. and BARFUSS, D. W. Membrane mechanisms for transepithelial amino acid absorption and secretion. *American Journal of Physiology*, **238**, F335–F346 (1980)

118 SCHNEIDER, J. A., SCHULMAN, J. D. and SEEGMILLER, J. E. Cystinosis and the Fanconi syndrome. In *The Metabolic Basis of Inherited Disease*, 4th edition, edited by J. B. Stanbury, J. B. Wyngaarden and D. S. Fredrickson, pp. 1660–1682. New York, McGraw-Hill (1978)

119 SCHOPF, J. W. The evolution of the earliest cells. *Scientific American*, **239** (3), 110–112, 114, 116–120, *passim* (1978)

120 SCRIVER, C. R. Vitamin D dependency. *Pediatrics*, **45**, 361–363 (1970)

121 SCRIVER, C. R. Rickets and the pathogenesis of impaired tubular transport of phosphate and other solutes. *American Journal of Medicine*, **57**, 43–49 (1974)

122 SCRIVER, C. R. The William Allan Memorial Award Address: on phosphate transport and genetic screening. 'Understanding backward – living forward' in human genetics. *American Journal of Human Genetics*, **31**, 243–263 (1979)

123 SCRIVER, C. R. Transepithelial transport of phosphate: perspectives from man and mouse. In *Pediatric Diseases Related to Calcium*, edited by H. F. DeLuca and C. S. Anast, pp. 165–177. New York, Elsevier (1980)

124 SCRIVER, C. R., CHESNEY, R. W. and McINNES, R. R. Genetic aspects of renal tubular transport: diversity and topology of carriers. *Kidney International*, **9**, 141–171 (1976)

125 SCRIVER, C. R., GLORIEUX, F. H., READE, T. M. and TENENHOUSE, H. S. X-linked hypophosphataemia and autosomal recessive vitamin D dependency: models for the resolution of vitamin D refractory rickets. In *Inborn Errors of Calcium and Bone Metabolism*, edited by H. Bickel and J. Stern, pp. 150–178. Baltimore, University Park Press (1976)

126 SCRIVER, C. R., GOLDBLOOM, R. B. and ROY, C. C. Hypophosphatemic rickets with renal hyperglycinuria, renal glucosuria and glycyl-prolinuria: a syndrome with evidence for renal tubular secretion of phosphorus. *Pediatrics*, **34**, 357–371 (1964)

127 SCRIVER, C. R., MacDONALD, W., READE, T., GLORIEUX, F. H. and NOGRADY, B. Hypophosphatemic nonrachitic bone disease: an entity distinct from X-linked hypophosphatemia in the renal defect, bone involvement and inheritance. *American Journal of Medical Genetics*, **1**, 101–117 (1977)

128 SCRIVER, C. R., READE, T. M., DeLUCA, H. F. and HAMSTRA, A. J. Serum 1,25-dihydroxyvitamin D levels in normal subjects and in patients with hereditary rickets or bone disease. *New England Journal of Medicine*, **299**, 976–979 (1978)

129 SCRIVER, C. R., READE, T., HALAL, F., COSTA, T. and COLE, D. E. C. Autosomal hypophosphataemic bone disease responds to $1,25(OH)_2D_3$. *Archives of Disease in Childhood*, **56**, 203–207 (1981)

130 SCRIVER, C., R., STACEY, T. E., TENENHOUSE, H. S. and MacDONALD, W. A. Transepithelial transport of phosphate anion in kidney. Potential mechanisms for hypophosphatemia. *Advances in Experimental Medicine and Biology*, **81**, 55–70 (1977)

131 SHORT, E., MORRIS, R. C., Jr., SEBASTIAN, A. and SPENCER, M. Exaggerated phosphaturic response to circulating parathyroid hormone in patients with familial X-linked hypophosphatemic rickets. *Journal of Clinical Investigation*, **58**, 152–163 (1976)

132 SHORT, E. M., BINDER, H. J. and ROSENBERG, L. E. Familial hypophosphatemic rickets: defective transport of inorganic phosphate by intestinal mucosa. *Science*, **179**, 700–702 (1973)

133 STAMP, T. C. B. and ROUND, J. M. Seasonal changes in human plasma levels of 25-hydroxyvitamin D. *Nature*, **247**, 563–565 (1974)

134 STEARNS, G. A guide to the adequacy of therapy in resistant rickets due to familial or essential hypophosphatemia. *Journal of Bone and Joint Surgery*, **46A**, 959–964 (1964)

135 STEENBOCK, H. and BLACK, A. Fat-soluble vitamins: XVII. The induction of growth-promoting and calcifying properties in a ration by exposure to ultraviolet light. *Journal of Biological Chemistry*, **61**, 405–422 (1924)

136 STEENDIJK, R. The effect of a continuous intravenous infusion of inorganic phosphate on the rachitic lesions in cystinosis. *Archives of Disease in Childhood*, **36**, 321–324 (1961)

137 STICKLER, G. B., BEABOUT, J. W. and RIGGS, B. L. Vitamin D-resistant rickets: clinical experience with 41 typical familial hypophosphatemic patients and 2 atypical nonfamilial cases. *Mayo Clinic Proceedings*, **45**, 197–218 (1970)

138 STICKLER, G. B., HAYLES, A. B. and ROSEVEAR, J. W. Familial hypophosphatemic vitamin D resistant rickets. *American Journal of Diseases of Children*, **110**, 664–667 (1965)

139 STOOP, J. W., SCHRAAGEN, M. J. C. and TIDDENS, H. A. W. M. Pseudo-vitamin D deficiency rickets: report of four new cases. *Acta Paediatrica Scandinavica*, **56**, 607–616 (1967)

140 STUMPF, W. E., SAR, M., NARBAITZ, R., REID, F. A., DeLUCA, H. F. and TANAKA, Y. Cellular and subcellular localization of 1,25(OH)$_2$-vitamin D$_3$ in rat kidney: comparison with localization of parathyroid hormone and estradiol. *Proceedings of the National Academy of Sciences of the United States of America*, **77**, 1149–1153 (1980)

141 TANFORD, C. The hydrophobic effect and the organization of living matter. *Science*, **200**, 1012–1018 (1978)

142 TENENHOUSE, H. S., COLE, D. E. C. and SCRIVER, C. R. Mendelian hypophosphataemias as probes of phosphate and sulphate transport by mammalian kidney. In *Inherited Problems of Transport*, edited by N. Belton and C. Toothill, 231–262. Baltimore, University Park Press (1981)

143 TENENHOUSE, H. S., FAST, D. K., SCRIVER, C. R. and NOLTAY, M. Intestinal transfer of phosphate anion is not impaired in the *Hyp* (hypophosphatemic) mouse. *Biochemical and Biophysical Research Communications*, **100**, 537–543 (1981)

144 TENENHOUSE, H. S. and SCRIVER, C. R. Orthophosphate transport in the erythrocyte of normal subjects and of patients with X-linked hypophosphatemia. *Journal of Clinical Investigation*, **55**, 644–645 (1975)

145 TENENHOUSE, H. S. and SCRIVER, C. R. The defect in transcellular transport of phosphate in the nephron is located in brush-border membranes in X-linked hypophosphatemia (*Hyp* mouse model). *Canadian Journal of Biochemistry*, **56**, 640–646 (1978)

146 TENENHOUSE, H. S. and SCRIVER, C. R. Effect of 1,25-dihydroxyvitamin D$_3$ on phosphate homeostasis in the X-linked hypophosphatemic (*Hyp*) mouse. *Endocrinology*, **109**, 658–660 (1981)

147 TENENHOUSE, H. S., SCRIVER, C. R., McINNES, R. R. and GLORIEUX, F. H. Renal handling of phosphate *in vivo* and *in vitro* by the X-linked hypophosphatemic male mouse: evidence for a defect in the brush-border membrane. *Kidney International*, **14**, 236–244 (1978)

148 TENENHOUSE, H. S., SCRIVER, C. R. and VIZEL, E. J., Alkaline phosphatase activity does not mediate phosphate transport in the renal–cortical brush-border membrane. *Biochemical Journal*, **190**, 473–476 (1980)

149 TSUCHIYA, Y., MATSUO, N., CHO, H., KUMAGAI, M., YASAKA, A., SUDA, T., ORIMO, H. and SHIRAKI, M. An unusual form of vitamin D-dependent rickets in a child: alopecia and marked end-organ hyposensitivity to biologically active vitamin D. *Journal of Clinical Endocrinology and Metabolism*, **51**, 685–690 (1980)

150 TUCKER, G. III, GAGNON, R. E. and HAUSSLER, M. R. Vitamin D$_3$-25-hydroxylase: tissue occurrence and apparent lack of regulation. *Archives of Biochemistry and Biophysics*, **155**, 47–57 (1973)

151 TURNER, R. T., PUZAS, J. E., FORTE, M. D., LESTER, G. E., GRAY, T. K., HOWARD, G. A. and BAYLINK, D. J. *In vitro* synthesis of 1α,25-dihydroxycholecalciferol and 24,25-dihydroxycholecalciferol by isolated calvarial cells. *Proceedings of the National Academy of Sciences of the United States of America*, **77**, 5720–5724 (1980)

152 VOGEL, F. and MOTULSKY, A. G. *Human Genetics: Problems and Approaches*. New York, Springer-Verlag (1979)

153 WALLING, M. W. and LEE, D. B. N. Theories on the mechanism of action of 1,25(OH)₂D₃ on active intestinal calcium and inorganic phosphate absorption: are the calcium and phosphate transport processes coupled, uncoupled or both? In *Vitamin D: Basic Research and its Clinical Application*, edited by A. W. Norman, K. Schaefer, D. V. Herrath, H. G. Grigoleit, E. B. Mawer, T. Suda, H. F. DeLuca and J. W. Coburn, pp. 687–692. New York, de Gruyter (1979)

154 WALTON, R. J. and BIJVOET, O. L. M. Nomogram for derivation of renal theshold phosphate concentration. *Lancet*, **2**, 309–310 (1975)

155 WASSERMAN, R. H. Molecular aspects of the intestinal absorption of calcium and phosphorus. In *Pediatric Diseases Related to Calcium*, edited by H. F. DeLuca and C. S. Anast, pp. 107–132. New York, Elsevier (1980)

156 WATTERSON, D. M. and VINCENZI, F. F. (editors). Calmodulin and cell functions. *Annals of the New York Academy of Sciences*, **356** (1980)

157 WEST, C. D., BLANTON, J. C., SILVERMAN, F. N. and HOLLAND, N. H. Use of phosphate salts as an adjunct to vitamin D in the treatment of hypophosphatemic vitamin D refractory rickets. *Journal of Pediatrics*, **64**, 469–477 (1964)

158 WILKE, R., HARMEYER, J., VON GRABE, C., HEHRMANN, R. and HESCH, R. D. Regulatory hyperparathyroidism in a pig breed with vitamin D dependency rickets. *Acta Endocrinology*, **92**, 294–308 (1979)

159 WINAVER, J. and PUSCHETT, J. B. Structural determinants of the renal tubular activity of vitamin D₃ derivatives: studies with 1α-hydroxy, 24R,25-dihydroxy and 1α,24R,25-trihydroxyvitamin D₃. *Proceedings of the Society for Experimental Biology and Medicine*, **159**, 204–209 (1978)

160 WINTERS, R. W., GRAHAM, J. B., WILLIAMS, T. F., McFALLS, V. W. and BURNETT, C. H. A genetic study of familial hypophosphatemia and vitamin D resistant rickets with a review of the literature. *Medicine*, **37**, 97–142 (1958)

161 ZERWEKH, J. E., GLASS, K., JOWSEY, J. and PAK, C. Y. C. An unique form of osteomalacia associated with end-organ refractoriness to 1,25-dihydroxyvitamin D and apparent defective synthesis of 25-hydroxyvitamin D. *Journal of Clinical Endocrinology and Metabolism*, **49**, 171–175 (1979)

2
The prevention of osteoporosis

J. M. Aitken

Osteoporosis is the most common abnormality of the adult skeleton and this abnormality becomes increasingly prevalent as people age. Osteoporotic bone is structurally weak and prone to fracture as a result of relatively trivial trauma. The female skeleton becomes osteoporotic much more readily than the male skeleton and after middle age Colles' fracture, vertebral body compression and fracture of the femoral neck occur at an almost exponential rate in the ageing female population. It would therefore be a distinct socioeconomic advantage to be able to prevent the development of osteoporosis and thereby remove a potential cause of considerable suffering in the elderly. However, in order to be able to prevent osteoporosis it is important to know how osteoporosis develops and the way in which different variables may affect this.

The term osteoporosis is interpreted in different ways by different people, but for the purpose of this chapter it will be defined as a significant reduction in skeletal mass. This reduction in skeletal mass may be localized or generalized, but the bony tissue present is assumed to show no qualitative differences from normal bone. A significant reduction in bone mass is defined by a value more than 2 SD below the mean value found in a normal population of either men or women at a time when skeletal mass is at its peak value. In both men and women skeletal mass reaches this peak value somewhere between the ages of 30 and 40 years. This sort of information has in the past been obtained from cross-sectional population surveys and the results of one of these is shown in *Figure 2.1*.

In this survey the parameter of bone mass was the Standardized Aluminium Equivalent (SAE) measured at the midpoint of the third metacarpal from a plain X-ray of the hand alongside an aluminium step wedge[12]. Using this method for measuring bone mass, the critical value 2 SD below the mean at the age of 35 years in women is 2.8 mmAl cm^{-1}, and hence any woman with a SAE of 2.8 mmAl cm^{-1} or less would be said to have osteoporosis. Although this definition is somewhat empirical it has been shown that the prevalence of vertebral crush fractures increases progressively as the SAE falls further below this critical value[88].

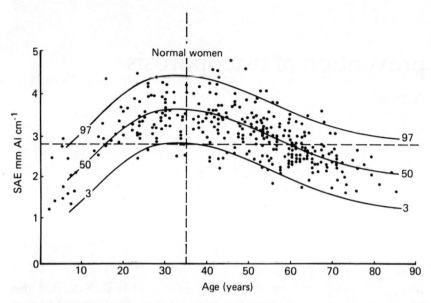

Figure 2.1 Relationship between metacarpal mineral content (SAE) and age in women. Mean ± 2 SD (3rd–97th percentile). (After Smith *et al.*[89])

Similar observations have been made by other investigators using different methods and different skeletal reference sites[36]. Johnston *et al.*[48] studied 526 normal Caucasian women using a γ-ray photon absorptiometric technique to measure bone mass at the midpoint of the radius. In their study a value 2 SD below the mean at the age of 35 years was found to be about 0.70 g bone mineral/cm. They found that there was a considerable overlap in the radius bone mass values between women with vertebral crush fractures and those without. However Mazess *et al.*[65] found that a mid-radius bone mineral value of 0.68 g/cm discriminated between 50 white women without evidence of skeletal failure, and 50 white women with spontaneous fractures of the vertebrae, femoral neck or radius.

The implicit assumption that osteoporotic bone is qualitatively indistinguishable from normal bone may not necessarily be wholly true, for although the ratio of calcium to phosphorus remains constant as skeletal mass declines, the ratios of calcium to zinc and calcium to magnesium fall both with age and bone mass[4] (*Figure 2.2*). It is therefore quite possible, if one were to look critically at other constituents of osteoporotic bone and compare these with those present in normal bone, that further biochemical differences would be found.

When one uses histomorphometric techniques to study osteoporotic bone obtained from the iliac crest, it is apparent that in about 10% of patients the resorption surfaces and the surface area covered by osteoid are increased. This suggests that in these patients there is increased bone turnover. Likewise, when bone samples from osteoporotic patients are examined after double tetracycline labelling, it has been found that about 37% have a low osteoblastic appositional rate[70].

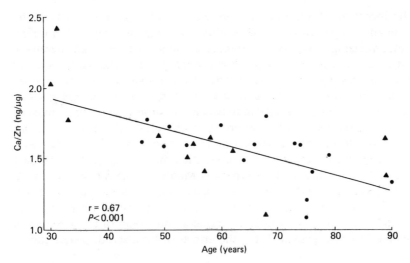

Figure 2.2 Relationship between trabecular bone calcium/zinc ratio and age in 12 female (▲) and 16 male (●) cadavers. (After Aitken[4])

Whereas serum calcium and phosphorus concentrations and urinary hydroxyproline excretion are within the normal range in patients with osteoporosis, there is a tendency for these values to be at the upper end of the normal range. Furthermore, using whole body retention of technetium-labelled (^{99m}Tc) diphosphonate as a measure of skeletal metabolic activity, patients with osteoporosis as a whole tend to have higher than normal values, although lower than those found in patients with osteomalacia, hyperparathyroidism and Paget's disease[19]

In spite of these minor differences, the diagnosis of osteoporosis is still made on the basis of a significantly reduced bone mass in association with normal values for serum calcium, phosphorus and alkaline phosphatase, normal urinary hydroxyproline excretion and normal bone histology using routine laboratory techniques. It is therefore important to exclude all other causes of metabolic bone disease associated with rarefaction of the skeleton including osteomalacia, hyperparathyroidism, multiple myeloma and carcinomatosis, since all these conditions occur with increasing frequency in the ageing population. In patients with these diseases radiotranslucency of the bone may be the result of the underlying condition or, in view of the increasing prevalence of osteoporosis with age, merely coincidental.

The diagnosis of osteoporosis initially rests upon establishing adequate radiological criteria to substantiate a deficiency of bone substance. The appearance of radiotranslucency of the skeleton is not enough and the diagnosis must be backed up by a quantitative measurement at an appropriate skeletal site. When osteoporosis is generalized bone mass measurements on peripheral bone sites, where cortical bone predominates, are preferable to measurements on the axial skeleton, where there is a higher proportion of trabecular bone, because the former are amenable to a much greater degree of precision and reproducibility. This is in spite of the fact that not all types of bone share the same degree of metabolic activity, and thus at the inception of a period of generalized bone loss, those parts of the skeleton with the most rapid turnover will be affected to a greater degree before the more slowly metabolizing parts. Hence trabecular bone, with its high metabolic activity, is lost to a much greater extent than cortical bone in the early stages of generalized skeletal wasting. However, in spite of this initial lack of synchronism between bone loss at trabecular and cortical sites, there is a surprisingly good *in vitro* correlation in the ageing population between measurements of bone mass at sites of widely varying structural composition[9]. Unfortunately this correlation is not good enough for one to be able to predict bone mass at a critical site, such as a vertebral body, from measurements at a non-critical but easily quantifiable site such as the midshaft of the radius. In this respect Madsen[61] found that about 15% of subjects with low *in vivo* spinal bone mass measurements had normal midshaft radius values. However, serial bone mass measurements at a peripheral site amenable to good reproducibility will give a reliable indication of the progress of generalized skeletal wasting provided that the effects of localized disorders can be excluded.

LOCALIZED OSTEOPOROSIS

On occasions osteoporosis is a local phenomenon affecting the bones in one limb or part of a limb or just part of a single bone. Localized osteoporosis can rarely be substantiated histologically since when it occurs it tends to affect areas of the skeleton not amenable to biopsy. Precise and careful radiographic techniques are therefore important, and knowledge of the degree of variation in bone density that one can expect to find at a particular site is essential, before an absolute difference in radiodensity can be assumed to be significant.

In this context limb dominance as a possible factor affecting bone mass should not be overlooked. Griffiths *et al.*[39] studied the distal radius of 31 normal subjects by photon absorptiometry and showed that the bone mass of the dominant arm was significantly greater than that of the non-dominant arm, with the difference averaging about 12%, but on occasions the difference was almost 25%. It would appear from this study that differences in bone mass would have to be in excess of 25% before one could begin to invoke a localized cause for osteoporosis. Furthermore, the radiographic changes of localized osteoporosis, which are loss of normal trabecular structure at the epiphyses and loss of cortical thickness in the diaphysis, must be reproducible and significantly different from normal before being accepted as pathological.

Aetiology

The most common aetiological factor in the development of localized osteoporosis is immobility, although other factors such as neurological damage and vascular changes may play a part quite independently of the immobilization. It was shown in dogs that the severity of the loss of bone substance appears to depend upon the degree of immobility rather than its cause[11]. Subsequent studies in man have tended to support these experiments and one early finding during the course of immobilization was of an increase in urinary calcium excretion[25].

Until the last two decades, when more accurate methods for the quantification of bone mass first became available, urinary calcium excretion alone or in combination with metabolic balance studies have been the mainstay of the investigation of immobilization osteoporosis. Deitrick *et al.*[28] showed that urinary calcium excretion may double in healthy male volunteers immobilized in plaster of paris casts from the waist downwards. Whedon and Shorr[94] examined urinary calcium excretion in patients with lower limb fractures and found values up to three times the normal, although even greater degrees of hypercalciuria were found in patients immobilized as a result of poliomyelitis. In patients with paralytic poliomyelitis urinary calcium excretion reached a peak value in the 5th week of immobilization and then persisted until just before ambulation became possible. The duration and magnitude of the hypercalciuria was found to be directly related to the severity of the paralysis, and the first macroscopic signs of osteoporosis appeared on standard radiographs of the paralysed limbs from 2 to 3½ months after the onset of the illness.

Nilsson[75] studied 90 men and women, aged 16–78 years, who had sustained a lower leg fracture of moderate severity from 6 months to 15 years previously. He showed, using a γ-ray photon absorptiometric method, that about 25% of the bone of the ipsilateral lower femoral epiphysis had been lost. This loss of trabecular bone appeared to occur within the period of plaster of paris immobilization (median 3½ months). It was apparent that even though half of these patients were under 45 years of age at the time of injury, the ipsilateral lower femoral epiphysis usually remained osteoporotic relative to the contralateral lower femoral epiphysis for up to 15 years after the injury.

Inflammatory joint disease is usually associated with loss of trabecular bone from the articulating epiphyses. This phenomenon is classically found in rheumatoid arthritis, but is also seen in chronic suppurative arthritis[87]. It is likely that this loss of bone substance is the result of more than just a reduction in limb mobility. Klein and Raisz[51] showed that prostaglandins, which are found in abundance in rheumatoid synovia, readily induce bone resorption in tissue culture. Kennedy *et al.*[50] demonstrated the presence of a substance, in the sera of some patients with rheumatoid arthritis, which was neither a prostaglandin nor parathyroid hormone, but which was capable of inducing bone resorption in tissue culture. These findings may well explain the increased prevalence of generalized osteoporosis that is found in patients with rheumatoid arthritis, irrespective of corticosteroid therapy.

There have been many hypotheses to explain the way in which immobilization induces localized osteoporosis. Burkhart and Jowsey[18] demonstrated an increase in P_{CO_2} and a fall in the pH of venous blood emerging from the immobilized tibiae of intact adult male dogs. However, where these dogs had previously been thyroidectomized, parathyroidectomized or both thyroidectomized and parathyroidectomized, there were no significant changes in the venous effluent P_{CO_2} or pH, nor unlike the intact animals did these animals develop osteoporosis in the immobilized limb. These findings would suggest that the changes in pH and P_{CO_2} were the result of increased bone destruction and not causally related to the subsequent osteoporosis. There is, however, no clear explanation as to how the immobilized limb of an intact animal becomes more sensitive than the non-immobilized limb to the effects of thyroid and parathyroid hormones.

Natural reversibility

Unlike the natural history of generalized osteoporosis, in some situations localized osteoporosis is reversible. Weightlessness, as occurs in astronauts during space travel, has been claimed to be a potent cause of localized osteoporosis. However studies by Mack and Vogt[60] in 12 astronauts, who were weightless for up to 14 days, revealed that the localized changes observed were reversible without recourse to medication or other special measures.

Transient osteoporosis, another form of localized osteoporosis which was first described in three pregnant women[24], usually resolves radiographically within a few weeks or, on occasions, a few years. Unfortunately the areas involved, especially the femoral head and neck, are not particularly amenable to quantification and an apparently normal radiograph is a poor endpoint[75].

Natural irreversibility

Strict immobilization of a limb is usually followed by localized skeletal wasting which does not regress when normal activity is restored. Where hypercalciuria has been used as a marker for the development of localized osteoporosis following enforced immobilization of healthy subjects, it has been possible to demonstrate a reduction in calcium excretion of about 50% by using an oscillating bed[93]. However the use of the oscillating bed for up to 8 hours daily, the adoption of the erect position for about 2 hours daily using a tilt table, and the employment of early assisted ambulation, have not been shown to have any material effect on the hypercalciuria found in patients with either traumatic paraplegia[97] or acute poliomyelitis[81, 94], nor have they prevented subsequent bone loss. It is only with the return of adequate muscle power sufficient to initiate active ambulation that the hypercalciuria is ameliorated. Unfortunately there have been no meaningful studies of bone mass during the acute and chronic stages of poliomyelitis to allow a proper assessment of the prophylactic effects of early ambulation in the prevention of the consequent localized osteoporosis. Furthermore, extrapolating the results of urinary calcium excretion to changes in bone mass can be misleading. In this context Rose[85] studied two patients during the hypercalciuric phase complicating immobilization for a fractured leg, and treated both with 10 mg bendrofluazide daily for 3 weeks. He found that whereas bendrofluazide therapy consistently lowered urinary calcium excretion, this was accompanied by an equivalent rise in faecal calcium excretion in one patient, due to a decrease in calcium absorption from the gut. It was suggested that bendrofluazide therapy might be useful in the prevention of localized osteoporosis complicating immobilization, but this has in fact never been substantiated.

Supplements of calcium and vitamin D were at one time recommended for patients whilst immobilized after fractures, but the main effect of this treatment was to increase the incidence of urolithiasis[91].

Treatment with a variety of diphosphonates has been shown to be effective in the prevention of the localization osteoporosis caused by immobilizing the hind limb of the rat[71], but treatment with calcitonin had no effect in this particular experimental model[74]. Neither diphosphonates nor calcitonin have been shown convincingly to inhibit the localized osteoporosis of immobilization in man, although Arnstein *et al.*[13] claimed that ethane-hydroxy-diphosphonate (EHDP) had a small effect in limiting bone mineral loss in paraplegic women.

Methods devised to simulate the piezo-electric effect of bony deformation, by exposing an immobilized limb to pulsating electromagnetic fields, have as yet not been shown to prevent the osteoporosis of immobilization, although this technique has been used with some success to stimulate bony union where fracture healing has been delayed[27].

GENERALIZED OSTEOPOROSIS

Generalized osteoporosis is usually completely symptomless until localized skeletal failure occurs. Lower forearm (Colles') fracture in a postmenopausal woman is a common presentation, but rarely does this situation stimulate the initiation of further investigation. This is an unfortunate state of affairs since many women under the age of 60 years would benefit from appropriate although slightly belated prophylaxis. Femoral neck fracture will usually attract the diagnosis of osteoporosis because of the well-established association between osteoporosis and femoral neck fracture in women over the age of 70 years, although efforts are rarely made to confirm this by appropriate skeletal quantification. In these patients further interest in the osteoporotic process quickly evaporates since skeletal wasting is usually far advanced and beyond the scope of prophylaxis. A postmenopausal woman with back pain, which has failed to respond to simple physical measures and analgesics, is probably the most familiar situation in which generalized osteoporosis is first considered, although unless vertebral deformity has occurred the pain is likely to be attributed to other causes. In this situation, if the spinal X-ray shows vertebral compression or wedging, particularly if this affects more than one vertebra, osteoporosis is the most likely diagnosis. Once other causes of metabolic bone disease have been excluded it is important to quantify the degree of osteoporosis present and ascertain the underlying cause for the osteoporosis.

The investigation and quantification of generalized osteoporosis have passed through a series of phases over the past 40 years. Metabolic balance studies were once the only tool available to assess perturbations in calcium homeostasis, but their results on occasions have been misleading and are insufficiently precise to be useful in monitoring the long-term efficacy of prophylactic measures.

Iliac crest histomorphometric measurement is useful as a method of investigating the cause of skeletal rarefaction, but only a few devoted exponents have used it to quantify the effects of treatment regimens, and this technique is clearly inappropriate for assessing the value of prophylactic therapy[17].

Radiographic morphometry is probably the most readily available and widely used tool for assessing the value of different regimens in subjects at risk from developing osteoporosis[15, 44].

Radiographic photodensitometry might be seen as a clever attempt to improve upon the accuracy and reproducibility of radiographic morphometry[12, 31]. However, where duplicate morphometric measurements are made on six metacarpals radiographic photodensitometry is both an inferior and a considerably more expensive method of investigation[44].

Photon absorptiometry is probably the most sophisticated method for skeletal quantification that is both within the purse and the available expertise of the average nuclear medicine department[64]. The accuracy and reproducibility of this method is somewhat superior to the most detailed radiographic morphometric method.

Neutron activation analysis[20] was introduced in an attempt to assess the whole skeleton rather than an isolated selected site, but its potential advantages are probably more than completely outweighed by the disadvantages of expense and unacceptable irradiation to the patient.

The above-mentioned non-invasive methods for making direct measurements on the skeleton may be used both to define osteoporosis and to monitor the progress of skeleton status. It is, however, essential to remember that bone mass may be reduced by other types of metabolic bone disease such as osteomalacia, hyperparathyroidism, myeloma and carcinomatosis, and it is implicit that these conditions should be excluded before making deductions from bone mass measurements in isolation.

Aetiology

There are a number of well-established potentially preventable causes of generalized osteoporosis. These include hypercortisolism (*see below*), hyperthyroidism, gastric surgery, alcoholism, heparin therapy and hypogonadism. The most common aetiological factor is hypogonadism and this is almost exclusively confined to women over the age of 45 years, in whom it is described as postmenopausal osteoporosis[10].

Hyperthyroidism

In 1891 Von Recklinghausen described skeletal wasting in a young woman dying of thyrotoxicosis. Aub *et al.*[14] showed that thyrotoxicosis can be associated with a severe degree of negative calcium balance. Smith *et al.*[90] found that in 92 patients with thyrotoxicosis, 5% were hypercalcaemic, 25% had hypercalciuria, 35% had hyperphosphatasia and 80% had increased urinary hydroxyproline excretion. Although these features are rather like those found in hyperparathyroidism, thyrotoxics differ in so far as the serum phosphorus tends to be at the upper end of the normal range or is raised, and renal tubular reabsorption of phosphate is increased. There has been some contention about the histological nature of the bone disease found in thyrotoxicosis, but the consensus of opinion is that osteomalacia and osteitis fibrosa are not a feature and that the bone merely shows evidence of osteoporosis as a result of increased bone turnover[2]. This hypermetabolic state of the skeleton can be detected on a plain X-ray of the hand, using industrial film, in 50% of thyrotoxics. The radiographic appearance is that of longitudinal intracortical striations in the metacarpals[68]. Fraser *et al.*[34] clearly demonstrated a significantly increased prevalence of osteoporosis in thyrotoxicosis, using a radiographic photodensitometric technique to measure metacarpal density and a photon absorptiometric technique to measure distal radius bone mass. Similar but less marked changes were described by Ikkos *et al.*[46] using radiographic morphometry of the second metacarpal. The difference between these two studies is probably explained by the failure of the morphometric technique to detect loss of bone substance caused by intracortical bone resorption. However, both studies appeared to show some restoration of bone mass after treatment of thyrotoxicosis, although this was less apparent in women over the age of 50 years. Bayley *et al.*[16], who performed partial body neutron activation analysis sequentially in 13 patients after ^{131}I therapy for thyrotoxicosis, found that in all patients there was an increment in body calcium and that this was greater in men than in women, but a return to a normal bone mass was not demonstrated.

The prevention of thyrotoxic osteoporosis depends to a large extent on early diagnosis, and for this a high degree of clinical awareness of thyroid disease is essential especially in older subjects in whom the classical symptoms and signs are often absent. In these patients treatment with radioactive iodine, which is usually the treatment of choice, should be expedited. The common practice of giving small and if necessary repeated doses of ^{131}I should be abandoned in preference for giving a once-and-for-all dose of ^{131}I in the knowledge that although subsequent hypothyroidism may occur both sooner and more frequently, at least the patient can be spared the ravages of a more severe degree of osteoporosis.

Gastric surgery

There is good evidence that partial gastrectomy is associated with a greater than normal prevalence of skeletal rarefaction, and this is particularly so in women[29, 73]. Hyperphosphatasia has been documented in about 15% of subjects after gastric surgery, and there is often a mild degree of hypocalcaemia[23, 30, 72]. These biochemical findings have led many observers to believe that the bony changes were caused by vitamin D deficiency, but histologically proven osteomalacia is rarely found (1% men, 3% women), and, except in the presence of osteomalacia, vitamin D therapy does not change any of these abnormal parameters[72].

Alcohol

Alcoholism is associated with accelerated skeletal wasting and this is not dependent upon the development of cirrhosis[76, 86]. Acute elevations of blood alcohol are attended by both hypercalciuria[49], and hypercortisolism[47, 69]. In certain patients the hypercortisolism may persist for several days after total abstinence from alcohol[83].

There is no known antidote to the osteolytic effects of alcohol and therefore abstinence is the only appropriate course to take. Unfortunately most female alcoholics are secretive about the habit, and therefore the true relevance of alcohol intake in the aetiology of osteoporosis is obscure. However, when a patient is at special risk from the development of osteoporosis one must be wary of permitting free access to alcohol.

Heparin

This uncommon cause of symptomatic osteoporosis is usually only seen in patients receiving more than 15 000 i.u. sodium heparin daily for more than 4 months, although some patients have received more than 20 000 i.u. daily for up to 27 months without any apparent deleterious effects[38]. Spearing *et al.*[92] have advocated the use of long-term heparin therapy during pregnancy for the prevention of venous thromboembolism. They reported no adverse effects during 22 pregnancies with heparin in doses exceeding 15 000 i.u. daily. However, two women have been described who sustained vertebral collapse after receiving similar amounts of heparin during pregnancy[1, 96].

It is clear that until more is known about the susceptibility of the skeleton to the accelerated bone loss caused by heparin, this drug should be used with great caution.

Sex hormone deficiency

The role of gonadal hormone insufficiency as a cause of osteoporosis was not fully enunciated until Fuller Albright drew attention to his observation that, in the absence of other known causes of metabolic bone disease, symptomatic osteoporosis was usually seen in postmenopausal women, especially after an early or artificial menopause[10]. However, although the term postmenopausal osteoporosis has enjoyed 40 years of respectability, proof of the causal relationship between loss of ovarian function and loss of bone mass was lacking. Various retrospective studies were reported but either lacked controls or were insufficiently searching in their attempts to exclude bias[66, 79].

In 1968 a project was set up in Glasgow with the intention of answering the various outstanding questions on this subject. In 1973 the first definitive publication, on the skeletal effects of hysterectomy and bilateral salpingo-oophorectomy compared with hysterectomy alone, was made[6]. Altogether 258 women who satisfied the criteria for inclusion were interviewed. All the women had been menstruating until the time of operation, which had been performed either 3 or 6 years prior to review. Bone mass was assessed from a hand X-ray by photodensitometry[12]. The bone mass of the women who underwent hysterectomy alone was in all respects found to be similar to that of a normal population of Glaswegian women[89]. Similarly premenopausal women who were oophorecto-mized after the age of 45 years did not appear to lose bone mineral faster than women who had undergone hysterectomy alone. However, where the ovaries had been removed from women before the age of 45 years, not only did the women become significantly more osteoporotic within 6 years of surgery as compared with their hysterectomized controls, but the degree of skeletal loss was greatest where oophorectomy had been performed in the youngest patients (*Figure 2.3*).

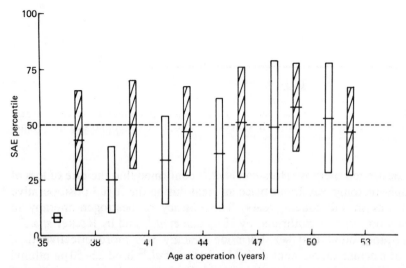

Figure 2.3 Relationship between metacarpal mineral content corrected for age (SAE percentile) 3–6 years after hysterectomy and bilateral oophorectomy (□) or hysterectomy alone (▨), and the age of the patient at the time of operation. Means ± 1 SD

At that time there was good reason to suppose that, of the various ovarian endocrine secretions, oestrogen would prove to be the most likely hormone responsible for maintaining the integrity of the premenopausal skeleton. There had been several attempts to confirm this, but none had been adequately controlled and all were open to the influence of bias[26, 67]. Consequently a double-blind controlled trial was set up to test the effect of an oestrogen (mestranol) against placebo in the prevention of further bone loss after oophorectomy.

The results after an average of 2[7], 5[52] and 9 years[54] observation confirmed the hypothesis that oestrogen replacement therapy was capable of preventing post-menopausal osteoporosis. Furthermore in some subjects, first treated 3 years after oophorectomy, a small increase in bone mineral content was found[52] (*Figure 2.4*). It was also noted that the rate of bone loss during the first 3 years after oophorectomy was about twice that seen in the postmenopausal population in general, and that this accelerated rate of loss of bone mineral could be completely

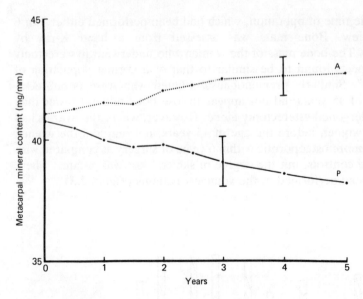

Figure 2.4 Effect of mestranol (A) or placebo (P) on metacarpal mineral content during 5 years of treatment starting 3 years after hysterectomy and bilateral oophorectomy. (After Lindsay *et al.*[52])

prevented by oestrogen therapy. Horsman *et al.*[45] confirmed that the rate of loss of bone after oophorectomy was about twice as great during the first 3 postoperative years than it was in subsequent years. The efficacy of oestrogen therapy in preventing osteoporosis was confirmed by Horsman *et al.*[42] and by Recker *et al.*[82]. Both these groups found that sex hormone therapy was more effective than 800–1200 mg of calcium supplement daily. Horsman *et al.*[42] used 25–50 µg ethinyl oestradiol daily for 21 days each month, whereas Recker *et al.*[82] used a mixture of 625 µg conjugated equine oestrogens plus 5 mg methyl testosterone daily for 21 days each month.

The withdrawal of oestrogen treatment after several years of continuous therapy has been claimed to be followed by accelerated bone loss[43, 56]. However Christiansen *et al.*[22], in a well-controlled study, failed to substantiate these claims.

The minimum daily dose of oestrogen required to achieve skeletal homeostasis is uncertain, but where 'continuous' daily treatment was given to 50 oophorectomized women, a dose in excess of 30 µg mestranol daily appeared to be less effective than 20 µg mestranol taken rather irregularly[8]. In adult male mice oestrogens appear to have a positive log linear effect on femoral whole bone density, suggesting that the larger the dose of oestrogen given the greater the effect on the skeleton[32]. Fogelman *et al.*[33] found a direct relationship between the 24-hour whole body retention of ^{99m}Tc diphosphonate and the rate of bone mineral loss measured by photon absorptiometry in a large group of postmenopausal women. In 11 oestrogen-treated oophorectomized women they also found an inverse relationship between oestrogen dosage and skeletal uptake of diphosphonate, such that the lowest rates of bone turnover were found in those women taking the largest doses of oestrogen (10–40 µg mestranol daily). However it does not necessarily follow that those women taking the largest doses of oestrogen would have had the lowest rates of bone mineral loss, and until this has been substantiated in a much larger group of women the question of optimum oestrogen dosage must remain in question.

It is known that a proportion of postmenopausal women produce significant amounts of oestrone by peripheral conversion from androstenedione[40, 59]. In theory these women might be sufficiently protected from the development of postmenopausal osteoporosis not to require exogenous oestrogen therapy. Initial studies in Glasgow using 24-hour total urinary oestrogen and gonadotrophin excretion, failed to document either an inverse correlation between urinary oestrogen excretion and the rate of bone loss, or a positive correlation between urinary gonadotrophin excretion and the rate of bone loss[3]. Nordin *et al.*[77] also failed to find a correlation between urinary total oestrogen excretion and bone loss in 33 postmenopausal women, although they found that patients excreting more than 15 µg (50 nmol) oestrogen daily had only very small rates of bone loss. With the advent of highly specific radioimmunoassay techniques to measure steroid hormone levels in plasma, it became possible to reassess the association between the oestrogen status of postmenopausal women and their current rate of bone loss. Lindsay *et al.*[53] first demonstrated an inverse correlation between plasma 17β-oestradiol, and both urinary calcium excretion and renal tubular reabsorption of phosphate in 44 oophorectomized women not receiving oestrogens. Subsequently a loose but significant correlation was demonstrated between the plasma 17β-oestradiol level and the rate of bone loss in 16 of these women, such that those women with the highest plasma oestrogen levels tended to be losing bone less rapidly than those with the lowest plasma oestrogen levels[57]. Unfortunately this correlation has not been substantiated in a larger group of women nor by other workers.

On the assumption that the single factor which distinguishes the postmenopausal woman, predisposed to develop symptomatic osteoporosis is the ability to convert an adequate quantity of androstenedione and related adrenal steroids to oestrogen, it is necessary to discover how some women achieve sufficient oestrogen synthesis after ovarian failure, whereas other women fail to rise to this metabolic challenge. Clearly many factors may be involved, but both the supply of adequate quantities of available substrate and the wherewithal to effect their aromatization to oestrogen are essential.

Marshall *et al.*[62] have explored several of these avenues and have produced some answers. Whereas plasma androstenedione and oestrone concentrations are lower in oophorectomized women than in postmenopausal women with intact ovaries, women with symptomatic spinal osteoporosis have the lowest levels of these steroids irrespective of the presence or absence of the ovaries. In fact only postmenopausal women on long-term corticosteroid therapy have lower plasma levels of androstenedione and oestrone[63]. This might infer that either adrenal androstenedione synthesis is impaired in women destined to develop symptomatic osteoporosis postmenopausally, or that reduced peripheral conversion of androstenedione to oestrone brings about a secondary reduction in sex hormone binding globulin (SHBG) synthesis with a consequent reduction in the capacity for the plasma to carry androstenedione, and hence a fall in the total plasma andros-tenedione concentration.

In either event one might expect there to be a direct relationship between plasma oestrone and androstenedione levels, and this has been confirmed[62, 63]. However, investigations into the conversion rate of androstenedione to oestrone using isotope dilution studies have failed to reveal a difference between osteoporotic and non-osteoporotic postmenopausal women[80].

Oestrogen is not the only steroid synthesized by the ovary. The biochemical properties of progesterone make it theoretically much more likely to have a direct effect on bone than oestrogen, since the latter appears to lack specific receptors on bone cells and fails to compete with corticosteroids for the corticoid receptors on bone cells, whereas progesterone is able to displace corticosteroids from these receptors[21]. Most *in vivo* experiments have been made using synthetic prog-estogens. In mature ovariectomized rats the progestogen ethynodiol diacetate appeared to increase periosteal new bone formation without affecting the increased endosteal resorption seen after oophorectomy[5].

In a small group of postmenopausal women, some of whom had been oophorectomized, Lindsay *et al.*[58] showed that gestronol, a progestogen with no apparent oestrogenic activity, was as effective as mestranol in preventing post-menopausal bone loss, but this medication failed to produce a significant reduction in urinary hydroxyproline excretion. Gallagher and Nordin[35] found that norethis-terone 5 mg daily reduced urinary hydroxyproline excretion to the same extent as 25 µg ethinyl oestradiol daily, and Nordin *et al.*[78] claimed that 5 mg norethisterone daily was as effective as 25 µg ethinyl oestradiol for 21 days each month in preventing postmenopausal bone loss.

Whether long-term progestogen therapy would be as effective as oestrogens in preventing postmenopausal osteoporosis is uncertain, but the issue is complicated in so far as all postmenopausal women with intact uteri given oestrogen therapy should have not less than 7 days progestogen therapy each month in order to prevent the small risk of developing endometrial cancer[95].

The use of synthetic anabolic steroids in the prevention and treatment of osteoporosis has enjoyed a rather chequered history. Reinfenstein[84], extrapolating from metabolic balance studies, made extravagant claims for the efficacy of anabolic steroids which were never substantiated by changes in bone mass. Gordan *et al.*[37] showed that a large variety of androgens and anabolic steroids were considerably less effective than oestrogens in the prevention of further spinal collapse in postmenopausal women. Henneman and Wallach[41] claimed that anabolic steroids were only effective in patients with osteoporosis if given in doses sufficient to cause virilization. However Lindsay *et al.*[55], using an anabolic steroid (tibolone), which has weak oestrogenic, progestational and androgenic properties, found that when 2.5 mg was taken daily for 2 years it was as effective as oestrogen in preventing bone loss in 33 postmenopausal women. Interestingly, about 12% of patients given 5 mg tibolone daily had uterine bleeding, suggesting that even at 2.5 mg daily the dominant effect may have been oestrogenic rather than purely 'anabolic'.

The prevention of osteoporosis caused by sex hormone deficiency should theoretically be simple if all postmenopausal women were to be assessed for sex hormone replacement therapy. However, in practice this ideal devolves upon approaching appropriately motivated women, making an initial estimate of bone mass and then discussing the value of treatment and/or regular follow-up with the person in question. Unfortunately many postmenopausal women with intact uteri are unhappy to resume regular menstruation, but if it were possible to predict accurately which women would eventually develop symptomatic postmenopausal osteoporosis, one could perhaps be more persuasive about the benefits of oestrogen therapy for those at risk.

Most women undergoing oophorectomy before the age of 45 years will have sufficiently troublesome vasomotor symptoms for them to seek medical attention at an early stage. Unless there are specific contraindications oestrogen therapy is the treatment of choice and one's aim is to give the smallest possible dose of oestrogen to achieve substantial relief of symptoms, but not necessarily complete abolition of vasomotor phenomena. Since these women usually have no uteri additional progestogen therapy is not essential. The author prescribes 10 µg ethinyl oestradiol daily with the exception of the first 7 days of the calendar month and increases the dose where necessary by 10 µg every 2 months to a maximum of 30 µg daily. This dose should be reviewed at least once a year, and an attempt made to reduce the dose to something between 10 µg and 20 µg daily. In this instance the dose will be dictated largely by the patient's symptoms, but one must bear in mind the possibility that the optimum osteotrophic dose of oestrogen may not be the same as the dose necessary to give the patient complete symptomatic relief from her vasomotor phenomena. It is for this reason that some parameter of bone mass should be measured before treatment is started, and thereafter at yearly intervals. The skeletal measurement selected will depend upon the facilities available, but the simplest satisfactory method is that of Horsman and Simpson[44]. The aim of treatment is to prevent the combined six metacarpal hand score (6MHS), in other words, the combined cortical thickness expressed as a percentage of the combined metacarpal diameter, from falling below 45%. A fall of the 6MHS by more than 5% in 2 years should alert the patient's medical attendant to review the treatment regimen, the patient's compliance with treatment and the possibility of other complicating factors causing skeletal wasting.

Postmenopausal women with intact uteri, who are symptom-free but present for assessment of their need for hormone replacement therapy, require a somewhat different approach. The author's practice is to measure the 6MHS and the 24-hour urinary oestrogen excretion before deciding upon the desirability for sex hormone therapy. Women with a 6MHS greater than 60% are considered not be at immediate risk of developing a significant degree of osteoporosis within the next 2 years and, unless there were some other indication for prescribing oestrogens, they would be left untreated but reassessed once a year. Women with a 6MHS less than 60% and urinary oestrogen excretion less than 7 nmol/mmol creatinine should be offered oestrogen therapy unless there are specific contraindications. Postmenopausal women excreting more than 7 nmol oestrogen/mmol creatinine are uncommon and may require special consideration. Regimens used for the prevention of postmenopausal osteoporosis in women with intact uteri tend to be a matter of personal taste rather than of proven efficacy, but the author prefers to prescribe oestrogens intermittently with a progestogen taken on the oestrogen-free days. Women requiring treatment are given 10 µg ethinyl oestradiol daily with the exception of the first 7 days of the calendar month when they are given 500 µg ethynodiol diacetate daily instead. On this regimen the patient can expect a menstrual period somewhere between the 7th and 12th day of the month, although the loss may not amount to much in some women. Many gynaecologists recommend that suction curettage should be performed once a year or whenever there is an unscheduled uterine bleed, but the risk of uterine neoplasia is so small with this sort of regimen that the author usually only requests curettage where there has been an unexpected and unscheduled uterine bleed. There are many other oestrogens and progestogens available for the treatment of postmenopausal women but they offer no practical advantage over the above-mentioned treatment schedule, and are all without exception considerably more expensive.

References

1 AARSKOG, D., AKSNES, L. and LEHMANN, V. Low 1,25-dihydroxyvitamin D in heparin-induced osteopenia. *Lancet*, **2**, 650–651 (1980)

2 ADAMS, P. H., JOWSEY, J., KELLY, P. J., RIGGS, L., KENNEY, V. R. and JONES, D. J. Effects of hyperthyroidism on bone and mineral metabolism in man. *Quarterly Journal of Medicine*, **36**, 1–15 (1967)

3 AITKEN, J. M. Mineral metabolism and the ovary. *MD thesis*, Cambridge University (1973)

4 AITKEN, J. M. Factors affecting the distribution of zinc in the human skeleton. *Calcified Tissue Research*, **20**, 23–30 (1976)

5 AITKEN, J. M., ARMSTRONG, E. and ANDERSON, J. B. Osteoporosis after oophorectomy in the mature female rat and the effect of oestrogen and/or progestogen replacement therapy in its prevention. *Journal of Endocrinology*, **55**, 79–87 (1972)

6 AITKEN, J. M., HART, D. M., ANDERSON, J. B., LINDSAY, R., SMITH, D. A. and SPEIRS, C. F. Osteoporosis after oophorectomy for non-malignant disease in premenopausal women. *British Medical Journal*, **2**, 325–328 (1973)

7 AITKEN, J. M., HART, D. M. and LINDSAY, R. Oestrogen replacement therapy for prevention of osteoporosis after oophorectomy. *British Medical Journal*, **3**, 515–518 (1973)

8 AITKEN, J. M., HART, D. M., LINDSAY, R. and MacDONALD, E. B. Oestrogen dosage in the treatment of post-menopausal osteoporosis. *Medikon International*, **8**, 3–5 (1974)

9 AITKEN, J. M., SMITH, C. B., HORTON, P. W., CLARK, D. L., BOYD, J. F. and SMITH, D. A. The interrelationships between bone mineral at different skeletal sites in male and female cadavers. *Journal of Bone and Joint Surgery*, **56B**, 370–375 (1974)

10 ALBRIGHT, F., SMITH, P. H. and RICHARDSON, A. M. Postmenopausal osteoporosis; its clinical features. *Journal of the American Medical Association*, **116**, 2465–2474 (1941)

11 ALLISON, N. and BROOKS, B. Bone atrophy. An experimental study of the changes in bone which result from non-use. *Surgery Gynecology and Obstetrics*, **33**, 250–260 (1921)

12 ANDERSON, J. B., SHIMMINS, J. and SMITH, D. A. A new technique for the measurement of metacarpal density. *British Journal of Radiology*, **39**, 443–450 (1966)

13 ARNSTEIN, A. R., BLUMENTHAL, F. S. and McCANN, D. S. The effects of diphosphonate (EHDP) therapy on immobilization osteoporosis. In *Proceedings of 55th Annual Meeting of the Endocrine Society*, A-183 (1973)

14 AUB, J. C., BAUER, W., HEATH, C. and ROPES, M. Studies of calcium and phosphorus metabolism III. The effects of thyroid hormone and thyroid disease. *Journal of Clinical Investigation*, **7**, 97–137 (1929)

15 BARNETT, E. and NORDIN, B. E. C. The radiological diagnosis of osteoporosis: a new approach. *Clinical Radiology*, **11**, 166–174 (1960)

16 BAYLEY, T. A., HARRISON, J. E., McNEILL, K. G. and MERNAGH, J. R. Effect of thyrotoxicosis and its treatment on bone mineral and muscle mass. *Journal of Clinical Endocrinology and Metabolism*, **50**, 916–922 (1980)

17 BORDIER, P. J. and TUN CHOT, S. Quantitative histology of metabolic bone disease. In *Clinics in Endocrinology and Metabolism*, **1**, 197–215. Philadelphia, Saunders and Co (1972)

18 BURKHART, J. M. and JOWSEY, J. Parathyroid and thyroid hormones in the development of immobilization osteoporosis. *Endocrinology*, **81**, 1053–1062 (1967)

19 CANIGGIA, A. and VATTIMO, A. Kinetics of ^{99m}technetium–tin–methylene–diphosphonate in normal subjects and pathological conditions: a simple index of bone metabolism. *Calcified Tissue International*, **30**, 5–13 (1980)

20 CHAMBERLAIN, M. J., FREMLIN, J. H., HOLLOWAY, I. and PETERS, D. K. Use of the cyclotron for whole body neutron activation analysis. Theoretical and practical considerations. *International Journal of Applied Radiation Isotopes*, **21**, 725–734 (1970)

21 CHEN, T. L., ARONOW, L. and FELDMAN, D. Glucocorticoid receptors and inhibition of bone cell growth in primary culture. *Endocrinology*, **100**, 619–628 (1977)

22 CHRISTIANSEN, C., CHRISTENSEN, M. S. and TRANSBØL, I. Bone mass in postmenopausal women after withdrawal of oestrogen/gestogen replacement therapy. *Lancet*, **1**, 459–461 (1981)

23 CLARK, C. G., CROOKS, J., DAWSON, A. A. and MITCHELL, P. E. G. Disordered calcium metabolism after Polya partial gastrectomy. *Lancet*, **1**, 734–738 (1964)

24 CURTISS, P. H. and KINCAID, W. E. Transitory demineralization of the hip in pregnancy: a report of three cases. *Journal of Bone and Joint Surgery*, **41A**, 1327–1333 (1959)

25 CUTHBERTSON, D. P. The influence of prolonged muscular rest on metabolism. *Biochemical Journal*, **23**, 1328–1345 (1929)

26 DAVIS, M. E., STRANDJORD, N. M. and LANZL, L. H. Estrogens and the aging process. *Journal of the American Medical Association*, **196**, 219–224 (1966)

27 DeHAAS, W. G., WATSON, J. and MORRISON, D. M. Non-invasive treatment of ununited fractures of the tibia using electrical stimulation. *Journal of Bone and Joint Surgery*, **62B**, 465–470 (1980)

28 DEITRICK, J. E., WHEDON, G. D. and SHORR, E. Effects of immobilization upon various metabolic and physiologic functions in normal men. *American Journal of Medicine*, **4,** 3–36 (1948)

29 DELLER, D. J. and BEGLEY, M. D. Calcium metabolism and the bones after partial gastrectomy. 1. Clinical features and radiology of the bones. *Australian Annals of Medicine*, **12,** 282–294 (1963)

30 DELLER, D. J., EDWARDS, R. G. and ADDISON, M. Calcium metabolism and the bones after partial gastrectomy. II. The nature and cause of the bone disorder. *Australian Annals of Medicine*, **12,** 295–309 (1963)

31 DOYLE, F. H. Ulnar bone mineral concentration in metabolic bone disease. *British Journal of Radiology*, **34,** 698–712 (1961)

32 EDGREN, R. A. and CALHOUN, D. W. Density as an index of the effects of estrogens on bone. *Endocrinology*, **59,** 631–636 (1956)

33 FOGELMAN, I., BESSENT, R. G., COHEN, H. N., HART, D. M. and LINDSAY, R. Skeletal uptake of diphosphonate. Method for prediction of post-menopausal osteoporosis. *Lancet*, **2,** 667–670 (1980)

34 FRASER, S. A., ANDERSON, J. B., SMITH, D. A. and WILSON, G. M. Osteoporosis and fractures following thyrotoxicosis. *Lancet*, **1,** 981–983 (1971)

35 GALLAGHER, J. C. and NORDIN, B. E. C. Effects of oestrogen and progestogen therapy on calcium metabolism in postmenopausal women. In *Estrogens in the Postmenopause*, edited by P. A. Van Keep and C. Lauritzen, *Frontiers of Hormone Research*, **3,** pp. 150–176 Basel, Karger (1975)

36 GOLDSMITH, N. F., JOHNSTON, J. O., PICETTI, G. and GARCIA, C. Bone mineral in the radius and vertebral osteoporosis in an insured population. *Journal of Bone and Joint Surgery*, **55A,** 1276–1293 (1973)

37 GORDAN, G. S., PICCHI, J. and ROOF, B. S. Antifracture efficacy of long-term estrogens for osteoporosis. *Transactions of the Association of American Physicians*, **86,** 326–332 (1973)

38 GRIFFITH, G. C., NICHOLS, G., ASHER, J. D. and FLANAGAN, B. Heparin osteoporosis. *Journal of the American Medical Association*, **193,** 91–94 (1965)

39 GRIFFITHS, H. J., D'ORSI, C. J. and ZIMMERMAN, R. E. Use of ^{125}I photon scanning in the evaluation of bone density in a group of patients with spinal cord injury. *Investigative Radiology*, **7,** 107–111 (1972)

40 GRODIN, J. M., SIITERI, P. K. and MacDONALD, P. C. Source of estrogen production in post-menopausal women. *Journal of Clinical Endocrinology and Metabolism*, **36,** 207–214 (1973)

41 HENNEMAN, P. H. and WALLACH, S. A review of the prolonged use of estrogens and androgens in postmenopausal and senile osteoporosis. *Archives of Internal Medicine*, **100,** 715–723 (1957)

42 HORSMAN, A., GALLAGHER, J. C., SIMPSON, M. and NORDIN, B. E. C. Prospective trial of oestrogen and calcium in post-menopausal women. *British Medical Journal*, **2,** 789–792 (1977)

43 HORSMAN, A., NORDIN, B. E. C. and CRILLY, R. G. Effect on bone of withdrawal of oestrogen therapy. *Lancet*, **2,** 33 (1979)

44 HORSMAN, A. and SIMPSON, M. The measurement of sequential changes in cortical bone geometry. *British Journal of Radiology*, **48,** 471–476 (1975)

45 HORSMAN, A., SIMPSON, M., KIRBY, P. A. and NORDIN, B. E. C. Non-linear bone loss in oophorectomized women. *British Journal of Radiology*, **50**, 504–507 (1977)

46 IKKOS, D. G., KATSICHTIS, P., NTALLES, K. and VALENTZAS, C. Osteoporosis in thyrotoxicosis. *Lancet*, **2**, 1159 (1971)

47 JENKINS, J. S. and CONNOLLY, J. Adrenocortical response to ethanol in man. *British Medical Journal*, **2**, 804–805 (1968)

48 JOHNSTON, C. C., SMITH, D. M., NANCE, W. E. and BEVAN, J. Evaluation of radial bone mass by the photon absorption technique. In *Clinical Aspects of Metabolic Bone Disease*, edited by B. Frame, A. M. Parfitt and H. Duncan, pp. 28–35. Amsterdam, Excerpta Medica (1973)

49 KALBFLEISCH, J. M., LINDEMAN, R. D., GINN, H. E. and SMITH, W. O. Effects of ethanol administration on urinary excretion of magnesium and other electrolytes in alcoholic and normal subjects. *Journal of Clinical Investigation*, **42**, 1471–1475 (1963)

50 KENNEDY, A. C., LINDSAY, R., BUCHANAN, W. W. and ALLAM, B. F. Bone resorbing activity in the sera of patients with rheumatoid arthritis. *Clinical Science and Molecular Medicine*, **51**, 205–207 (1976)

51 KLEIN, D. C. and RAISZ, L. G. Prostaglandins: stimulation of bone resorption in tissue culture. *Endocrinology*, **86**, 1436–1440 (1970)

52 LINDSAY, R., AITKEN, J. M., ANDERSON, J. B., HART, D. M., MacDONALD, E. B. and CLARKE, A. C. Long-term prevention of postmenopausal osteoporosis by oestrogen. *Lancet*, **1**, 1038–1041 (1976)

53 LINDSAY, R., COUTTS, J. R. T. and HART, D. M. The effect of endogenous oestrogen on plasma and urinary calcium and phosphate in oophorectomized women. *Clinical Endocrinology*, **6**, 87–93 (1977)

54 LINDSAY, R., HART, D. M., FORREST, C. and BAIRD, C. Prevention of spinal osteoporosis in oophorectomized women. *Lancet*, **2**, 1151–1154 (1980)

55 LINDSAY, R., HART, D.McK. and KRASZEWSKI, A. Prospective double-blind trial of synthetic steroid (Org OD 14) for preventing postmenopausal osteoporosis. *British Medical Journal*, **1**, 1207–1209 (1980)

56 LINDSAY, R., HART, D. M., MacLEAN, A., CLARK, A. C., KRASZEWSKI, A. and GARWOOD, J. Bone response to termination of oestrogen treatment. *Lancet*, **1**, 1325–1327 (1978)

57 LINDSAY, R., HART, D. M., MacLEAN, A., GARWOOD, J., AITKEN, J. M., and CLARK, A. C. Pathogenesis and prevention of post-menopausal osteoporosis. In *The Role of Estrogen/Progestogen in the Management of the Menopause*, edited by I. D. Cooke, pp. 9–25. Lancaster, MTP Press (1978)

58 LINDSAY, R., HART, D. M., PURDIE, D., FERGUSON, M. M., CLARK, A. C. and KRASZEWSKI, A. Comparative effects of oestrogen and a progestogen on bone loss in postmenopausal women. *Clinical Science and Molecular Medicine*, **54**, 193–195 (1978)

59 MacDONALD, P. C., ROMBAUT, R. P. and SIITERI, P. K. Extent of conversion of plasma androstenedione to estrone in normal males and nonpregnant normal, castrate and adrenalectomised females. *Journal of Clinical Endocrinology*, **27**, 1103–1111 (1967)

60 MACK, P. E. and VOGT, F. B. Roentgenographic bone density changes in astronauts during representative Apollo space flight. *American Journal of Roentgenology*, **113**, 621–633 (1971)

61 MADSEN, M. Vertebral and peripheral bone mineral content by photon absorptiometry. *Investigative Radiology*, **12**, 185–188 (1977)

62 MARSHALL, D. H., CRILLY, R. G. and NORDIN, B. E. C. Plasma androstenedione and oestrone levels in normal and osteoporotic postmenopausal women. *British Medical Journal*, **2**, 1177–1179 (1977)

63 MARSHALL, D. H., CRILLY, R. and NORDIN, B. E. C. The relation between plasma androstenedione and oestrone levels in untreated and corticosteroid-treated post-menopausal women. *Clinical Endocrinology*, **9**, 407–412 (1978)

64 MAZESS, R. B. Non-invasive measurement of bone. In *Osteoporosis II*, edited by U. Barzel, pp. 5–26. New York, Grune and Stratton (1979)

65 MAZESS, R. B., JUDY, P. F. WILSON, C. R. and CAMERON, J. R. Progress in clinical use of photon absorptiometry. In *Clinical Aspects of Metabolic Bone Disease*, edited by B. Frame, A. M. Parfitt and H. Duncan, pp. 37–42. Amsterdam, Excerpta Medica (1973)

66 MEEMA, H. E., BUNKER, M. L. and MEEMA, S. Loss of compact bone due to menopause. *Obstetrics and Gynecology*, **26**, 333–343 (1965)

67 MEEMA, H. E. and MEEMA, S. Prevention of postmenopausal osteoporosis by hormone treatment of the menopause. *Canadian Medical Association Journal*, **99**, 248–251 (1968)

68 MEEMA, H. E. and SCHATZ, D. L. Simple radiologic demonstration of cortical bone loss in thyrotoxicosis. *Radiology*, **97**, 9–15 (1970)

69 MENDELSON, J. M., OGATA, M. and MELLO, N. K. Adrenal function and alcoholism 1. Serum cortisol. *Psychosomatic Medicine*, **33**, 145–157 (1971)

70 MEUNIER, P. J., COURPRON, P., EDOUARD, C., BERNARD, J., BRINGUIER, J. and VIGNON, G. Physiological senile involution and pathological rarefaction of bone. Quantitative and comparative histological data. *Clinics in Endocrinology and Metabolism*, **2**, 239–256 (1973)

71 MICHAEL, W. R., KING, W. R. and FRANCIS, M. D. Effectiveness of diphosphonates in preventing 'osteoporosis' of disuse in the rat. *Clinical Orthopaedics*, **78**, 271–276 (1971)

72 MORGAN, D. B., PATERSON, C. R., WOODS, C. G., PULVERTAFT, C. N. and FOURMAN, P. Search for osteomalacia in 1228 patients after gastrectomy and other operations on the stomach. *Lancet*, **2**, 1085–1088 (1965)

73 MORGAN, D. B., PULVERTAFT, C. N. and FOURMAN, P. Effects of age on the loss of bone after gastric surgery. *Lancet*, **2**, 772–773 (1966)

74 MUHLBAUER, R. C., RUSSELL, R. G. G., WILLIAMS, D. A. and FLEISCH, H. The effects of diphosphonates, polyphosphates and calcitonin on 'immobilisation osteoporosis' in rats. *European Journal of Clinical Investigation*, **1**, 336–344 (1971)

75 NILSSON, B. E. R. Post-traumatic osteopenia. *Acta Orthopaedica Scandinavica*, Supplement 91 (1966)

76 NILSSON, B. E. and WESTLIN, N. E. Changes in bone mass in alcoholics. *Clinical Orthopaedics*, **90**, 229–232 (1973)

77 NORDIN, B. E. C., GALLAGHER, J. C., AARON, J. C. and HORSMAN, A. Post-menopausal osteopenia and osteoporosis. In *Estrogens in the Postmenopause*, edited by P. A. Van Keep and C. Lauritzen, *Frontiers of Hormone Research*, **3**, pp. 131–149. Basel, Karger (1975)

78 NORDIN, B. E. C., HORSMAN, A., CRILLY, R. G., MARSHALL, D. H. and SIMPSON, M. Treatment of spinal osteoporosis in postmenopausal woman. *British Medical Journal*, **1**, 451–454 (1980)

79 NORDIN, B. E. C., YOUNG, M. M., BENTLEY, B., ORMONDROYD, P. and SYKES, J. Lumbar spine densitometry methodology and results in relation to the menopause. *Clinical Radiology*, **19**, 459–464 (1968)

80 PELC, B., MARSHALL, D. H., GUHA, P., KHAN, M. Y. and NORDIN, B. E. C. The relation between plasma androstenedione, plasma oestrone and androstenedione to oestrone conversion rates in postmenopausal women with and without fractures. *Clinical Science and Molecular Medicine*, **54**, 125–131 (1978)

81 PLUM, F. and DUNNING, M. F. The effect of therapeutic mobilization on hypercalciuria following acute poliomyelitis. *Archives of Internal Medicine*, **101**, 528–536 (1958)

82 RECKER, R. R., SAVILLE, P. D. and HEANEY, R. P. Effect of estrogens and calcium carbonate on bone loss in postmenopausal women. *Annals of Internal Medicine*, **87**, 649–655 (1977)

83 REES, L. H., BESSER, G. M., JEFFCOATE, W. J., GOLDIE, D. J. and MARKS, V. Alcohol-induced pseudo-Cushing's syndrome. *Lancet*, **1**, 726–728 (1977)

84 REIFENSTEIN, E. C. The relationships of steroid hormones to the development and management of osteoporosis in aging people. *Clinical Orthopaedics*, **10**, 206–253 (1957)

85 ROSE, G. A. Immobilization osteoporosis. A study of the extent, severity and treatment with bendrofluazide. *British Journal of Surgery*, **53**, 769–774 (1966)

86 SAVILLE, P. D. Changes in bone mass with age and alcoholism. *Journal of Bone and Joint Surgery*, **47A**, 492–499 (1965)

87 SISSONS, H. A. Osteoporosis and epiphysial arrest in joint tuberculosis. *Journal of Bone and Joint Surgery*, **34B**, 275–290 (1952)

88 SMITH, D. A., ANDERSON, J. B., SHIMMINS, J., SPEIRS, C. F. and BARNETT, E. Mineral and density changes in bone with age in normal and pathological states. In *Progress in Methods of Bone Mineral Measurement*, US Department of Health NIH, pp. 177–191 (1968)

89 SMITH, D. A., ANDERSON, J. B., SHIMMINS, J., SPEIRS, C. F. and BARNETT, E. Changes in metacarpal mineral content and density in normal male and female subjects with age. *Clinical Radiology*, **20**, 23–31 (1969)

90 SMITH, D. A., FRASER, S. A. and WILSON, G. M. Hyperthyroidism and calcium metabolism. *Clinics in Endocrinology and Metabolism*, **2**, 333–354 (1973)

91 SNAPPER, I. Osteoporosis. *Medical Clinics of North America*, **36**, 847–863 (1952)

92 SPEARING, G., FRASER, I., TURNER, G. and DIXON, G. Long-term self-administered subcutaneous heparin in pregnancy. *British Medical Journal*, **1**, 1457–1458 (1978)

93 WHEDON, G. D., DEITRICK, J. E. and SHORR, E. Modification of the effects of immobilization upon metabolic and physiologic functions of normal men by the use of an oscillating bed. *American Journal of Medicine*, **6**, 684–711 (1949)

94 WHEDON, G. D. and SHORR, E. Metabolic studies in paralytic acute anterior poliomyelitis. II Alterations in calcium and phosphorus metabolism. *Journal of Clinical Investigation*, **36**, 966–981 (1957)

95 WHITEHEAD, M. I., McQUEEN, J., MINARDI, J. and CAMPBELL, S. Progestogen modification of estrogen-induced endometrial proliferation in climacteric women. In *The Role of Estrogen/Progestogen in the Management of the Menopause*, edited by I. D. Cooke, pp. 121–133. Lancaster, MTP Press (1978)

96 WISE, P. H. and HALL, A. J. Heparin-induced osteopenia in pregnancy. *British Medical Journal*, **281**, 110–111 (1980)

97 WYSE, D. M. and PATTEE, C. J. Effect of the oscillating bed and tilt table on calcium, phosphorus and nitrogen metabolism in paraplegia. *American Journal of Medicine*, **17**, 645–661 (1954)

3
The treatment of postmenopausal and senile osteoporosis
Ego Seeman and B. Lawrence Riggs

INTRODUCTION

Osteoporosis is a multifactorial and heterogeneous disorder that affects 4 million older Americans. Among women older than 65 years of age, 30% have suffered a vertebral fracture[75]. The incidence of hip fracture doubles every 5 years after the age of 60, so that by the age of 90 years, 30% of women have suffered a hip fracture and 15% of these patients die within 6 months. Osteoporosis is clearly a major health problem in the United States, costing 1 billion dollars annually in short-term medical care.

In this chapter, we review the current forms of treatment of osteoporosis. We discuss the underlying pathogenesis of the disorder only insofar as it gives us insight and a rational basis for treatment.

CALCIUM

The rationale underlying calcium supplementation in the treatment of osteoporosis is four-fold. First, intestinal calcium absorption decreases with aging[3, 10, 32, 115] and is lower in patients with osteoporosis than in age-matched controls[32]. Second, osteoporotic or elderly subjects (older than 65 years) cannot adapt to a low calcium intake by increasing fractional calcium absorption[32], the principal mechanism preventing a negative calcium balance[76]. Without this increased absorption, the body cannot offset obligatory calcium loss in stool and urine, and serum calcium must be maintained at the expense of the skeleton. Third, superimposed on these age-related defects, the menopause is associated with a decrease in calcium absorption and a more negative calcium balance. The dietary calcium requirement needed to prevent negative calcium balance increases after the menopause from 0.98–1.45 g/day[43]. Fourth, the calcium intake in patients with osteoporosis approximates 600 mg/day and has frequently been reported to be less than that of age-matched controls[101] and less than that needed to prevent a negative calcium balance.

Although no definitive epidemiological evidence demonstrates that a low dietary calcium uptake *per se* causes osteoporosis, bone mineral content has been found to be lower in subjects with a more negative calcium balance[84]. Most studies suggest that the amount of calcium required to prevent a negative calcium balance is 0.9–1.5 g/day. Nordin *et al.*[86] evaluated the calcium intake and balance in 212 studies of 84 postmenopausal normal subjects. For 95% of subjects to be in positive balance, an intake of 900 mg/day was required. Heaney *et al.*[42] found a calcium intake of 1.24 g/day was necessary to prevent a negative calcium balance in 130 middle-aged women. Others[52, 83, 88, 113, 117] have reported similar dietary requirements, most of which were more than the 800 mg/day stipulated by the recommended dietary allowances[82].

Calcium supplementation initially results in a more positive calcium balance[84] and a decrease in bone resorption[57]. During prolonged treatment, calcium balance becomes less positive and bone formation decreases[108]. The close coupling of bone resorption and bone formation limits the therapeutic value of calcium; bone mass cannot be increased.

The effect of calcium supplementation on bone mineral mass varies according to the method used for evaluation and skeletal area examined. At present, no studies have examined the effect of calcium supplements on trabecular bone mineral density of the axial skeleton or hip, the sites of the clinically important fractures. Nordin *et al.*[85] found that bone loss, as assessed by serial measurements of metacarpal cortical area, decreases in postmenopausal patients treated with 1.2 g of calcium daily. Similarly, Recker *et al.*[94] treated patients for 2 years with 1.5 g of elemental calcium and found a substantial reduction in metacarpal cortical bone loss and a smaller reduction in the rate of bone loss measured by photon densitometry of the radius. In contrast, Horsman *et al.*[48] conducted a controlled prospective study of 24 postmenopausal women treated with 800 mg of elemental calcium daily for 2–3 years. The rate of metacarpal bone loss was unaffected by calcium supplementation. The decreased rate of bone loss measured at the distal radius and ulna by using photon densitometry reached statistical significance at the latter site only. These changes suggest that calcium supplements do have a beneficial effect on bone mineral, albeit less than the effects of estrogen therapy (which were also examined in these studies).

Few studies have specifically addressed the effect of calcium supplementation on fracture rate. Nordin *et al.*[85] reported a reduction in vertebral fracture rate with use of 1.2 g of calcium daily. In our studies[103], calcium carbonate 1.5 g/day, with or without vitamin D 50 000 u twice a week, reduced the vertebral fracture rate to half that found in untreated controls.

Thus, the preponderance of evidence suggests that dietary calcium supplementation improves calcium balance, decreases the rate of bone loss by decreasing bone resorption, helps meet the increased calcium requirement imposed by menopause, and may decrease the incidence of vertebral fractures.

ESTROGEN

Research during the last 40 years has documented a central role for estrogen deficiency in the pathogenesis of postmenopausal osteoporosis and has affirmed the therapeutic efficacy of estrogen replacement.

Estrogen replacement retards the rate of bone loss from the appendicular skeleton. Aitken *et al.*[1] measured the bone mineral content of the third metacarpal by using photon densitometry; they found that patients treated with mestranol 23 µg/day, within 2 months after oophorectomy had considerably reduced rates of bone loss when compared with untreated control patients. In women treated 6 or more years after artificial menopause, bone loss persisted at a rate similar to that in untreated control patients. The results published by Lindsay *et al.*[66, 68] after 5 and 9 years of treatment demonstrate continued protection against bone loss and spinal deformity. During the last 2 years bone mineral decreased, an indication that resistance to estrogen may have developed.

The prevention of bone loss may necessitate continued estrogen replacement. Lindsay *et al.*[70] observed the effect of discontinuing the use of estrogen supplements in 14 patients treated for 4 years. Bone loss accelerated during the 4 years after cessation of therapy, and the beneficial effects of treatment for 4 years were lost. Horsman *et al.*[49] confirmed their observations. More recently, Christiansen *et al.*[19] found that the annual rate of bone loss after discontinuation of hormone therapy was not accelerated; thus, a beneficial effect of temporary estrogen replacement was seen. These patients were receiving calcium supplementation, however, which may have partially protected against the effects of estrogen withdrawal[20, 67].

Estrogen deficiency is associated with increased bone resorption when measured by microradiography[100] or radiocalcium kinetics[44]. Estrogen replacement is associated with a decrease in bone resorption. Riggs *et al.*[100], using quantitative microradiography, found normalization of bone resorption in 17 patients treated cyclically with conjugated estrogen (Premarin) 2.5 mg daily. In most patients, bone resorption normalized within 2–4 months after institution of treatment. After 26–42 months, resorbing surfaces increased but remained appreciably below pretreatment values. Bone-forming surfaces remained unchanged initially and then decreased after long-term therapy. Estrogen effectively decreased bone resorption when it had been increased before initiation of treatment. The effect was sustained for up to 42 months and was associated with a secondary decline in bone formation – an explanation of the failure of estrogens to increase bone mass substantially. In addition, Recker *et al.*[94], using radiocalcium kinetics, demonstrated a decrease in overall bone turnover; however, because the reduction in bone resorption was greater than the decrease in bone formation, net bone balance improved.

The menopause is associated with a decline in intestinal calcium absorption and a more negative calcium balance[43]. The major regulator of intestinal calcium absorption[25] is 1,25-dihydroxyvitamin D (1,25(OH)$_2$D), and the serum concentration of this metabolite is lower in postmenopausal osteoporotic patients than in age-matched controls[32]. Estrogen replacement improves calcium absorption[30, 32] and results in a more positive calcium balance[28]. Gallagher *et al.*[30] treated 12 patients with conjugated estrogen 1.25–2.5 mg/day for 6 months. Both intestinal calcium absorption and serum 1,25(OH)$_2$D concentrations increased. In addition, the serum immunoreactive parathyroid hormone (iPTH) level increased, whereas serum calcium and phosphate concentrations declined. The changes in calcium absorption and 1,25(OH)$_2$D found with estrogen replacement were similar to those seen in 10 patients treated with physiological doses of $1,25(OH)_2D_3$. Alterations in serum D-binding protein induced by estrogen therapy could explain in part the increase in serum $1,25(OH)_2D$ but not the increase in calcium absorption.

The morbid event in osteoporosis is fracture. Gordan *et al.*[37] reported a reduction in the occurrence of vertebral fractures in patients who were treated with conjugated estrogen (Premarin) 1.25–2.5 mg/day for up to 25 years. Wallach and Henneman[120] studied 292 patients who were under surveillance for a total of 1480 patient-years. Although the patients received a variety of estrogen preparations, after 1945 most received Premarin (1.25–5 mg/day) or diethylstilbestrol (1–3 mg/ day) administered cyclically; loss of height (an index of vertebral fracture) was prevented. Burch *et al.*[11] reviewed the results of estrogen treatment in 1000 hysterectomized women for 14 318 patient-years and found 12 Colles' fractures. On the basis of actuarial tables, 40 would be predicted. We have found a substantial reduction in vertebral fracture rate to a quarter that seen in untreated patients with osteoporosis[103]. Retrospective studies also suggest that administration of estrogens prevents hip and Colles' fractures. This protective effect was greater in patients treated within 5 years after the menopause[53] and in those patients receiving estrogens for more than 5 years[53, 123]. There was no difference in the protective effect of either 0.625 mg or 1.25 mg of conjugated estrogen[123].

Numerous case-control studies suggest that estrogen replacement increases by eight-fold the mean relative risk of developing endometrial carcinoma[50, 54, 79, 112, 121, 122]. The estimated incidence of endometrial carcinoma in the at-risk population of women in the age range 50–74 years is approximately one to two per 1000 persons annually[118]. With such a low incidence, it is not surprising that the occurrence of endometrial carcinoma in prospective studies is low[37, 81] and it is impossible to ignore the conclusions made by the case-control studies. The risk is greater in women who receive prolonged (more than 10 years), continuous, high-dose estrogen therapy without a progestational agent. The type of carcinoma regarded as being estrogen-related is believed to be a low-grade malignant lesion that is associated with a good prognosis[116].

Mammary changes occurring with estrogen treatment consist of benign, bilateral, reversible cystic or epithelial (or both) alterations[38]. These occur in 1–5% of patients who receive estrogen replacement[89]. Some[124], but not all[47], studies suggest that estrogen use may confer protection against breast cancer.

Other complications such as thromboembolism, gallbladder disease, myocardial infarction, hypertension, and clotting factor defects have primarily been studied in relationship to contraception rather than in relationship to estrogen treatment of osteoporosis. An increased risk of gallbladder disease[8] has been reported. The occurrence of other complications remains very controversial.

The ideal estrogen should have the greatest potency with respect to decreased bone loss and a minimal effect on the endometrial mucosa. The relative efficacy of several estrogens has been compared by Gallagher and Nordin[29]. They found that daily administered conjugated estrogens (Premarin 0.625 mg) and ethinyl estradiol (0.025 mg) were equipotent with respect to reducing serum calcium, hydroxyproline, and renal tubular reabsorption of phosphate. Premarin (0.625–1.25 mg), ethinyl estradiol (0.025 mg), and mestranol (25–50 μg) have been commonly used in practice and found to decrease bone loss effectively. Provisional data from Cann and Genant[14] suggest that Premarin in doses of less than 0.625 mg daily may be ineffective in reducing bone loss. In addition, Lindsay et al.[71] have shown that estriol hemisuccinate did not prevent bone loss in 28 postmenopausal women who were followed up for 2 years unless doses of 12 mg daily were used, an amount that negated the value of its weaker effect on the endometrium.

For minimization of the possibility of untoward endometrial effects, estrogens may be administered at lower doses in conjunction with calcium supplements and given cyclically, with or without a progestational agent in the last 10 days. The progestational agents reduce the proliferative effects of estrogen on the endometrium.

ANDROGENS AND SYNTHETIC ANABOLIC AGENTS

Androgens have received little attention because of their virilizing effects. The development of synthetic analogs with potent anabolic activity and reduced virilizing potency has resulted in suggestions from numerous studies that these agents may be effective in decreasing bone loss.

Riggs et al.[99] treated 12 postmenopausal patients with oxandrolone 10–20 mg daily. Bone-forming and resorbing surfaces, measured by quantitative microradiography, decreased after 9–15 months of treatment. The local apposition rate, measured by tetracycline double-labeling, remained unchanged. This finding was associated with a reduction in bone resorption and accretion (measured by using radiocalcium kinetics). Similar radiokinetic data have been reported by Lafferty et al.[63] The failure to observe an appreciable decrease in bone-resorbing surfaces may have been due to the greater proportion of patients having normal values for bone resorption; the decrease in bone resorption is more notable when the pretreatment value for bone resorption is higher.

For 26 months, Chesnut et al.[17] treated 13 patients with methandrostenolone (Dianabol) 5 mg daily cyclically for 3 out of 4 weeks. Total body calcium, measured by neutron activation, increased by 2% in the treated group and decreased by 3% in the placebo group. Serum calcium, phosphate, and alkaline phosphatase values remained unchanged. Apart from transitory elevations in serum glutamic-oxaloacetic transaminase, no side-effects of treatment, and in particular no masculinizing effects, were noted. More recently, Chesnut et al.[16] reported the results of 2 years of treatment with stanozolol 6 mg daily for 3 out of 4 weeks. Total body calcium increased by 4.4% in the 15 patients who received treatment but showed no substantial change in the control subjects. Because free hydroxyproline excretion increased without a change in the total fraction, an increase in bone formation was suggested (unlike the effect of estrogens). In the six biopsies done, bone resorption surfaces decreased by 70.7%; additionally, serum calcium increased and iPTH and urinary calcium decreased.

These studies suggest that the use of anabolic agents with decreased virilizing potency may have a role in the treatment of osteoporosis, particularly in those patients in whom use of estrogens is contraindicated.

PROGESTOGENS

In some studies progestogens have been used in the last 7–13 days of each estrogen treatment cycle to minimize the occurrence of endometrial hyperplasia and the risk of endometrial carcinoma. Medroxyprogesterone acetate 10 mg/day, and norethisterone 5–10 mg/day (for 7–13 days), have commonly been used. Recently two studies suggested that progestational agents may be useful alternatives for estrogen replacement in the prevention of bone loss.

Gallagher and Nordin[29] showed that norethisterone 5 mg daily decreased plasma and urine calcium and hydroxyproline to an extent similar to that seen with estrogen replacement. Lindsay *et al.*[72] treated 10 patients with gestronol hexanoate 200 mg monthly by intramuscular injection for 3 months and then on a 3-monthly basis. After 12 months, the 10 placebo-treated patients lost 3.6% metacarpal bone mineral as measured by photon absorptiometry. Bone mineral in the gestronol-treated group was considerably greater than that in the placebo-treated patients and similar to that in 10 mestranol-treated control patients. Hydroxyproline excretion decreased in the mestranol-treated group but remained unaltered in placebo-treated or gestronol-treated patients. These findings suggest that the progestogens and estrogens have a different mode of action. Lindsay *et al.*[69] also studied the effect of Org OD14, a synthetic compound with estrogenic, anabolic and progestational properties. Bone loss was prevented in the three patients who completed 2 years of treatment. The 30 placebo-treated patients continued to lose bone. On aspiration curettage, 20 patients had no endometrial hyperplasia.

These studies suggest that progestational agents have potential value in the prevention of bone loss.

FLUORIDE

Increased bone mineral deposition resulting in osteosclerosis of the skeleton and calcification of the ligaments and tendons was described in 1937 in workers exposed to sodium aluminum fluoride dust[105]. Similar changes were found in parts of India where the potable water contains large amounts of fluoride. A decreased incidence of osteoporosis has been reported in naturally fluoridated areas, whereas an increased incidence of osteoporosis has been described in communities where the fluoride content of the drinking water is low[7, 110]. These observations led Rich and Ensinck[97] to use sodium fluoride in patients with osteoporosis in an attempt to induce subclinical fluorosis, in the hope that bone mass could be increased without severe side-effects.

Fluoride avidly seeks bone and substitutes isomorphically for the hydroxyl ion of hydroxyapatite to form the less soluble fluoroapatite crystal[90]. Using X-ray crystallography of bone specimens obtained from the iliac crest, Bernstein and Cohen[6] demonstrated enlargement and improvement of the crystal lattice structure of bone in patients treated with 10–66 mg of sodium fluoride daily for up to 12 months. The improvement in lattice structure correlated with the fluoride concentration in the bone.

The effects of fluoride are predominantly on bone formation and result in an increase in trabecular bone surface, thickness, and volume[87]. The increased osteoid matrix remains poorly mineralized when fluoride is used alone[59]. The defective mineralization of matrix is partially prevented when fluoride is used in conjunction with vitamin D and calcium. Our group[57] treated patients with 45 mg of fluoride daily, 600 mg of calcium carbonate daily, and 50 000 u of vitamin D twice weekly and found increased bone formation in 10 out of 11 subjects. The increase correlated with the dose of fluoride used. Unmineralized osteoid was present in eight patients and correlated inversely with the calcium × phosphorus product. Bone resorption decreased in eight subjects and correlated inversely with the calcium intake. Meunier *et al.*[80] treated 55 patients with a similar therapeutic regimen for up to 2 years. Total bone volume, total osteoid volume, seam thickness, and surfaces covered by osteoid increased. The calcification rate, as measured by tetracycline double-labeling, was unaltered. Bone resorption surfaces did not increase. Rosenquist *et al.*[106] treated 20 male patients with 0.8 mg/kg of sodium fluoride for 107 weeks; alkaline phosphatase and non-dialyzable hydroxy-proline increased, an indication that bone formation increased.

Prolonged treatment with fluoride and calcium is needed to increase bone mass. The increase in trabecular bone mass is detectable roentgenographically as sclerosis and thickening of the vertical trabeculae and end-plate regions. These changes may take from 1 to 3 years to be evident in the 60% of patients who respond to therapy[98, 102]. Harrison *et al.*[41] treated 13 patients with 50 mg of sodium fluoride daily, 1 g of calcium carbonate daily, and 50 000 u of vitamin D twice weekly for 3 years. Bone mineral density of the trunk and proximal femurs increased 12.7% in the eight patients with adequate fluoride retention, whereas bone loss was noted in the five patients with inadequate fluoride retention. The changes in bone mineral were detectable after 12 months, although histological evidence of fluorosis was found 6 months after the onset of treatment. Increases in trabecular bone mineral of the third and fourth lumbar vertebrae have been reported by Hansson and Roos[40] in eight out of nine patients treated for 1.5–2 years with 30–50 mg of sodium fluoride, 1 g calcium, and 0.6 mg of dihydrotachysterol daily. No roentgenological changes were detected. Manzke *et al.*[77] found that fluoride treatment for 2 years reduced the rate of appendicular bone loss. Bone mineral measurements were based on photometric analysis of standard roentgenograms of the middle phalanx of the small finger. Some studies have suggested that decreased bone mineral of the appendicular skeleton is detected in patients receiving fluoride when the more accurate technique of direct photon absorptiometry in the forearm or femur is used[23, 104].

Sodium fluoride therapy has been shown to reduce the vertebral fracture rate. Riggs *et al.*[103] studied 45 patients who were not treated (91 person-years of observation), 59 who were treated conventionally with calcium (alone or combined with estrogen) or vitamin D or both (218 years), and 61 who were treated with sodium fluoride combined with conventional therapy (251 years). The fracture rate (per 1000 person-years) was 834 in untreated patients, 419 in those given calcium with or without vitamin D, 304 in those given fluoride and calcium with or without vitamin D, 181 in those given estrogen and calcium with or without vitamin D, and 53 in those given fluoride, estrogen and calcium with or without vitamin D. The vertebral fracture rate was reduced in all treatment groups ($P < 0.001$ for calcium and $P < 0.01 \times 10^{-6}$ for other combinations); fluoride (1 year of treatment) and estrogen, but not vitamin D, independently reduced the rate from that observed with calcium alone ($P < 0.001$). The combination of calcium, fluoride and estrogen was more effective than any other combination ($P < 0.001$).

Side-effects of fluoride therapy – including synovial irritation, plantar fasciitis, epigastric pain, nausea, vomiting, iron-deficiency anemia from occult gastrointestinal bleeding, and hair loss – occur in 30–50% of subjects[98] and frequently necessitate cessation of therapy.

Thus, sodium fluoride is an agent that can potentially increase bone mass, which is the ultimate goal in the treatment of osteoporosis. Before sodium fluoride can be widely used in the treatment of osteoporosis, several serious problems require resolution. When administered alone, sodium fluoride results in poorly mineralized new bone. To some degree, this problem has been resolved by the concurrent use of vitamin D and calcium supplements. Side-effects are frequent and severe and often require withdrawal of therapy. Not all patients respond to fluoride therapy; usually 1 year of treatment, and often up to 5 years of treatment, is necessary to induce a response. Guidelines identifying patients who will respond to treatment with sodium fluoride have not been established but are needed before patients are subjected to prolonged and potentially hazardous treatment. Finally, some evidence has indicated that although trabecular bone mass is increased with sodium fluoride therapy, this may be at the price of decreased appendicular bone mineral.

VITAMIN D AND VITAMIN D METABOLITES

Currently, the major, if not the sole, indication for the use of vitamin D metabolites in the treatment of osteoporosis is low intestinal calcium absorption. Calcium absorption decreases with age in both sexes, particularly after 70 years of age[3, 10]. Compared with age-matched controls, patients with osteoporosis have low normal[115] or low[10, 13, 61] calcium absorption.

The physiologically active form of vitamin D, $1,25(OH)_2D$, is the major determinant of intestinal calcium absorption[25] and mediates the adaptive increase in calcium absorption when dietary calcium intake is low. Vitamin D deficiency, reflected in low serum 25-hydroxyvitamin D concentrations, has been found in patients with osteoporosis in northern Europe[74]. This does not parallel the findings in patients with osteoporosis in the United States, where dietary fortification with vitamin D is adequate and where skin reception of ultraviolet solar radiation is more abundant[28].

Pharmacological doses of vitamin D are required to overcome the defect in calcium absorption found in patients with osteoporosis. Gallagher et al.[28] found that the mean dose of vitamin D required to normalize calcium absorption was 20 000 u daily. The response was variable; some patients required as little as 1000 u daily and others require 40 000 u daily.

Gallagher et al.[32] demonstrated that intestinal calcium absorption and serum $1,25(OH)_2D$ concentration decreased with aging and were lower in patients with osteoporosis than in age-matched controls. The decline in calcium absorption correlates with the decline in serum $1,25(OH)_2D$ concentration and can be reversed by administration of low doses of synthetic $1,25(OH)_2D_3$. These studies suggest the presence of an underlying abnormality of $1,25(OH)_2D$ production or degradation.

Synthetic $1,25(OH)_2D_3$ and 1α-hydroxyvitamin D_3 ($1\alpha(OH)D_3$) have both been found to increase intestinal calcium absorption effectively in short-term studies [21, 24, 31, 78, 114]; however, the effects of these agents are exceedingly dose-dependent, and hypercalcemia and hypercalciuria frequently complicate therapy[9, 65, 73]. Furthermore, Gallagher *et al.*[31] found that the beneficial short-term effect of $1,25(OH)_2D$ on calcium balance declined with prolonged treatment.

Vitamin D metabolites, especially in higher doses, have no effect or a detrimental effect on the skeleton. Nordin *et al.*[85] found that treatment of 25 patients for 56.8 patient-years with 10 000 to 50 000 u of vitamin D daily accelerated the rate of metacarpal bone loss and increased the incidence of fractures. In 23 patients who received calcium supplements in addition to vitamin D, bone loss was appreciably retarded but not considerably different from the rate of bone loss in untreated patients. Moreover, the 20 patients who received only calcium supplements had a lower rate of bone loss than those receiving calcium and vitamin D. For 2 years, Shapiro *et al.*[111] treated 10 patients with 2.4 g of calcium daily and 50 000 u of vitamin D three times a week and found no increase in bone mineral of the radius, as measured by photon absorptiometry. Buring *et al.*[12] treated 23 patients for 1 year with 35 000 u of vitamin D and 1 g of calcium daily and found no changes in appendicular bone mineral by using photon absorptiometry.

Nordin *et al.*[85] found that vitamin D treatment had an adverse effect on the rate of spinal fractures. No spinal deterioration was noted in the calcium-treated patients, and only a very slow deterioration was seen in those treated with calcium and vitamin D. In our own work[103], we have been unable to demonstrate that vitamin D, 7000 to 15 000 u/day, substantially adds to the protective effect of calcium carbonate (1–2.5 g/day) alone or in combination with conjugated estrogen 0.625–2.5 mg/day, or sodium fluoride (50–70 mg/day).

No studies have determined the effect of $1,25(OH)_2D_3$ on bone mineral. Although increased appendicular bone mineral density measured by photon absorptiometry has been reported with $1\alpha(OH)D_3$ therapy[73, 114], this is an inconsistent finding[18]. In addition, Nordin *et al.*[85] treated 21 patients with $1\alpha(OH)_2D_3$ and found that the rate of metacarpal bone loss was the same as in untreated controls. Moreover, they documented a deterioration in spinal score, a measure of fracture occurrence.

CALCITONIN

A definitive role for calcitonin in skeletal remodeling and mineral homeostasis in humans has not been established. Calcitonin effectively inhibits bone resorption *in vitro*[91] and has been used in the treatment of osteoporosis in an attempt to decrease bone resorption. Interpretation of many clinical trials using calcitonin is difficult because most studies have been short-term analyses, have used small numbers of patients, and have not been controlled. Patients with heterogeneous forms of osteoporosis have been studied, and varying doses, frequency of administration, and types of calcitonin have been used.

The use of calcitonin without calcium or vitamin D supplements may result in secondary hyperparathyroidism with increased bone resorption. Our group[55] found that the increase in serum iPTH correlated with the increase in bone resorption seen in four patients after treatment with 100–500 µg of porcine calcitonin daily for 3–4 months. To combat the effects of secondary hyperparathyroidism, our group[58] examined the effect of salmon calcitonin (50–100 MRC u/day), calcium carbonate (1 g/day), and vitamin D (50 000 u twice weekly) in 26 subjects. After 3 months of treatment with calcium and calcitonin, bone resorption surfaces, measured by using quantitative microradiography, decreased in 20 out of 26 patients, but not to normal. Bone formation surfaces remained unaffected. The results of treatment with calcitonin added to calcium and vitamin D were no better than with calcium and vitamin D alone, and those investigators concluded that calcitonin is unlikely to have any additional desirable effect.

Three reported studies that used the technique of total-body neutron activation suggested an overall increase in total body calcium after combined therapy with calcium and calcitonin. Wallach *et al.*[119] treated 12 patients with porcine calcitonin 50–100 MRC u three times weekly and calcium carbonate 1.5 g daily. After 10–29 months, total body calcium increased by 9%. The increase reached a maximum after 6–8 months and remained stable thereafter. Smaller increases (2–3%) have been reported by Chesnut *et al.*[16] in their study of 24 patients with osteoporosis who received salmon calcitonin 100 MRC u daily and calcium carbonate 1.2 g daily for 24 months. Cohn *et al.*[22] found that after 3 months of therapy with porcine calcitonin (1 MRC u/kg twice daily) and calcium supplements (1.5 g daily), total body calcium increased in three of the seven patients. Moreover, because of the short duration of most of these studies, documentation of a meaningful effect of calcitonin treatment on fracture rates was not feasible.

DIPHOSPHONATES

The synthetic diphosphonates have a P-C-P bond replacing the P-O-P bond of the pyrophosphate, which renders them more stable. In addition to inhibiting hydroxy-apatite crystal formation and dissolution, these agents inhibit bone resorption. Ethane-1-hydroxy-1,1-diphosphonate (EHDP), dichloromethane diphosphonate (Cl_2MDP), and 3-amino-1-hydroxypropane-1,1-diphosphonate (AHPDP) have received attention.

These agents inhibit bone resorption both *in vivo* and *in vitro*[96, 107], increase calcium content of bone in the rat[33], and decrease bone turnover[45]. The compounds are cleared rapidly from the blood and absorbed onto hydroxyapatite crystals[60]. They enter osteoclasts and alter their morphological features selectively[27]. Although osteomalacia complicates therapy with EHDP, this condition is reversible on withdrawal of the drug and is not seen with the currently recommended dose of 5 mg/kg that is effective in the treatment of Paget's disease.

The results of two studies that used EHDP in patients with osteoporosis are disappointing. Our group[56] treated four patients with osteoporosis with 10–20 mg/kg of EHDP daily for 3 months. Hyperphosphatemia decreased serum ionized calcium, and secondary hyperparathyroidism complicated treatment. The most striking feature found on bone biopsy specimens was the increase in poorly mineralized osteoid. Heaney and Saville[45] treated 10 patients with osteoporosis with 20 mg/kg of EHDP daily for 6–12 months and found a substantial reduction in overall bone turnover, bone resorption, and mineralization by using radiocalcium kinetic techniques. No published studies have yet reported the use of AHPDP or Cl_2MDP in the treatment of osteoporosis.

PARATHYROID HORMONE

On the basis of experimental work in animals, Reeve *et al.*[95] administered 500 u daily of human parathyroid hormone (PTH (1–34)) by intramuscular injection to 23 patients with osteoporosis. After an observation period of 6–24 months, substantial increases in trabecular bone volume from the iliac crest biopsy samples were found. In addition, indices of bone formation – mineral accretion rate, trabecular osteoid surfaces, and serum alkaline phosphatase activity – increased. Bone resorption surfaces, osteoclast number, and hydroxyproline excretion increased; however, the rate of mineralization, determined by using tetracycline double-labeling, remained normal. Calcium balance and radiokinetically determined calcium absorption did not increase. This finding is important because the mineral content of trabecular bone may increase at the expense of cortical bone. Hesp *et al.*[46] recently found that the bone mineral content of the proximal femoral shaft, measured by photon densitometry, decreased in several subjects. Alterations in mineral content correlated with calcium balance; patients with a more negative calcium balance had a lower bone mineral content.

Rasmussen *et al.*[93] found that stimulation of endogenous PTH in patients with osteoporosis by using orally administered phosphate (1.5 g daily) and parenterally administered calcitonin (50 iu daily for 5 days every 3 weeks) resulted in increased trabecular bone volume and bone formation surfaces of iliac crest biopsy samples. Parameters of bone resorption – resorption surfaces, osteoclast number, and hydroxyproline excretion – remained unchanged.

Although the results of these studies are provocative, at this time the use of PTH in the treatment of osteoporosis remains experimental.

INORGANIC PHOSPHATE

The addition of phosphate to bone cultures decreases the release of prelabeled calcium-45 (^{45}Ca) and prevents PTH-mediated bone resorption[92]. Oral and intravenously administered phosphate has been used to treat hypercalcemia[35] and idiopathic hypercalciuria[34] and has been found to improve calcium balance in animal studies[64]. These observations suggest that phosphate may be useful in the treatment of osteoporosis.

In animal experiments, phosphate supplementation induces hyperphosphatemia, hypocalcemia, secondary hyperparathyroidism, increased bone resorption, and osteoporosis[62]. Limited evidence in humans suggests that phosphate is ineffective in osteoporosis. Goldsmith *et al.*[36] found that phosphate supplementation resulted in increased bone resorption surfaces and decreased bone-forming surfaces by using the technique of quantitative microradiography on iliac crest bone biopsy specimens. In addition, the occurrence of soft tissue deposition increased skeletal porosity[64], and the failure of orally administered phosphate to prevent osteoporosis as a complication of immobilization[51] suggests that phosphate supplementation is unsuitable in the treatment of osteoporosis.

GROWTH HORMONE

Acromegaly has traditionally been associated with osteoporosis[2]. More recent studies using photon absorptiometry of the appendicular skeleton[102], dual photon absorptiometry of the axial skeleton[109], quantitative microradiography of iliac crest bone biopsy samples[39], and total-body calcium measurements with neutron activation[4] suggest that bone mass is increased in acromegaly. These observations have resulted in one study of the efficacy of growth hormone in the treatment of osteoporosis. Aloia *et al.*[4] treated seven patients with growth hormone for 6 months. Small increases in bone turnover were reflected in an increase in bone formation, bone resorption, hydroxyproline excretion, and serum alkaline phosphatase. Trabecular bone volume remained unchanged, and total-body calcium measured by neutron activation did not increase. Measurements of appendicular bone mineral with use of photon absorptiometry remained unaltered. Moreover, hyperglycemia, hypertension, arthralgias, and carpal tunnel syndrome complicated therapy. Thus, growth hormone therapy for osteoporosis does not appear to hold promise at this time.

AN APPROACH TO TREATMENT OF THE INDIVIDUAL PATIENT

In a given patient, postmenopausal osteoporosis lacks definitive biochemical or clinical characteristics and therefore is a diagnosis of exclusion. The following classification, which is intentionally incomplete, emphasizes the more commonly encountered diseases that may be difficult to diagnose when osteoporosis is the sole clinical manifestation.

Commonly encountered
  Postmenopausal or senile
  Glucocorticoid excess

Uncommonly encountered
  Genetic (such as osteogenesis imperfecta)
  Idiopathic (in young adults and juveniles)

Common secondary forms
  Glucocorticosteroid excess (endogenous, exogenous)
  Gastrointestinal surgery
  Malabsorption
  Hematological disorder (multiple myeloma and so forth)
  Primary hyperparathyroidism
  Thyrotoxicosis
  Immobilization
  Others[5]

A more complete list can be found elsewhere[5].

The biochemical tests that should be performed in the evaluation of osteoporosis are the following.

Assessment of severity
   Thoracolumbar roentgenography (lateral and posteroanterior views)
   Photon absorptiometry (forearm and, when available, lumbar spine)
   Accurate measurement of height

Assessment of causes
   Serum calcium, phosphate, alkaline phosphatase, protein electrophoresis
   Serum 25-hydroxyvitamin D (especially for patients in Great Britain and
      northern Europe)
   Urinary excretion of calcium, creatinine clearance, urinary protein electro-
      phoresis
   Blood film, erythrocyte sedimentation rate
   When indicated – immunoelectrophoresis, thyroxine, cortisol (a.m. and p.m.),
      immunoreactive parathyroid hormone, carotene
   History – estimated calcium intake, age at onset of menopause

Precise assessment of the number, location, and degree of vertebral compressions should be clearly documented at diagnosis.

Single photon absorptiometry to measure appendicular bone mineral density at the midradius or distal radius distinguishes patients with osteoporosis from normals poorly but may be of value in longitudinal evaluation of appendicular bone mineral. Dual photon absorptiometry can measure bone mineral density at the clinically important sites of fracture: the spine and hip[26]. Although presently available in only a few medical centers, this procedure can provide accurate quantitative and non-invasive measurement of bone mineral density; fracture threshold can be used in followup to determine response to therapy. Quantitative computed tomography also appears to be a useful means of measuring bone mineral density in the axial skeleton[15].

Measurements of serum calcium, phosphate, and alkaline phosphatase are of value primarily in suggesting the presence of another underlying illness. An elevated serum alkaline phosphatase level suggests the recent occurrence of a fracture, metastatic disease, Paget's disease, osteomalacia, or primary hyperparathyroidism.

General measures

All patients with osteoporosis should receive supportive measures in addition to drug therapy. The treatment of acute pain from vertebral fracture and the accompanying muscle spasm should include analgesia, bedrest, immobilization, local deep heat delivered by heat lamp, and repeated hot baths.

In the long-term course of osteoporosis, continued chronic back pain results from the postural and mechanical changes that occur with spinal deformity; severe muscle spasms can occur intermittently and may be incapacitating. Posture training, graded spinal extensor muscle exercises conducted in collaboration with a physiotherapist, and the use of a back brace are also helpful. The patient should be instructed to avoid carrying heavy objects, to avoid sudden or asymmetric mechanical stress, and to use care when walking in obstructed or poorly lit areas. Falls must be assiduously avoided; stair-rails and bathroom grab-rails are invaluable. Weight reduction, use of a firm mattress, and exercises such as swimming and walking will also sometimes provide symptomatic relief.

Drug treatment

In an elderly patient who has only one or two vertebral fractures from mild osteoporosis, calcium supplementation alone may be sufficient, especially when the patient is very elderly. To attain a calcium intake of 1.0–1.5 g daily may be difficult for some elderly persons. A normal daily diet excluding dairy products contains 300 mg of elemental calcium. An 230 ml (8 oz) glass of milk contains 240 mg of calcium, and five slices of American cheese contain 600 mg of calcium. Supplementary calcium can also be given as medicinal tablets*, one method of avoiding the calorie excess of a high intake of milk.

In a patient with more severe disease, low daily doses of estrogen – conjugated estrogen (Premarin 0.625 mg), ethinyl estradiol (25 µg), or mestranol (25 µg), administered in 21-day cycles and withdrawn for 10 days – should be added to the calcium supplements. If clinical progression and additional fractures are evident, the dose of estrogen should be doubled, and a progestational agent such as medroxyprogesterone acetate (10 mg/day) or norethisterone (5 mg/day) should be given for 10–13 days of each month to decrease the proliferative effect of estrogens on the endometrium. The value of an annual gynecological examination has never been established but is advisable. Any uterine bleeding must be investigated. Untoward effects such as breast swelling, hypertension, hyperlipidemia, cholecystitis, or thrombophlebitis should be sought during followup. The duration of treatment should be indefinite, and further disease progression should be monitored by accurate determination of height, thoracolumbar roentgenography, and bone mineral measurement in the spine and forearm (if available).

The use of sodium fluoride for osteoporosis has not been approved by the US Food and Drug Administration. A dose of 45–60 mg daily is commonly used in research protocols in combination with calcium supplements.

Probably the most effective treatment regimens combine calcium, estrogen, sodium fluoride, and possibly vitamin D[103]. Elderly patients who do not object to the possibility of some degree of masculinization, and who prefer to avoid the possibility of bleeding with use of cyclic estrogen, may use androgens such as oxandrolone (10–20 mg/day) as a reasonable alternative to estrogen.

Osteoporosis can occur in men and should be investigated in the same manner as outlined for women. Hypogonadism may cause osteoporosis in men; although

---

* Tablets: calcium carbonate 650 mg (260 mg Ca^{2+}); calcium gluconate 650 mg (58.5 mg Ca^{2+}) or 1 g (90 mg Ca^{2+}); calcium lactate 650 mg (94.5 mg Ca^{2+})

present only in a minority of cases, it must be sought and treated if found. Androgens can be administered orally as methyltestosterone (5–10 mg/day) or fluoxymesterone (Halotestin 5–10 mg/day) or monthly by intramuscular injections of 200 mg of testosterone enanthate (Delatestryl). Calcium, vitamin D supplements, and sodium fluoride (pending approval) should be administered as described above.

References

1 AITKEN, J. M., HART, D. M. and LINDSAY, R. Oestrogen replacement therapy for prevention of osteoporosis after oophorectomy. *British Medical Journal*, **3**, 515–518 (1973)

2 ALBRIGHT, F. and REIFENSTEIN, E. C., Jr. *The Parathyroid Glands and Metabolic Bone Disease: Selected Studies*, p. 188. Baltimore, Williams and Wilkins Company (1948)

3 ALEVIZAKI, C. C., IKKOS, D. G. and SINGHELAKIS, P. Progressive decrease of true intestinal calcium absorption with age in normal man. *Journal of Nuclear Medicine*, **14**, 760–762 (1973)

4 ALOIA, J. F., ZANZI, I., ELLIS, K., JOWSEY, J., ROGINSKY, M., WALLACH, S. and COHN, S. H. Effects of growth hormone in osteoporosis. *Journal of Clinical Endocrinology and Metabolism*, **43**, 992–999 (1976)

5 AVIOLI, L. V. Osteoporosis: pathogenesis and therapy. In *Metabolic Bone Disease*, **1**, edited by L. V. Avioli and S. M. Krane, pp. 333–355. New York, Academic Press (1977)

6 BERNSTEIN, D. S. and COHEN, P. Use of sodium fluoride in the treatment of osteoporosis. *Journal of Clinical Endocrinology and Metabolism*, **27**, 197–210 (1967)

7 BERNSTEIN, D. S., SADOWSKY, N., HEGSTED, D. M., GURI, C. D. and STARE, F. J. Prevalence of osteoporosis in high- and low-fluoride areas in North Dakota. *Journal of the American Medical Association*, **198**, 499–504 (1966)

8 BOSTON COLLABORATIVE DRUG SURVEILLANCE PROGRAM. Surgically confirmed gallbladder disease, venous thromboembolism, and breast tumors in relation to postmenopausal estrogen therapy. *New England Journal of Medicine*, **290**, 15–19 (1974)

9 BRICKMAN, A. S., COBURN, J. W., MASSRY, S. G. and NORMAN, A. W. 1,25 Dihydroxyvitamin D_3 in normal man and patients with renal failure. *Annals of Internal Medicine*, **80**, 161–168 (1974)

10 BULLAMORE, J. R., GALLAGHER, J. C., WILKINSON, R., NORDIN, B. E. C. and MARSHALL, D. H. Effect of age on calcium absorption. *Lancet*, **2**, 535–537 (1970)

11 BURCH, J. C., BYRD, B. F. and VAUGHN, W. K. Results of estrogen treatment in one thousand hysterectomized women for 14 318 years. In *Consensus on Menopause Research: A Summary of International Opinion*, edited by P. A. Van Keep, R. B. Greenblatt and M. Albeaux-Fernet, pp. 164–169. Baltimore, University Park Press (1976)

12 BURING, K., HULTH, A. G., NILSSON, B. E., WESTLIN, N. E. and WIKLUND, P. E. Treatment of osteoporosis with vitamin D. *Acta Medica Scandinavica*, **195**, 471–472 (1974)

13 CANIGGIA, A., GENNARI, C., BIANCHI, V. and GUIDERI, R. Intestinal absorption of ^{45}Ca in senile osteoporosis. *Acta Medica Scandinavica*, **173**, 613–617 (1963)

14 CANN, C. E. and GENANT, H. K. Comparison of cancellous and integral spinal mineral loss in oophorectomized women using quantitative computed tomography *Calcified Tissue International*, **33**, 307 (1981)

15 CANN, C. E., GENANT, H. K., ETTINGER, B. and GORDAN, G. S. Spinal mineral loss in oophorectomized women: determination by quantitative computed tomography. *Journal of the American Medical Association*, **244**, 2056–2059 (1980)

16 CHESNUT, C. H., III, BAYLINK, D. J. and NELP, W. B. Bone mass change with calcitonin therapy in osteoporosis, as assessed by total body activation analysis (abstract). *Journal of Nuclear Medicine*, **20**, 677 (1979)

17 CHESNUT, C. H., III, NELP, W. B., BAYLINK, D. J. and DENNY, J. D. Effect of methandrostenolone on postmenopausal bone wasting as assessed by changes in total bone mineral mass. *Metabolism*, **26**, 267–277 (1977)

18 CHRISTIANSEN, C., CHRISTENSEN, M. S., McNAIR, P., HAGEN, C., STOCKLUND, K. and TRANSBØL, I. Prevention of early postmenopausal bone loss: controlled 2-year study in 315 normal females. *European Journal of Clinical Investigation*, **10**, 273–279 (1980)

19 CHRISTIANSEN, C., CHRISTENSEN, M. S. and TRANSBØL, I. Bone mass in postmenopausal women after withdrawal of oestrogen/gestagen replacement therapy. *Lancet*, **1**, 459–461 (1981)

20 CHRISTIANSEN, C., CHRISTENSEN, M. S. and TRANSBØL, I. Bone mass after withdrawal of oestrogen replacement (letter to the editor). *Lancet*, **1**, 1053–1054 (1981)

21 COHEN, H. N., FARRAH, D., FOGELMAN, I., GOLL, C. C., BEASTALL, G. H., McINTOSH, W. B., FLETCHER, M. and BOYLE, I. T. A low dose regime of 1α-hydroxyvitamin D_3 in the management of senile osteoporosis: a pilot study. *Clinical Endocrinology (Oxford)*, **12**, 537–542 (1980)

22 COHN, S. H., DOMBROWSKI, C. S., HAUSER, W., KLOPPER, J. and ATKINS, H. L. Effects of porcine calcitonin on calcium metabolism in osteoporosis. *Journal of Clinical Endocrinology and Metabolism*, **33**, 719–728 (1971)

23 DAMBACHER, M. A., LAUFFENBURGER, T., LÄMMLE, B. and HAAS, H. G. Long-term effects of sodium fluoride in osteoporosis. In *Fluoride and Bone*, edited by B. Courvoisier, A. Donath and C. A. Baud, pp. 238–241. Bern, Switzerland, Hans Huber Publishers (1978)

24 DAVIES, M., MAWER, E. B. and ADAMS, P. H. Vitamin D metabolism and the response to 1,25-dihydroxycholecalciferol in osteoporosis. *Journal of Clinical Endocrinology and Metabolism*, **45**, 199–208 (1975)

25 DeLUCA, H. F. Recent advances in our understanding of the vitamin D endocrine system. *Journal of Laboratory and Clinical Medicine*, **87**, 7–26 (1976)

26 DUNN, W. L., WAHNER, H. W. and RIGGS, B. L. Measurement of bone mineral content in human vertebrae and hip by dual photon absorptiometry. *Radiology*, **136**, 485–487 (1980)

27 FAST, D. K., FELIX, R., DOWSE, C., NEUMAN, W. F. and FLEISCH, H. The effects of diphosphonates on the growth and glycolysis of connective-tissue cells in culture. *Biochemical Journal*, **172**, 97–107 (1978)

28 GALLAGHER, J. C., AARON, J., HORSMAN, A., MARSHALL, D. H., WILKINSON, R. and NORDIN, B.E.C. The crush fracture syndrome in postmenopausal women. *Clinics in Endocrinology and Metabolism*, **2**, 293–315 (1973)

29 GALLAGHER, J. C. and NORDIN, B. E. C. Effects of oestrogen and progestogen therapy on calcium metabolism in postmenopausal women. *Frontiers of Hormone Research*, **3**, 150–176 (1975)

30 GALLAGHER, J. C., RIGGS, B. L. and DeLUCA, H. F. Effect of estrogen on calcium absorption and serum vitamin D metabolites in postmenopausal osteoporosis. *Journal of Clinical Endocrinology and Metabolism*, **51**, 1359–1364 (1980)

31 GALLAGHER, J. C., RIGGS, B. L. and DeLUCA, H. F. Effect of long-term treatment with synthetic 1,25-dihydroxyvitamin D_3 in postmenopausal osteoporosis (abstract). *Clinical Research*, **28**, 777A (1980)

32 GALLAGHER, J. C., RIGGS, B. L., EISMAN, J., HAMSTRA, A., ARNAUD, S. B. and DeLUCA, H. F. Intestinal calcium absorption and serum vitamin D metabolites in normal subjects and osteoporotic patients: effect of age and dietary calcium. *Journal of Clinical Investigation*, **64**, 729–736 (1979)

33 GASSER, A. B., MORGAN, D. B., FLEISCH, H. A. and RICHELLE, L. J. The influence of two diphosphonates on calcium metabolism in the rat. *Clinical Science*, **43**, 31–45 (1972)

34 GOLDSMITH, R. S. Multiple effects of phosphate therapy (editorial). *New England Journal of Medicine*, **282**, 927–928 (1970)

35 GOLDSMITH, R. S. and INGBAR, S. H. Inorganic phosphate treatment of hypercalcemia of diverse etiologies. *New England Journal of Medicine*, **274**, 1–7 (1966)

36 GOLDSMITH, R. S., JOWSEY, J., DUBÉ, W. J., RIGGS, B. L., ARNAUD, C. D. and KELLY, P. J. Effects of phosphorus supplementation on serum parathyroid hormone and bone morphology in osteoporosis. *Journal of Clinical Endocrinology and Metabolism*, **43**, 523–532 (1976)

37 GORDAN, G. S., PICCHI, J. and ROOF, B. S. Antifracture efficacy of long-term estrogens for osteoporosis. *Transactions of the Association of American Physicians*, **86**, 326–331 (1973)

38 GRAY, L. A. and ROBERTSON, R. W., Jr. Estrogens, the pill, and the breast. In *Early Breast Cancer: Detection and Treatment*, edited by H. S. Gallagher, pp. 28–36. New York, John Wiley and Sons (1975)

39 HALSE, J., MELSEN, F. and MOSEKILDE, L. Iliac crest bone mass and remodelling in acromegaly. *Acta Endocrinologica (Copenhagen)*, **97**, 18–22 (1981)

40 HANSSON, T. and ROOS, B. Effect of combined therapy with sodium fluoride, calcium, and vitamin D on the lumbar spine in osteoporosis. *American Journal of Roentgenology*, **126**, 1294–1296 (1976)

41 HARRISON, J. E., McNEILL, K. G., STURTRIDGE, W. C., BAYLEY, T. A., MURRAY, T. M., WILLIAMS, C., TAM, C. and FORNASIER, V. Three-year changes in bone mineral mass of postmenopausal osteoporotic patients based on neutron activation analysis of the central third of the skeleton. *Journal of Clinical Endocrinology and Metabolism*, **52**, 751–758 (1981)

42 HEANEY, R. P., RECKER, R. R. and SAVILLE, P. D. Calcium balance and calcium requirements in middle-aged women. *American Journal of Clinical Nutrition*, **30**, 1603–1611 (1977)

43 HEANEY, R. P., RECKER, R. R. and SAVILLE, P. D. Menopausal changes in calcium balance performance. *Journal of Laboratory and Clinical Medicine*, **92**, 953–963 (1978)

44 HEANEY, R. P., RECKER, R. R. and SAVILLE, P. D. Menopausal changes in bone remodeling. *Journal of Laboratory and Clinical Medicine*, **92**, 964–970 (1978)

45 HEANEY, R. P. and SAVILLE, P. D. Etidronate disodium in postmenopausal osteoporosis. *Clinical Pharmacology and Therapeutics*, **20**, 593–604 (1976)

46 HESP, R., HULME, P., WILLIAMS, D. and REEVE, J. The relationship between changes in femoral bone density and calcium balance in patients with involutional osteoporosis treated with human parathyroid hormone fragment (hPTH 1-34). *Metabolic Bone Disease and Related Research*, **2**, 331–334 (1981)

47 HOOVER, R., GRAY, L. A., Sr, COLE, P. and MacMAHON, B. Menopausal estrogens and breast cancer. *New England Journal of Medicine*, **295**, 401–405 (1976)

48 HORSMAN, A., GALLAGHER, J. C., SIMPSON, M. and NORDIN, B. E. C. Prospective trial of oestrogen and calcium in postmenopausal women. *British Medical Journal*, **2**, 789–792 (1977)

49 HORSMAN, A., NORDIN, B. E. C. and CRILLY, R. G. Effect on bone of withdrawal of oestrogen therapy (letter to the editor). *Lancet*, **2**, 33 (1979)

50 HULKA, B. S., FOWLER, W. C., Jr., KAUFMAN, D. G., GRIMSON, R. C., GREENBERG, B. G., HOGUE, C. J. R., BERGER, G. S. and PULLIAM, C. C. Estrogen and endometrial cancer: cases and two control groups from North Carolina. *American Journal of Obstetrics and Gynecology*, **137**, 92–101 (1980)

51 HULLEY, S. B., VOGEL, J. M., DONALDSON, C. L., BAYERS, J. H., FRIEDMAN, R. J. and ROSEN, S. N. The effect of supplemental oral phosphate on the bone mineral changes during prolonged bed rest. *Journal of Clinical Investigation*, **50**, 2506–2518 (1971)

52 HURXTHAL, L. M. and VOSE, G. P. The relationship of dietary calcium intake to radiographic bone density in normal and osteoporotic persons. *Calcified Tissue Research*, **4**, 245–256 (1969)

53 HUTCHINSON, T. A., POLANSKY, S. M. and FEINSTEIN, A. R. Post-menopausal oestrogens protect against fractures of hip and distal radius: a case-control study. *Lancet*, **2**, 706–709 (1979)

54 JICK, H., WATKINS, R. N., HUNTER, J. R., DINAN, B. J., MADSEN, S., ROTHMAN, K. J. and WALKER, A. M. Replacement estrogens and endometrial cancer. *New England Journal of Medicine*, **300**, 218–222 (1979)

55 JOWSEY, J., RIGGS, B. L., GOLDSMITH, R. S., KELLY, P. J. and ARNAUD, C. D. Effects of prolonged administration of porcine calcitonin in postmenopausal osteoporosis. *Journal of Clinical Endocrinology and Metabolism*, **33**, 752–758 (1971)

56 JOWSEY, J., RIGGS, B. L., KELLY, P. J., HOFFMAN, D. L. and BORDIER, P. The treatment of osteoporosis with disodium ethane-1-hydroxy-1,1-diphosphonate. *Journal of Laboratory and Clinical Medicine*, **78**, 574–584 (1971)

57 JOWSEY, J., RIGGS, B. L., KELLY, P. J. and HOFFMAN, D. L. Effect of combined therapy with sodium fluoride, vitamin D and calcium in osteoporosis. *American Journal of Medicine*, **53**, 43–49 (1972)

58 JOWSEY, J., RIGGS, B. L., KELLY, P. J. and HOFFMAN, D. L. Calcium and salmon calcitonin in treatment of osteoporosis. *Journal of Clinical Endocrinology and Metabolism*, **47**, 633–639 (1978)

59 JOWSEY, J., SCHENK, R. K. and REUTTER, F. W. Some results of the effect of fluoride on bone tissue in osteoporosis. *Journal of Clinical Endocrinology and Metabolism*, **28**, 869–874 (1968)

60 JUNG, A., BISAZ, S. and FLEISCH, H. The binding of pyrophosphate and two diphosphonates by hydroxyapatite crystals. *Calcified Tissue Research*, **11**, 269–280 (1973)

61 KINNEY, V. R., TAUXE, W. N. and DEARING, W. H. Isotopic tracer studies of intestinal calcium absorption. *Journal of Laboratory and Clinical Medicine*, **66**, 187–203 (1965)

62 KROOK, L., BARRETT, R. B., USUI, K. and WOLKE, R. E. Nutritional secondary hyperparathyroidism in the cat. *Cornell Veterinarian*, **53**, 224–240 (1963)

63 LAFFERTY, F. W., SPENCER, G. E., Jr and PEARSON, O. H. Effects of androgens, estrogens and high calcium intakes on bone formation and resorption in osteoporosis. *American Journal of Medicine*, **36**, 514–528 (1964)

64 LAFLAMME, G. H. and JOWSEY, J. Bone and soft tissue changes with oral phosphate supplements. *Journal of Clinical Investigation*, **51**, 2834–2840 (1972)

65 LINDHOLM, T. S., SEVASTIKOGLOU, J. A. and LINDGREN, U. Treatment of patients with senile, post-menopausal and corticosteroid-induced osteoporosis with 1α-hydroxyvitamin D_3 and calcium: short- and long-term effects. *Clinical Endocrinology (Oxford)*, **7** (Suppl.), 183S–189S (1977)

66 LINDSAY, R., HART, D. M., AITKEN, J. M., MacDONALD, E. B., ANDERSON, J. B. and CLARK, A. C. Long-term prevention of postmenopausal osteoporosis by oestrogen: evidence for an increased bone mass after delayed onset of oestrogen treatment. *Lancet*, **1**, 1038–1041 (1976)

67 LINDSAY, R., HART, D. M. and FOGELMAN, I. Bone mass after withdrawal of oestrogen replacement (letter to the editor). *Lancet*, **1**, 729 (1981)

68 LINDSAY, R., HART, D. M., FORREST, C. and BAIRD, C. Prevention of spinal osteoporosis in oophorectomised women. *Lancet*, **2**, 1151–1154 (1980)

69 LINDSAY, R., HART, D. M. and KRASZEWSKI, A. Prospective double-blind trial of synthetic steroid (Org OD14) for preventing postmenopausal osteoporosis. *British Medical Journal*, **280**, 1207–1209 (1980)

70 LINDSAY, R., HART, D. M., MacLEAN, A., CLARK, A. C., KRASZEWSKI, A. and GARWOOD, J. Bone response to termination of oestrogen treatment. *Lancet*, **1**, 1325–1327 (1978)

71 LINDSAY, R., HART, D. M., MacLEAN, A., GARWOOD, J., CLARK, A. C. and KRASZEWSKI, A. Bone loss during oestriol therapy in postmenopausal women. *Maturitas*, **1**, 279–285 (1979)

72 LINDSAY, R., HART, D. M., PURDIE, D., FERGUSON, M. M., CLARK, A. S. and KRASZEWSKI, A. Comparative effects of oestrogen and a progestogen on bone loss in postmenopausal women. *Clinical Science and Molecular Medicine*, **54**, 193–195 (1978)

73 LUND, B., HJORTH, L., KJAER, I., REIMANN, I., FRIIS, T., ANDERSEN, R. B. and SØRENSEN, O. H. Treatment of osteoporosis of ageing with 1α-hydroxycholecalciferol. *Lancet*, **2**, 1168–1171 (1975)

74 LUND, B., SØRENSEN, O. H. and CHRISTENSEN, A. B. 25-Hydroxycholecalciferol and fractures of the proximal femur. *Lancet*, **2,** 300–302 (1975)

75 LUTWAK, L. and WHEDON, G. D. Osteoporosis. *Disease-A-Month*, **April,** 1–39 (1963)

76 MALM, O. J. Calcium requirement and adaption in adult men. *Scandinavian Journal of Clinical and Laboratory Investigation*, **10** (Suppl. 36), 1–280 (1958)

77 MANZKE, E., RAWLEY, R., VOSE, G., ROGINSKY, M., RADER, J. I. and BAYLINK, D. J. Effect of fluoride therapy on nondialyzable urinary hydroxyproline, serum alkaline phosphatase, parathyroid hormone, and 25-hydroxyvitamin D. *Metabolism*, **26,** 1005–1010 (1977)

78 MARSHALL, D. M., GALLAGHER, J. C., GUHA, P., HANES, F., OLDFIELD, W. and NORDIN, B. E. C. The effect of 1α-hydroxycholecalciferol and hormone therapy on the calcium balance of post-menopausal osteoporosis. *Calcified Tissue Research*, **22,** 78–84 (1977)

79 McDONALD, T. W., ANNEGERS, J. F., O'FALLON, W. M., DOCKERTY, M. B., MALKASIAN, G. D., Jr and KURLAND, L. T. Exogenous estrogen and endometrial carcinoma: case-control and incidence study. *American Journal of Obstetrics and Gynecology*, **127,** 572–580 (1977)

80 MEUNIER, P. J., BRESSOT, C., VIGNON, E., EDOUARD, C., ALEXANDER, C., COURPRON, P. and LAURENT, J. Radiological and histological evolution of post-menopausal osteoporosis treated with sodium fluoride–vitamin D–calcium: preliminary results. In *Fluoride and Bone*, edited by B. Courvoisier, A. Donath and C. A. Baud, pp. 263–276. Bern, Switzerland, Hans Huber Publishers (1978)

81 NACHTIGALL, L. E., NACHTIGALL, R. H., NACHTIGALL, R. D. and BECKMAN, E. M. Estrogen replacement therapy. II. A prospective study in the relationship to carcinoma and cardiovascular and metabolic problems. *Obstetrics and Gynecology*, **54,** 74–79 (1979)

82 NATIONAL RESEARCH COUNCIL, FOOD AND NUTRITION BOARD. *Recommended Dietary Allowances, 8th revised edition.* Washington, DC, National Academy of Sciences (1974)

83 NORDIN, B. E. C. The pathogenesis of osteoporosis. *Lancet*, **1,** 1011–1014 (1961)

84 NORDIN, B. E. C. Calcium balance and calcium requirement in spinal osteoporosis. *American Journal of Clinical Nutrition*, **10,** 384–390 (1962)

85 NORDIN, B. E. C., HORSMAN, A., CRILLY, R. G., MARSHALL, D. H. and SIMPSON, M. Treatment of spinal osteoporosis in postmenopausal women. *British Medical Journal*, **280,** 451–455 (1980)

86 NORDIN, B. E. C., HORSMAN, A., MARSHALL, D. H., SIMPSON, M. and WATERHOUSE, G. M. Calcium requirement and calcium therapy. *Clinical Orthopaedics and Related Research*, **140,** 216–239 (1979)

87 OLAH, A. J., REUTTER, F. W. and SCHENK, R. K. Histological bone changes after long-term treatment with sodium fluoride. In *Calcium Metabolism, Bone and Metabolic Bone Diseases* (Tenth European Symposium on Calcified Tissues), edited by F. Kuhlencordt and H.-P. Kruse, pp. 146–150. Berlin, Springer-Verlag (1975)

88 OWEN, E. C., IRVING, J. T. and LYALL, A. The calcium requirements of older male subjects with special reference to the genesis of senile osteoporosis. *Acta Medica Scandinavica*, **103,** 235–250 (1940)

89 PECK, D. R. and LOWMAN, R. M. Estrogen and the postmenopausal breast: mammographic considerations. *Journal of the American Medical Association*, **240**, 1733–1735 (1978)

90 POSNER, A. S., EANES, E. D. and ZIPKIN, I. X-ray diffraction analysis of the effect of fluoride on bone. In *Proceedings of the Second European Symposium on Calcified Tissues*, edited by L. J. Richelle and M. J. Dallemagne, pp. 79–88. Liège, Belgium, Université de Liège (1965)

91 RAISZ, L. G., AU, W. Y. W., FRIEDMAN, J. and NIEMANN, I. Thyrocalcitonin and bone resorption: studies employing a tissue culture bioassay. *American Journal of Medicine*, **43**, 684–690 (1967)

92 RAISZ, L. G. and NIEMANN, I. Effect of phosphate, calcium, and magnesium on bone resorption and hormonal responses in tissue culture. *Endocrinology*, **85**, 446–452 (1969)

93 RASMUSSEN, H., BORDIER, P., MARIE, P., AUQUIER, L., EISINGER, J. B., and KUNTZ, D., *et al.* Effect of combined therapy with phosphate and calcitonin on bone volume in osteoporosis. *Metabolic Bone Disease and Related Research*, **2**, 107–111 (1980)

94 RECKER, R. R., SAVILLE, P. D. and HEANEY, R. P. Effect of estrogens and calcium carbonate on bone loss in postmenopausal women. *Annals of Internal Medicine*, **87**, 649–655 (1977)

95 REEVE, J., MEUNIER, P. J., PARSONS, J. A., BERNAT, M., BIJVOET, O. L. M., and COURPRON, P., *et al.* Anabolic effect of human parathyroid hormone fragment on trabecular bone in involutional osteoporosis: a multicentre trial. *British Medical Journal*, **280**, 1340–1344 (1980)

96 REYNOLDS, J. J., MINKIN, C., MORGAN, D. B., SPYCHER, D. and FLEISCH, H. The effect of two diphosphonates on the resorption of mouse calvaria *in vitro*. *Calcified Tissue Research*, **10**, 302–313 (1972)

97 RICH, C. and ENSINCK, J. Effect of sodium fluoride on calcium metabolism of human beings (letter to the editor). *Nature*, **191**, 184–185 (1961)

98 RIGGS, B. L., HODGSON, S. F., HOFFMAN, D. L., KELLY, P. J., JOHNSON, K. A. and TAVES, D. Treatment of primary osteoporosis with fluoride and calcium: clinical tolerance and fracture occurrence. *Journal of the American Medical Association*, **243**, 446–449 (1980)

99 RIGGS, B. L., JOWSEY, J., GOLDSMITH, R. S., KELLY, P. J., HOFFMAN, D. L. and ARNAUD, C. D. Short- and long-term effects of estrogen and synthetic anabolic hormone in postmenopausal osteoporosis. *Journal of Clinical Investigation*, **51**, 1659–1663 (1972)

100 RIGGS, B. L., JOWSEY, J., KELLY, P. J., JONES, J. D. and MAHEN, F. T. Effect of sex hormones on bone in primary osteoporosis. *Journal of Clinical Investigation*, **48**, 1065–1072 (1969)

101 RIGGS, B. L., KELLY, P. J., KINNEY, V. R., SCHOLZ, D. A. and BIANCO, A. J., Jr. Calcium deficiency and osteoporosis: observations in one hundred and sixty-six patients and critical review of the literature. *Journal of Bone and Joint Surgery. American Volume*, **49**, 915–924 (1967)

102 RIGGS, B. L., RANDALL, R. V., WAHNER, H. W., JOWSEY, J., KELLY, P. J. and SINGH, M. The nature of the metabolic bone disorder in acromegaly. *Journal of Clinical Endocrinology and Metabolism*, **34**, 911–918 (1972)

103 RIGGS, B. L., SEEMAN, E., HODGSON, S. F., TABES, D. R. and O'FALLON, W. M. Effect of the fluoride/calcium regime on vertebral fracture occurrence in postmenopausal osteoporosis. *New England Journal of Medicine,* **306**, 446–450 (1982)

104 RINGE, J. D., KRUSE, H. P. and KUHLENCORDT, F. Long term treatment of primary osteoporosis by sodium fluoride. In *Fluoride and Bone*, edited by B. Courvoisier, A. Donath and C. A. Baud, pp. 228–232. Bern, Switzerland, Hans Huber Publishers (1978)

105 ROHOLM, K. *Fluorine Intoxication: A Clinical-Hygienic Study*; *With a Review of the Literature and Some Experimental Investigations*. London, H. K. Lewis and Co. Ltd (1937)

106 ROSENQUIST, J., MANZKE, E., BAYLINK, D., WERGEDAL, J., RAWLEY, R. and VOSE, G. Increased urine non-dialyzable hydroxyproline (NDH) in sodium fluoride (NaF) treated patients with osteoporosis. *Clinical Research*, **24**, 369A (1976) (Abstract)

107 SCHENK, R., MERZ, W. A., MÜHLBAUER, R., RUSSELL, R. G. G. and FLEISCH, H. Effect of ethane-1-hydroxy-1,1-diphosphonate (EHDP) and dichloromethylene diphosphonate (Cl_2MDP) on the calcification and resorption of cartilage and bone in the tibial epiphysis and metaphysis of rats. *Calcified Tissue Research*, **11**, 196–214 (1973)

108 SCHWARTZ, E., PANARIELLO, V. A. and SAELI, J. Radioactive calcium kinetics during high calcium intake in osteoporosis. *Journal of Clinical Investigation*, **44**, 1547–1560 (1965)

109 SEEMAN, E., WAHNER, H. W., OFFORD, K.P., KUMAR, R., JOHNSON, W. J. and RIGGS, B. L. Differential effects of endocrine dysfunction on the axial and appendicular skeleton. *Journal of Clinical Investigation* (in press)

110 SHAMBAUGH, G. E., Jr and SCOTT, A. Sodium fluoride for arrest of osteoporosis: theoretical considerations. *Archives of Otolaryngology*, **80**, 263–270 (1964)

111 SHAPIRO, J. R., MOORE, W. T., JORGENSEN, H., REID, J., EPPS, C. H. and WHEDON, D. Osteoporosis: evaluation of diagnosis and therapy. *Archives of Internal Medicine*, **135**, 563–567 (1975)

112 SHAPIRO, S., KAUFMAN, D. W., SLONE, D., ROSENBERG, L., MIETTINEN, O. S., STOLLEY, P. D., ROSENSHEIN, N. B., WATRING, W. G., LEAVITT, T., Jr and KNAPP, R. C. Recent and past use of conjugated estrogens in relation to adenocarcinoma of the endometrium. *New England Journal of Medicine*, **303**, 485–489 (1980)

113 SMITH, D. A. and NORDIN, B.E.C. The relation between calcium balance and hydroxyproline excretion in osteoporosis. *Proceedings of the Royal Society of Medicine*, **57**, 868–870 (1964)

114 SØRENSEN, O. H., ANDERSEN, R. B., CHRISTENSEN, M. S., FRIIS, T., HJORTH, L., JØRGENSEN, F. S., LUND, B., MELSEN, F. and MOSEKILDE, L. Treatment of senile osteoporosis with 1α-hydroxyvitamin D_3. *Clinical Endocrinology (Oxford)*, 7 (Suppl.) 169S–175S (1977)

115 SZYMENDERA, J., HEANEY, R. P. and SAVILLE, P. D. Intestinal calcium absorption: concurrent use of oral and intravenous tracers and calculation by the inverse convolution method. *Journal of Laboratory and Clinical Medicine*, **79**, 570–578 (1972)

116 UNDERWOOD, P. B., MILLER, M. C., KREUTNER, A., Jr., JOYNER, C. A. and LUTZ, M. H. Endometrial carcinoma: the effect of estrogens. *Gynecologic Oncology*, **8,** 60–73 (1979)

117 VINTHER-PAULSEN, N. Calcium and phosphorus intake in senile osteoporosis. *Geriatrics*, **8,** 76–79 (1953)

118 WALKER, A. M. and JICK, H. Declining rates of endometrial cancer. *Obstetrics and Gynecology*, **56,** 733–736 (1980)

119 WALLACH, S., COHN, S. H., ATKINS, H. L., ELLIS, K. J., KOHBERGER, R., ALOIA, J. F. and ZANZI, I. Effect of salmon calcitonin on skeletal mass in osteoporosis. *Current Therapeutic Research*, **22,** 556–572 (1977)

120 WALLACH, S. and HENNEMAN, P. H. Prolonged estrogen therapy in postmenopausal women. *Journal of the American Medical Association*, **171,** 1637–1642 (1959)

121 WEISS, N. S., SZEKELY, D. R. and AUSTIN, D. F. Increasing incidence of endometrial cancer in the United States. *New England Journal of Medicine*, **294,** 1259–1262 (1976)

122 WEISS, N. S., SZEKELY, D. R., ENGLISH, D. R. and SCHWEID, A. I. Endometrial cancer in relation to patterns of menopausal estrogen use. *Journal of the American Medical Association*, **242,** 261–264 (1979)

123 WEISS, N. S., URE, C. L., BALLARD, J. H., WILLIAMS, A. R. and DALING, J. R. Decreased risk of fractures of the hip and lower forearm with postmenopausal use of estrogen. *New England Journal of Medicine*, **303,** 1195–1198 (1980)

124 WILSON, R. A. The roles of estrogen and progesterone in breast and genital cancer. *Journal of the American Medical Association*, **182,** 327–331 (1962)

4
The assessment of parathyroid function

P. A. Lucas and J. S. Woodhead

INTRODUCTION

The parathyroids play a central role in regulating the calcium concentration of extracellular fluid. As long ago as 1925 their endocrine function was recognized when it was shown that extracts of bovine parathyroid tissue would prevent hypocalcaemia and its associated tetany in parathyroidectomized dogs[22]. Furthermore, the pathology associated with hormone excess was revealed when it was shown that administration of the extracts to healthy dogs resulted in hypercalcaemia and death[23]. Parathyroid hormone (PTH) acts primarily to conserve body calcium. This is achieved both by restriction of calcium excretion and by increased input of calcium into extracellular fluid. However, in addition to its stimulation of renal tubular reabsorption of calcium and bone mineral resorption, parathyroid hormone also interacts with the vitamin D endocrine system by increasing the activity of 25-hydroxycholecalciferol 1α-hydroxylase. The increased output of 1,25-dihydroxycholecalciferol which results from this leads in turn to stimulation of intestinal calcium absorption.

Disorders of calcium metabolism are common, and range from simple dietary vitamin D insufficiency to rare enzyme defects as in hereditary vitamin D-dependent rickets. Complex metabolic disorders such as chronic renal failure may also have a profound effect on calcium metabolism. Because of the close interactions between the parathyroid and vitamin D endocrine systems, it is apparent that parathyroid function may be altered by a wide spectrum of diseases. Assessment of parathyroid function may thus be crucial both to the diagnosis and management of many disorders. In this chapter we consider various methods for assessing parathyroid function and the interpretation of that assessment in the light of current knowledge of parathyroid physiology and pathology.

PARATHYROID HORMONE

Chemistry

Detailed understanding of the chemistry and molecular biology of parathyroid hormone has emerged from considerable research efforts of the last 10 years.

Purified hormones have been isolated from bovine[45], porcine[84] and human[46] species, which exhibit minor sequence differences[47]. While the purified peptides each comprise a single chain of 84 amino acids, work with fragments and structural analogues has identified the first 30 residues as being necessary for biological activity. Nevertheless, the difficulty in defining structure-activity relationships is exemplified by the observation that substitution of alanine (bovine parathyroid hormone) for serine (porcine and human parathyroid hormone) produces profound potency differences in certain biological assay systems[64].

Secretion

As with other secreted polypeptides, the major extracted form of parathyroid hormone represents only a single stage in a complex sequence of proteolytic degradations. The ability to study the translation of parathyroid hormone messenger RNA in cell-free systems[44] and experiments on synthesis in parathyroid slices using pulse labels[37] have led to the identification of a 115 residue prohormone (preproparathyroid hormone). The hydrophobic nature of the N-terminal extension is consistent with its role as a signal peptide, responsible for the attachment of the nascent polypeptide to the endoplasmic reticulum and its subsequent transport into the cisternal space[12]. Within one minute of synthesis, the initial 25 residues are cleaved to produce proparathyroid hormone, a further basic hexapeptide being removed in the subsequent 15 minutes during the packaging process[38]. Biochemical technology has now advanced to the stage where the preprohormone has been synthesized chemically[40] and also produced from cloned DNA in *Escherichia coli*[50].

Sequential proteolytic degradation of parathyroid hormone is not only a presecretory phenomenon. In some of the earliest immunoassay studies of circulating parathyroid hormone, Berson and Yalow[9] noted that the apparent rate of clearance of exogenously administered hormone varied according to the particular antiserum used, implying the existence of molecular heterogeneity. Studies with region specific immunoassays[41, 71] have established that secreted parathyroid hormone is catabolized rapidly in the peripheral circulation with the preferential removal of a biologically active N-terminal sequence. The remaining biologically inert portion of the molecule disappears more slowly from the circulation. While it is likely that specific molecular cleavages occur at the biological receptor sites, the Kupffer cells of the liver have been shown to be capable of taking up and metabolizing intact parathyroid hormone[72]. It is not clear whether hepatic cleavage represents a degradative pathway for hormone not utilized in the target tissue[70] or is important as an activation stage in the regulation of hormonal activity[58]. However, further understanding of these complex proteolytic pathways is crucial to the interpretation of tests based on the immunological measurement of hormone sequences.

Control of secretion

Secretion of parathyroid hormone is controlled primarily by the concentration of extracellular calcium. One of the first immunoassays to be established demonstrated a clear reciprocal relationship between serum calcium and immunoreactive hormone[73]. Direct measurement of secretion rates of perfused bovine parathyroids has revealed a large capacity for release in response to hypocalcaemia and also continued low-level secretion in the face of hypercalcaemia[39]. Since the storage capacity of the parathyroids is low compared with some endocrine tissues, it has been suggested that secretion reflects a calcium-sensitive regulation of intracellular parathyroid hormone breakdown[36].

Magnesium has an inhibitory effect on parathyroid secretion, both *in vitro*[39] and *in vivo*[16], though only at high concentrations. It is important to note that low extracellular magnesium levels can inhibit parathyroid activity[5, 67, 77] and also affect target organ responsiveness[67]. The importance of magnesium measurement in the investigation of parathyroid function is discussed further below.

The identification in parathyroid tissue of a cytoplasmic binding protein for 1,25-dihydroxycholecalciferol[14] suggests the possibility of regulation by vitamin D metabolites. Results in this area have been so far confusing[17, 18] and it is difficult at present to assess the importance of vitamin D metabolites as regulators of parathyroid activity.

Biological actions

Several discrete biological actions of parathyroid hormone are recognized and each of these can be used as a guide to parathyroid activity. The ability of parathyroid hormone to stimulate bone resorption was first demonstrated by Barnicot[6] using parathyroid tissue implanted into skull-bones of mice. The mechanism involves hormonal stimulation of osteoclasts which release lysosomal enzymes[78]. Under acidic conditions, these digest both matrix and bone mineral. Since the cells contain a parathyroid hormone-sensitive adenylate cyclase[21] it is likely that this activity is mediated via cyclic AMP.

Bone formation is also stimulated by parathyroid hormone, administration of exogenous hormone to parathyroidectomized rats resulting in a net increase in bone mass[43], and this has led to attempts to treat osteoporosis with low doses of synthetic (1–34) parathyroid hormone[66]. In hyperparathyroidism, where both mineralization and resorption are stimulated, there is a net loss of bone mineral which implies that stimulation of osteoclastic activity is the main action of parathyroid hormone on bone.

The renal actions of parathyroid hormone are more acute. The phosphaturic action was first noted by Albright and Ellsworth[2] when they administered parathyroid extract to a child with idiopathic hypoparathyroidism. At one stage phosphaturia was considered to be the primary response to the hormone, the reciprocal changes in serum phosphate and calcium resulting from some unspecified physicochemical interaction[3]. Changes in calcium excretion in response to parathyroid hormone are more difficult to identify, though expression of calcium excretion as a function of the filtered load shows that parathyroid hormone has a marked effect on renal calcium handling[48, 65].

Hormonally sensitive reabsorption of phosphate occurs mainly in the proximal tubule[69] while that of calcium is in the distal tubule[55, 82]. Both regions of the tubule have parathyroid hormone-sensitive adenylate cyclase mechanisms[19] suggesting that cyclic AMP is a mediator of both actions of the hormone. Other tubular actions of parathyroid hormone include the inhibition of sodium reabsorption[35] and stimulation of bicarbonate excretion[30, 59], though these offer little help as specific indices of parathyroid activity.

The parathyroids can also influence intestinal absorption of calcium, though not directly. This process is regulated by 1,25-dihydroxycholecalciferol $(1,25\text{-}(OH)_2D_3)$ whose renal synthesis is stimulated by parathyroid hormone[32, 34].

MEASUREMENT OF PARATHYROID HORMONE

In 1963, a radioimmunoassay was developed for the measurement of bovine parathyroid hormone[10] which was used to establish the important relationship between circulating hormone levels and serum calcium[73]. The cross-reactivity of some antisera with human parathyroid hormone led to the first clinical application of the assay in differentiating patients with hyperparathyroidism from those with hypercalcaemia associated with bronchogenic carcinoma[8]. It is, however, ironic that while parathyroid hormone assays provide vital information in a variety of clinical disorders of calcium metabolism, the laboratory performance of these assays may leave much to be desired. There are several reasons for this. Firstly, the reduced affinity of most antibovine parathyroid hormone antisera for the human hormone has frequently limited the sensitivity of assays, such that hormone measurement in normal subjects is not practical. The increased availability of human parathyroid hormone synthetic fragments has enabled the development of assays based on homologous antisera, though this approach still presents problems.

A second disadvantage stems from the difficulty of preparing labelled antigen of satisfactory quality. Like many other peptides, parathyroid hormone appears sensitive to iodination or the conditions under which it is carried out. The need for frequent preparation of labelled reagent is an important factor in controlling long-term performance of parathyroid hormone assays. It is not clear why parathyroid hormone is particularly problematic in this respect, especially since performance of the label appears to some extent to relate to individual batches of purified peptide. The familiar problem of aggregation of the hormone, either during preparation or labelling, which results in high non-specific binding in conventional immunoassay systems, can be overcome by further purification of the labelled derivative by gel filtration or other conventional methods.

In our experience the variable binding of parathyroid hormone to antibody in different matrices necessitates the use of hormone-free plasma as a diluent for the standards. In practice such plasma may be difficult to obtain and our own system relies on a small group of regular donors who consistently have low levels of circulating immunoreactive parathyroid hormone.

Two further difficulties make it virtually impossible to compare immunoassay data from different laboratories. In the first place there is no reference preparation of human parathyroid hormone. More importantly, the heterogeneous nature of the circulating hormone and the relative specificities of antisera used in quantitation lead to considerable interpretive problems.

In practical terms we have found that immunoradiometric assay, which employs an excess of labelled antibody rather than labelled antigen[54] offers considerable advantages in terms of technical performance compared with conventional immunoassay procedures. The original method[1] proved labour-intensive, but subsequent automation of this procedure using the Kemtek 3000 immunoassay system[85] enables us to carry out large numbers of assays to a consistent level of performance. The method consists essentially of reacting affinity purified, ^{125}I-labelled antibodies overnight with samples and standards. Cellulose-linked parathyroid hormone is then added to bind unreacted labelled antibody and this fraction is removed some 30 min later by automated filtration. Iodinated antibodies to parathyroid hormone have been found to perform satisfactorily for periods of up to 9 weeks[83].

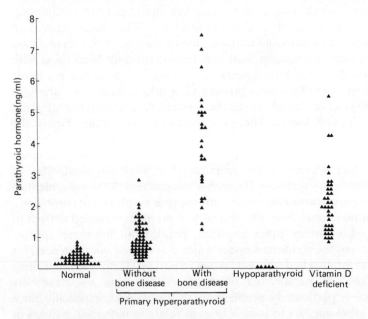

Figure 4.1 Immunoreactive parathyroid hormone in normal subjects and patients with disorders of calcium metabolism

However, despite the technical advantages of this approach there still remains the problem of interpretation. As shown in *Figure 4.1* a high proportion of patients with hyperparathyroidism have circulating levels of immunoreactive parathyroid hormone within the normal range. This phenomenon is well known[86], and though there may be a physiological basis for the observation, there is evidence to suggest that it relates in part at least to the specificity of the antisera used. Recent studies using region-specific immunoradiometric assays[52, 63] claim better discrimination between normal and abnormal parathyroid secretion, thus extending the diagnostic potential of these assays. Because of the difficulties associated with parathyroid hormone measurement, and the fact that it is not readily available to all clinicians, attempts continue to find indirect procedures for the assessment of parathyroid function. To date, however, none supersedes a parathyroid hormone estimation in a reliable assay.

INDIRECT ASSESSMENT OF PARATHYROID ACTIVITY

The physiological and pathological responses to altered parathyroid activity involve several well-characterized biochemical changes, all of which may be used to assess that activity. Thus the combination of a raised plasma calcium and a reduced plasma phosphate is suggestive of primary hyperparathyroidism and the reverse combination of hypoparathyroidism. These basic biochemical measurements are of course crucial to the investigation of any suspected disorder of calcium metabolism. Nevertheless, the subtlety and complexity of the mechanisms controlling calcium homeostasis account for the fact that marked metabolic disturbances may exist with no obvious derangement of plasma calcium or phosphate. For example, a normal plasma phosphate in a patient with chronic renal failure does not exclude the existence of hyperparathyroidism, because of the combination of factors influencing excretion. For this reason it is often more useful to consider renal handling of calcium and phosphate since these are of major importance in determining the ionic concentrations in plasma.

PHOSPHATE EXCRETION

The renal reabsorption of filtered phosphate occurs primarily in the proximal tubule[69], the process being regulated by parathyroid hormone. Many attempts have been made over the years to use phosphate excretion as a monitor of parathyroid function including such derivations as the phosphate excretion index[60]. However, indices such as this are subject to variations in phosphate intake, urine volume and glomerular filtration rate (GFR). The most useful index of phosphate handling is the derived maximum tubular reabsorption capacity for phosphate relative to the glomerular filtration rate (TmP/GFR). This derivation may be calculated from a plot of phosphate clearance relative to the plasma phosphate concentration[11], obtained during a phosphate infusion. This procedure, which involves frequent blood samples and urine collections, may be difficult to carry out in practice. We have found that the nomogram derived by Walton and Bijvoet[80] provides a satisfactory alternative. The nomogram relates TmP/GFR to plasma phosphate and its excretion relative to creatinine (*Figure 4.2*) and enables the parameter to be derived from data based on a single urine collection, and a mid-collection plasma measurement.

In practice a 2-hour collection is sufficient for clearance to be calculated from the formula:

$$\frac{\text{Urine phosphate} \times \text{plasma creatinine}}{\text{Plasma phosphate} \times \text{urine creatinine}} = \frac{\text{Clearance of phosphate } (C_p)}{\text{Clearance of creatinine } (C_{cr})}$$

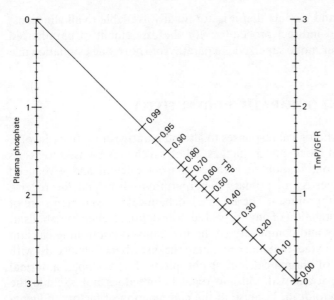

Figure 4.2 Nomogram for the derivation of the maximum renal tubular reabsorption capacity for phosphate (TmP/GFR). *Note*: Tubular reabsorption of phosphate (TRP) = $1 - C_p/C_{cr}$. (From Walton and Bijvoet[80], courtesy of the Editor and Publishers, *Lancet*)

In normal subjects TmP/GFR ranges from 0.75–1.4 mmol/l of glomerular filtrate. It is usually low in primary hyperparathyroidism[79] and may therefore provide diagnostic information. It has been possible to show that the nomogram may be used to detect small changes in phosphate reabsorption in response to near physiological doses of exogenous parathyroid hormone by sequential monitoring of urine and plasma[79]. The major drawback of TmP/GFR as a diagnostic test is the fact that it does not differentiate between malignancy and hyperparathyroidism, being low in both[76], and that its setting can be influenced by other factors such as oestrogens, growth hormone and glucocorticoids[11]. Thus, while a low TmP/GFR may provide additional evidence in a patient suspected of having hyperparathyroidism, as an independent observation it may be of relatively little value.

CALCIUM EXCRETION

Under normal circumstances, calcium excretion reflects intestinal absorption. Since the latter is normally regulated to meet body requirements, changes in excretion pattern may be helpful in the diagnosis of disorders of calcium metabolism. For example, a raised 24-hour urine calcium in a patient with normal plasma biochemistry is suggestive of calcium hyperabsorption, a well-recognized cause of renal stone disease. However, the complexity of the actions of parathyroid hormone may make calcium excretion a difficult parameter to interpret. The basic problem is that while parathyroid hormone exerts control over the reabsorption of calcium mainly in the distal tubule[55, 82], it also regulates the delivery of calcium to the tubule by influencing bone resorption and, indirectly, intestinal absorption. Thus, while total calcium excretion may be raised by increased parathyroid hormone secretion, a more meaningful assessment of parathyroid activity may be the level of excretion relative to the filtered load[65]. Thus fractional calcium excretion is reduced in hyperparathyroidism and raised in hypoparathyroidism.

By analogy to TmP/GFR, it is possible to calculate a similar parameter for calcium handling (TmCa/GFR) based on simultaneous measurement of plasma calcium and calcium clearance[53]. In normal subjects TmCa/GFR ranges from 1.6 to 2.1 mmol/l. It is frequently elevated in patients with hyperparathyroidism, though in our experience there is overlap with the normal range. As with TmP/GFR, this may be due in part to error consequent upon the use of a single calculated value derived from a nomogram. However, the added complication of having to calculate the ultrafiltrable fraction of plasma calcium in order to derive a measure of tubular reabsorption introduces further inaccuracy into the calculation. Finally, the setting of TmCa/GFR is not controlled by parathyroid hormone alone, tubular reabsorption being increased by thiazide diuretics[13] and lithium[24] for example. Thus, as with TmP/GFR, this index of renal tubular function is of limited diagnostic value.

CYCLIC AMP EXCRETION

The identification of a parathyroid hormone-sensitive adenylate cyclase in the renal cortex[20] first implicated cyclic AMP as a mediator of hormonal activity. While the detailed biochemistry of calcium and phosphate reabsorption is poorly understood, the localization of anatomically distinct regions of the tubule, corresponding to sites of maximum ion transport, which contain parathyroid hormone-sensitive cyclase systems suggests that both tubular activities of the hormone are mediated through these systems[19]. It has also been demonstrated that the parathyroid hormone-stimulated osteoclastic activity is mediated by adenylate cyclase stimulation[21].

Increased cyclic AMP excretion occurs in many patients with hyperparathyroidism[57] so that its measurement provides a means of assessing parathyroid function. As with other means of assessment, there is no clear-cut distinction between normal excretion and that found in mild hyperparathyroidism. Indeed we have found using low-dose parathyroid hormone infusions in man that changes in renal phosphate handling can provide a more sensitive index of hormonal response than excreted cyclic AMP[79]. This may result in part from the fact that under basal conditions less than half of the excreted cyclic AMP is of renal origin. It was suggested, therefore, that the calculation of the nephrogenous component from simultaneous measurement of plasma and urine cyclic AMP could provide a more reliable index of parathyroid activity[28]. In a recent study, for example[49], a good correlation was found between nephrogenous cyclic AMP and immunoreactive PTH in patients with mild renal failure, suggesting its usefulness as a means of monitoring developing renal osteodystrophy.

Rude *et al.*[68] found a considerable overlap between normal subjects and patients with hyperparathyroidism. They also found that hypercalcaemic malignant states produced, on the whole, similar values to hyperparathyroid patients. Broadus *et al.*[15] have developed a classical endocrine suppression test by measuring nephrogenous cyclic AMP before and after an oral calcium load. In normal subjects an oral calcium load suppressed cyclic AMP excretion but this did not occur in patients with mild hyperparathyroidism (*see Figure 4.4*). It would therefore appear that total urinary cyclic AMP and nephrogenous cyclic AMP are poor tests in the differentiation between various hypercalcaemic states and between normal and mildly hyperparathyroid subjects. Suppression tests, however, may produce more useful information.

STEROID SUPPRESSION TEST

The observation that hypercalcaemia of non-parathyroid origin can be suppressed by corticosteroids forms the basis of the steroid suppression test[25]. A high degree of diagnostic accuracy has been claimed for this test though patients with osteitis fibrosa may yield false-positive results[81].

Although the biochemical basis for the test is not fully understood it still remains of considerable value in the occasional patient. In the original test a positive response was judged to be a fall of serum calcium (corrected for serum albumin) of more than 0.25 mmol/l (1.0 mg/100 ml). Such changes can occur from day to day in some untreated hypercalcaemic patients and a better definition of response, therefore, is that the elevated calcium falls to within the normal range. Such a response is exceptional in hyperparathyroidism but may occur in other hypercalcaemic states. Patients with malignancy, however, sometimes fail to respond. A fall in calcium to the normal range makes hyperparathyroidism very unlikely but a failure to respond does not prove the existence of a hyperparathyroid state.

MULTIVARIANT ANALYSIS

In the differential diagnosis of hypercalcaemia, a multivariant analysis of several biochemical measurements including plasma bicarbonate and phosphate has been used[31, 81]. In the case of primary hyperparathyroidism, however, it is difficult to imagine that diagnostic accuracy based on this technique is greater than that based on accurate measurement of serum calcium and PTH.

PARATHYROID FUNCTION IN HYPERCALCAEMIA

Parathyroid function is most frequently assessed in patients with hypercalcaemia. Of these, the vast majority have either malignant disease or primary hyperparathyroidism. Each forms the subject of a separate chapter, so discussion of these conditions will be restricted to areas where problems of diagnosis or management may occur. It should be stressed that in most cases diagnosis is not particularly difficult. In the diagnosis of primary hyperparathyroidism the development and widespread availability of parathyroid hormone assays have rendered unnecessary many of the indirect tests. For the most part a raised serum calcium and a measurable parathyroid hormone level is diagnostic of hyperparathyroidism. The problem of overlap in parathyroid hormone values between patients with hyperparathyroidism and normal subjects has been discussed above, and it is too early to say whether or not it will be resolved by improvements in assay specificity.

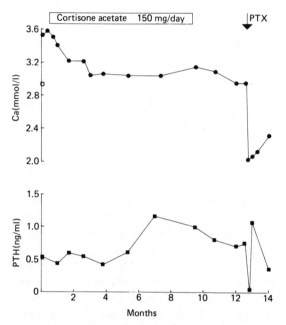

Figure 4.3 Plasma calcium and immunoreactive parathyroid hormone (PTH) levels in a patient with sarcoidosis and primary hyperparathyroidism. Note that normocalcaemia follows parathyroidectomy (PTX) but not corticosteroid administration

Recent surveys[42, 56] stress that the high incidence of hyperparathyroidism seen today stems from the finding of mild hypercalcaemia in largely asymptomatic patients subject to biochemical screening. The attempt to reach a diagnosis in cases with the mildest degree of disease provides a challenge to the accuracy and precision of laboratory technology. Reliability of the parathyroid hormone assay is crucial. *Figure 4.3* shows an example of a patient who presented with hypercalcaemia and sarcoidosis. The presence of a low but measurable serum parathyroid hormone suggested hyperparathyroidism as a cause of the hypercalcaemia. This was supported by a low TmP/GFR (0.67 mmol/l) and the failure of the serum calcium to normalize during steroid therapy. Biochemical normality was finally restored following removal of a parathyroid adenoma.

Reliable quantitation of serum calcium is equally important. Measurement of total calcium can sometimes be misleading and corrections applied to take into account serum protein binding are not necessarily reliable[61]. It remains to be seen

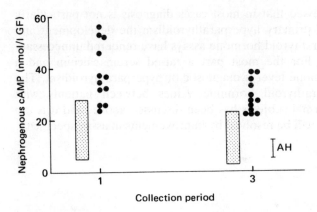

Figure 4.4 Nephrogenous cyclic AMP excretion in response to an oral calcium load in normal subjects, patients with absorptive hypercalciuria and patients with primary hyperparathyroidism with intermittent hypercalcaemia. ▨ = Values obtained in normal subjects; AH = range of values in 4 patients with absorptive hypercalciuria. (Data from Broadus *et al.*[15])

whether advances in the technology of ionized calcium determination can resolve problems of apparently intermittent hypercalcaemia. An alternative approach to the problem presented by patients with renal stones and intermittent hypercalcaemia has been adopted by Broadus *et al.*[15] based on suppression of nephrogenous cyclic AMP excretion by oral calcium loading. The limited data so far available (*Figure 4.4*) suggests that it is possible to identify patients with subtle primary hyperparathyroidism. It may be that nephrogenous cyclic AMP estimation is most useful when reliable parathyroid hormone assays are not readily available, though there is evidence which suggests particular value in differentiating various types of renal stone disease[4, 62]. In this context it should be stressed that a raised parathyroid hormone level in a renal stone-former who is normocalcaemic may be secondary to a tubular calcium leak, and should not therefore be taken as an indication for parathyroid surgery.

The reported presence of immunoreactive parathyroid hormone in the circulation of patients with malignant disease and hypercalcaemia gives grounds for confusion. Though this has been reported as a frequent finding[7], more recent studies reveal a low incidence[68, 76]. It is not readily apparent whether such findings reflect coincidental hyperparathyroidism, renal impairment or ectopic production of immunoreactive peptide. However, the severity of malignant disease usually associated with hypercalcaemia allows little room for diagnostic difficulty.

PARATHYROID FUNCTION IN CHRONIC RENAL FAILURE

Virtually all patients with chronic renal failure develop abnormal calcium metabolism. Hypocalcaemia occurs frequently and stimulates secondary hyperparathyroidism. Measurements of immunoreactive parathyroid hormone, particularly in the early stages of renal failure, may be difficult to interpret, since it may not be possible to assess the relative contributions of increased secretion of intact parathyroid hormone and impaired clearance of molecular fragments. At such stages measurement of cyclic AMP excretion or TmP/GFR may provide a more reliable estimate of parathyroid activity, though the development of immunoassays specific for the biologically active N-terminal region of parathyroid hormone may prove useful in the future[52].

From a clinical point of view the assessment of parathyroid function in renal failure is more important when hypercalcaemia develops. It is necessary to distinguish tertiary hyperparathyroidism from other causes of hypercalcaemia. We have recently studied a patient with longstanding renal failure and sarcoidosis. Sudden deterioration in renal function coincided with the finding of a serum calcium of 3.1 mmol/l and a parathyroid hormone of 0.44 ng/ml. In general, a patient with tertiary hyperparathyroidism would have been expected to have had values in excess of 3 ng/ml in our assay, suggesting sarcoidosis as the probable cause of hypercalcaemia. Subsequently, serum calcium fell and renal function improved in response to corticosteroid therapy. This example serves to illustrate the need for careful interpretation of parathyroid hormone levels in renal disease.

It should be remembered that renal impairment is a potential consequence of hypercalcaemia. It is relatively uncommon in patients with primary hyperparathyroidism, occurring mainly in those with overt bone disease[51]. It does occur, however, in a significant proportion of patients with hypercalcaemia associated with malignancy, and diagnostic problems may arise in the admittedly infrequent cases where the neoplasm is occult.

PARATHYROID FUNCTION IN HYPOCALCAEMIA

Hypocalcaemia is a less common problem than hypercalcaemia. It is important to differentiate between patients with parathyroid insufficiency (hypoparathyroidism), those lacking responsiveness to parathyroid hormone (pseudohypoparathyroidism) and those with non-parathyroid calcium disease who have appropriate parathyroid responses. Measurement of immunoreactive parathyroid hormone together with plasma phosphate, or perhaps better TmP/GFR, allows this distinction to be made. Clearly renal function should be taken into account.

Idiopathic hypoparathyroidism is rare and can occur in association with other endocrine abnormalities and candidiasis[26]. Hypocalcaemia is usually profound, the plasma phosphate raised and immunoreactive parathyroid hormone undetectable. In contrast, parathyroid hormone is invariably elevated in pseudohypoparathyroidism, and in this context provides the diagnosis. This condition is rare and may be associated with mental and skeletal abnormalities, for example shortened metacarpals. It is current practice to confirm the diagnosis by studying responsiveness to an infusion of exogenous parathyroid hormone since such patients show absent or minimal increases in the excretion of cyclic AMP and phosphate (*Figure 4.5*). On the basis of such a test a form of pseudohypoparathyroidism has been identified in which the urinary cyclic AMP is present but the phosphaturic response is absent[27].

In the past hypoparathyroidism was a not infrequent complication of thyroid surgery though this is less common nowadays. However, hypocalcaemia is a

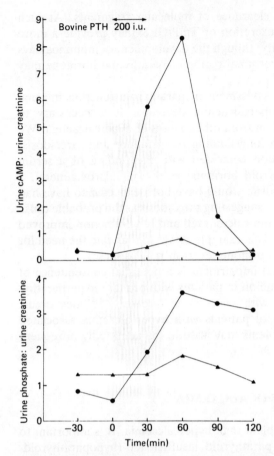

Figure 4.5 Excretion of cyclic AMP and phosphate in response to an infusion of bovine parathyroid hormone in a normal subject (●) and a patient with pseudohypoparathyroidism (▲)

common transient consequence of effective parathyroid surgery and maybe particularly profound when osteitis fibrosa is present. Long-term hypoparathyroidism may occasionally occur. The effectiveness of parathyroid surgery and the postoperative recovery of normal parathyroid activity has been monitored by measurement of urinary cyclic AMP[74, 75]. Interestingly, the normal suppressed parathyroids may respond rapidly to sudden hypocalcaemia (*Figure 4.6*) though it should be noted that the TmP/GFR may remain high in the postoperative period irrespective of the parathyroid hormone level. Clearly the relationship between these parameters at this stage is complex, and interpretation of biochemical data may be difficult.

Hypocalcaemia can be caused by magnesium depletion which occurs most commonly in alcoholism and various gastrointestinal disorders. It appears that hypomagnesaemia can inhibit both parathyroid secretion and target organ responsiveness[67]. It is thus difficult to interpret data relating to parathyroid function in such circumstances. Serum magnesium, or better still a 24-hour urine

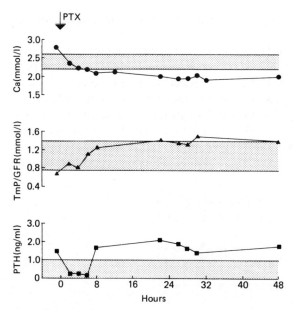

Figure 4.6 Changes in plasma calcium, TmP/GFR and immunoreactive parathyroid hormone in a patient undergoing parathyroid surgery (*see* text)

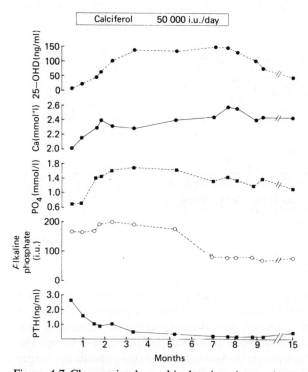

Figure 4.7 Changes in plasma biochemistry in a patient treated for severe osteomalacia with a large dose of calciferol (*see* text)

magnesium[29] should therefore be measured in patients with unexplained hypocalcaemia.

There are many causes of vitamin D insufficiency, most of which are associated
with secondary hyperparathyroidism, which may compensate for a tendency
towards hypocalcaemia. In most cases, therefore, parathyroid hormone is elevated
and TmP/GFR is low. The value of assessment of parathyroid function relates more
to monitoring of therapeutic response rather than to diagnosis itself. *Figure 4.7*
shows an example of a patient with dietary osteomalacia being treated with
calciferol. The rise in serum calcium following vitamin D administration suppresses
parathyroid activity, which is reflected by a rise in phosphate and subsequent
healing of the bones.

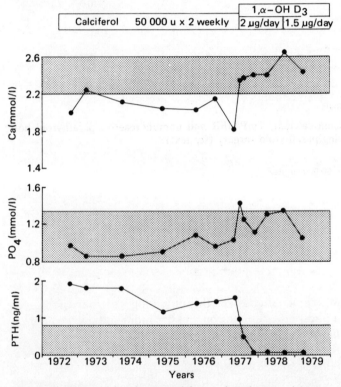

Figure 4.8 Changes in plasma calcium, phosphate and immunoreactive parathyroid hormone in a patient with vitamin D-dependent rickets

The importance of monitoring parathyroid function is illustrated in *Figure 4.8*
which relates biochemical changes to vitamin D therapy in a patient with vitamin
D-dependent rickets. Lack of response to adequate doses of calciferol was
indicated by the continued elevation of immunoreactive parathyroid hormone. The
efficacy of a small dose of 1α-hydroxycholecalciferol in this condition where
endogenous 1α-hydroxylase activity is defective[33], is shown by the prompt suppression of parathyroid activity.

Through rarely encountered, hereditary hypophosphataemic rickets is unusual in that parathyroid function is normal.

Hypocalcaemia is frequently seen in patients with malabsorption syndromes. Vitamin D deficiency and osteomalacia are common in such patients but assessment of parathyroid function may be complicated by coexisting magnesium depletion.

CONCLUSIONS

Parathyroid function is frequently assessed in patients with disorders of calcium metabolism. There is no doubt that the advent of parathyroid hormone immunoassay has made an enormous impact both on diagnosis and on the understanding of the often complex mechanisms of these diseases. We have attempted to indicate where other means of assessment of parathyroid activity may be useful. It may be that the application of these alternative investigations in general reflects the lack of availability of reliable parathyroid hormone immunoassays. It is likely that improvements in specificity and simplicity of these immunoassays will ultimately reduce the number of investigations carried out.

Acknowledgements

For the data taken from our own studies we are grateful to our colleagues Richard Brown, Joyce Davies, Hilary Foster, Roy Ghose and David Walker.

References

1 ADDISON, G. M., HALES, C. N., WOODHEAD, J. S. and O'RIORDAN, J. L. H. Immunoradiometric assay of parathyroid hormone. *Journal of Endocrinology*, **49**, 521–530 (1971)

2 ALBRIGHT, F. and ELLSWORTH, R. Studies on the physiology of the parathyroid glands. I. Calcium and phosphorus studies on a case of idiopathic hypoparathyroidism. *Journal of Clinical Investigation*, **7**, 183–201 (1929)

3 ALBRIGHT, F. and REIFENSTEIN, E. C. *The Parathyroid Glands and Metabolic Bone Disease.* Baltimore, Williams and Wilkins (1948)

4 ALSTON, W. C., ALLEN, K. R. and TOVEY, J. E. A comparison of nephrogenous cyclic AMP, total urinary cyclic AMP and the renal tubular maximum reabsorptive capacity for phosphate in the diagnosis of primary hyperparathyroidism. *Clinical Endocrinology*, **13**, 17–25 (1980)

5 ANAST, C. S., MOHS, J. M., BURNS, T. W. and KAPLAN, S. L. Evidence for parathyroid failure in magnesium deficiency. *Science*, **177**, 606–608 (1972)

6 BARNICOT, N. A. The local action of parathyroid hormone and other tissues on the bone in intracerebral grafts. *Journal of Anatomy (London)*, **82**, 233–248 (1948)

7 BENSON, R. C., RIGGS, B. L., PICKARD, B. M. and ARNAUD, C.D. Radioimmunoassay of parathyroid hormone in hypercalcaemic patients with malignant disease. *American Journal of Medicine*, **56**, 821–826 (1974)

8 BERSON, S. A. and YALOW, R. S. (1966) Parathyroid hormone in plasma in adenomatous hyperparathyroidism, uraemia and bronchogenic carcinoma. *Science*, **154**, 907–909 (1966)

9 BERSON, S. A. and YALOW, R. S. Immunochemical heterogeneity of parathyroid hormone in plasma. *Journal of Clinical Endocrinology*, **28**, 1037–1047 (1968)

10 BERSON, S. A., YALOW, R. S., AURBACH, G. D. and POTTS, J. T. Immunoassay of bovine and human parathyroid hormone. *Proceedings of the National Academy of Sciences USA*, **49**, 613–617 (1963)

11 BIJVOET, O. L. M., MORGAN, D. B. and FOURMAN, P. The assessment of phosphate reabsorption. *Clinica Chimica Acta*, **26**, 15–24 (1969)

12 BLOBEL, G. and DOBBERSTEIN, B. Transfer of proteins across membranes. 11. Reconstitution of functional rough microsomes from heterologous components. *Journal of Cellular Biology*, **67**, 852–862 (1975)

13 BRICKMAN, A. S., MASSRY, S. G. and COBURN, J. W. Changes in serum and urinary calcium during treatment with hydrochlorothiazide. Studies on mechanisms. *Journal of Clinical Investigation*, **51**, 945–954 (1972)

14 BRUMBAUGH, P. F., HUGHES, M. R. and HAUSSLER, M. R. Cytoplasmic and nuclear binding components for 1α, 25-dihydroxy-vitamin D_3 in chick parathyroid glands. *Proceedings of the National Academy of Sciences USA*, **72**, 4871–4875 (1975)

15 BROADUS, A. E., HORST, R. L., LITTLEDIKE, E. T., MAHAFFEY, J. E. and RASMUSSEN, H. Primary hyperparathyroidism with intermittent hypercalcaemia: serial observations and simple diagnosis by means of oral calcium tolerance test. *Clinical Endocrinology*, **12**, 225–235 (1980)

16 BUCKLE, R. M., CARE, A. D., COOPER, C. W. and GITELMAN, H. J. The influence of plasma magnesium concentration on parathyroid hormone secretion. *Journal of Endocrinology*, **42**, 529–534 (1968)

17 CANTERBURY, J. M., LERMAN, S., CLAFLIN, A. J., HENRY, H., NORMAN, A. and REISS, E. Inhibition of parathyroid hormone secretion by 25-hydroxycholecalciferol and 24,25 dihydroxycholecalciferol in the dog. *Journal of Clinical Investigation*, **61**, 1375–1383 (1978)

18 CARE, A. D., BATES, R. F. L., PICKARD, D. W., PEACOCK, M., TOMLINSON, S., O'RIORDAN, J. L. H., MAWER, E. B., TAYLOR, C. M., DeLUCA, H. F. and NORMAN, A. W. The effects of vitamin D metabolites and their analogues on the secretion of parathyroid hormone. *Calcified Tissue Research*, **21**, Suppl. 142–146 (1976)

19 CHABARDES, D., IMBERT, M. and MOREL, F. Localisation of PTH action sites along the rabbit nephron. In *Phosphate Metabolism, Kidney and Bone*, edited by L. Avioli, P. Bordier, H. Fleisch, S. Massry and E. Slatopolsky, pp. 123–131. Paris, Armour Montagu, (1975)

20 CHASE, L. R. and AURBACH, G. D. Renal adenyl cyclase: anatomically separate sites for parathyroid hormone and vasopressin. *Science*, **159**, 545–546 (1968)

21 CHASE, L. R., FEDAK, S. A. and AURBACH, G. D. Activation of skeletal adenyl cyclase by parathyroid hormone *in vitro*. *Endocrinology*, **84**, 761–768 (1969)

22 COLLIP, J. B. The extraction of a parathyroid hormone which will prevent or control parathyroid tetany and which regulates the level of blood calcium. *Journal of Biological Chemistry*, **63**, 395–438 (1925)

23 COLLIP, J. B., CLARK, E. P. and SCOTT, J. W. The effect of a parathyroid hormone on normal animals. *Journal of Biological Chemistry*, **63**, 439–460 (1925)

24 DAVIES, C. J., LAZARUS, J. H., WALKER, D. A., WALKER, S. and WOODHEAD, J. S. Effect of lithium on the renal tubular handling of calcium and phosphate in man. *Clinical Science and Molecular Medicine*, **55**, 8 p. (Abstract) (1978)

25 DENT, C. E. and WATSON, L. The hydrocortisone test in primary and tertiary hyperparathyroidism. *Lancet*, **2**, 662–664 (1968)

26 DIMICH, A., BEDROSSIAN, P. and WALLACH, S. Hypoparathyroidism: clinical observations in 34 patients. *Medicine (Chicago)*, **120**, 449–458 (1967)

27 DREZNER, M. K., NEELON, F. A. and LEBOVITZ, H. E. Pseudohypoparathyroidism type II: a possible defect in the reception of the cyclic AMP signal. *New England Journal of Medicine*, **289**, 1056–1060 (1973)

28 DREZNER, M. K., NEELON, F. A., CURTIS, H. B. and LEBOVITZ, H. E. Renal cyclic adenosine monophosphate: an accurate index of parathyroid function. *Metabolism*, **25**, 1103–1112 (1976)

29 EDITORIAL Magnesium deficiency *Lancet*, **1**, 523–524 (1976)

30 ELLSWORTH, R. and NICHOLSON, W. M. Further observations upon the changes in electrolytes of the urine following the injection of parathyroid extract. *Journal of Clinical Investigation*, **14**, 823–827 (1935)

31 FRASER, P., HEALY, M. and WATSON, L. Further experience with discriminant functions in differential diagnosis of hypercalcaemia. *Postgraduate Medical Journal*, **52**, 254–257 (1976)

32 FRASER, D. R. and KODICEK, E. Regulation of 25-hydroxycholecalciferol 1-hydrolyase activity in kidney by parathyroid hormone. *Nature New Biology*, **241**, 163–166 (1973)

33 FRASER, D., KOOH, S. W., KIND, H. P., HOLICK, M. F., TANAKA, Y. and De LUCA, H. F. Pathogenesis of hereditary vitamin-D dependent rickets. *New England Journal of Medicine*, **289**, 817–822 (1973)

34 GARABEDIAN, M., HOLICK, M. F., DeLUCA, H. F. and BOYLE, I. T. Control of 25-hydroxycholecalciferol metabolism by parathyroid glands. *Proceedings of the National Academy of Sciences USA*, **69**, 1673–1676 (1972)

35 GOLDBERG, M., AGUS, Z. S., PUSCHETT, J. B. and SENESKY, S. Mode of phosphaturic action of parathyroid hormone: micropuncture studies. In *Calcium, Parathyroid Hormone and the Calcitonins*, edited by R. V. Talmage and P. L. Munson. pp. 273–283. Amsterdam, Excerpta Medica (1972)

36 HABENER, J. F., KEMPER, B. and POTTS, J. T. Jr. Calcium-dependent intracellular degradation of parathyroid hormone: a possible mechanism for the regulation of hormone stores. *Endocrinology*, **97**, 431–441 (1975)

37 HABENER, J. F., KEMPER, B. W., POTTS, J. T. and RICH, A. Preproparathyroid hormone identified by cell-free translation of messenger RNA from hyperplastic human parathyroid tissue. *Journal of Clinical Investigation*, **56**, 1328–1333 (1975)

38 HABENER, J. F., KEMPER, B. W., RICH, A. and POTTS, J. T. Biosynthesis of parathyroid hormone. *Recent Progress in Hormone Research*, **33**, 249–308 (1977)

39 HABENER, J. F. and POTTS, J. T. Jr. Relative effectiveness of magnesium and calcium in the control of parathyroid hormone secretion and biosynthesis. *Endocrinology*, **98**, 209–214 (1976)

40 HABENER, J. F., ROSENBLATT, M., KEMPER, B., KRONENBERG, H. M., RICH, A. and POTTS, J. T. Pre-proparathyroid hormone: amino acid sequence, chemical synthesis, and some biological studies of the precursor region. *Proceedings of the National Academy of Sciences USA*, **75**, 2626–2620 (1978)

41 HABENER, J. R., SEGRE, G. V., POWELL, D., MURRAY, T. M. and POTTS, J. T. Jr. Immunoreactive parathyroid hormone in circulation of man. *Nature New Biology*, **238**, 152–154 (1972)

42 HEATH, H., HODGSON, S. F. and KENNEDY, M. A. Primary hyperparathyroidism: incidence, morbidity and potential economic impact in a community. *New England Journal of Medicine*, **302**, 189–193 (1980)

43 KALU, D. N., PENNOCK, S., DOYLE, F. H. and FOSTER, G. V. Parathyroid hormone and experimental osteosclerosis. *Lancet*, **1**, 1363–1366 (1970)

44 KEMPER, B., HABENER, J. F., MULLIGAN, R. C., POTTS, J. T. Jr and RICH, A. Pre-proparathyroid hormone: a direct translation product of parathyroid messenger RNA. *Proceedings of the National Academy of Sciences USA*, **71**, 3731–3735 (1974)

45 KEUTMANN, H. T., AURBACH, G. D., DAWSON, B. F., NIALL, H. D., DEFTOS, L. J. and POTTS., J. T. Jr. Isolation and characterization of the bovine parathyroid isohormones. *Biochemistry*, **10**, 2779–2787 (1971)

46 KEUTMANN, H. T., BARLING, P. M., HENDY, G. N., SEGRE, G. V., NIALL, H. D., AURBACH, G. *et al*. Isolation of human pararhyroid hormone. *Biochemistry*, **13**, 1646–1652 (1974)

47 KEUTMANN, H. T., SAUER, M. M. HENDY, G. N., O'RIORDAN, J. L. H. and POTTS, J. T. Jr. Complete amino acid sequence of human parathyroid hormone. *Biochemistry*, **17**, 5723–5729 (1978)

48 KLEEMAN, C. R., BERNSTEIN, D., ROCKNEY, R., DOWLING, J. T. and MAXWELL, M. H. Studies on the renal clearance of diffusible calcium and the role of the parathyroid glands in its regulation. *Yale Journal of Biological Medicine*, **34**, 1–30 (1961)

49 KRENSKY, A. M., HARMON, W. E., INGELFINGER, J. R., KIRKPATRICK, J. A. and GRUPE, W. E. Elevated nephrogenous cyclic adenosine monophosphate to monitor early renal osteodystrophy. *Clinical Nephrology*, **16**, 245–250 (1981)

50 KRONENBERG, H. M., McDEVITT, B. E., MAJZOUT, J. A., NATHANS, J., SHARP, P. A., POTTS, J. T. and RICH, A. Cloning and nucleotide sequence of DNA coding for bovine parathyroid hormone. *Proceedings of the National Academy of Sciences USA*, **76**, 4981–4985 (1979)

51 MALLETTE, L. E., BILEZIKIAN, J. P., HEATH, D. A. and AURBACH, G. D. Primary hyperparathyroidism: clinical and biochemical features. *Medicine (Baltimore)*, **53**, 127–146 (1974)

52 MANNING, R. M., ADAMI, S., PAPAPOULOS, S. E., GLEED, J. H., HENDY, G. N., ROSENBLATT, M. and O'RIORDAN, J. C. H. A carboxy-terminal specific assay for human parathyroid hormone. *Clinical Endocrinology*, **15**, 439–449 (1981)

53 MARSHALL, D. H. Calcium and phosphate kinetics. In *Calcium, Phosphate and Magnesium Metabolism*, edited by B. E. C. Nordin, pp. 257–297, Edinburgh, Churchill Livingstone (1977)

54 MILES, L. E. M. and HALES, C. N. Labelled antibodies and immunological assay systems. *Nature*, **219**, 186–187 (1968)

55 MIONI, G., D'ANGELO, A., OSSI, E., BERTAGLIA, E., MARCON, G. and MASCHIO, G. The renal handling of calcium in normal subjects and in renal disease. *European Journal of Clinical and Biological Research*, **16**, 881–887 (1971)

56 MUNDY, G. R., COVE, D. H., FISKEN, R., HEATH, D. A. and SOMERS, S. Primary hyperparathyroidism: changes in the pattern of clinical presentation. *Lancet*, **1**, 1317 –1320 (1980)

57 NEELON, F. A., DREZNER, M. and BIRCH, B. M. Urinary cyclic adenosine monophosphate as an aid in the diagnosis of hyperparathyroidism. *Lancet*, **1**, 631–633 (1973)

58 NEUMAN, W. F., SCHNEIDER, N. and DOOLITTLE, R. The peripheral metabolism of parathyroid hormone. In *Hormonal Control of Calcium Metabolism*, edited by D. V. Cohn, R. V. Talmage and J. L. Matthews, pp. 55–63. Amsterdam, Excerpta Medica (1981)

59 NORDIN, B. E. C. The effect of intravenous parathyroid extract on urinary pH, bicarbonate and electrolyte excretion. *Clinical Science*, **19**, 311–319 (1960)

60 NORDIN, B. E. C. and FRASER, R. Assessment of urinary phosphate excretion. *Lancet*, **1**, 947–950 (1960)

61 PAIN, R. W., ROWLAND, K. M., PHILLIPS, P. J. and DUNCAN, B. McL. Current 'corrected' calcium concept challenged. *British Medical Journal*, **4**, 617–619 (1975)

62 PAK, C. Y. C., KAPLAN, R. A., BONE, H., TOWNSEND, J. and WATERS, O. A simple test for the diagnosis of absorptive, resorptive and renal hypercalciurias. *New England Journal of Medicine*, **292**, 497–500 (1975)

63 PAPAPOULOS, S. E., MANNING, R. M., HENDY, G. N., LEWIN, I. G. and O'RIORDAN, J. L. H. Studies of circulating parathyroid hormone in man using a homologous aminoterminal specific immunoradiometric assay. *Clinical Endocrinology*, **13**, 57–67 (1980)

64 PARSONS, J. A., RAFFERTY, B., GRAY, D., REIT, B., ZANELLI, J. M., KEUTMANN, H. T., TREGEAR, G. W., CALLAHAN, E. N. and POTTS, J. T. Pharmacology of parathyroid hormone and some of its fragments and analogues. In *Calcium Regulating Hormones*, edited by R. V. Talmage, M. Owen and J. A. Parsons, pp. 33–39. Amsterdam, Excerpta Medica (1975)

65 PEACOCK, M., ROBERTSON, W. G. and NORDIN, B. E. C. Relation between serum and urinary calcium with particular reference to parathyroid hormone. *Lancet*, **1**, 384–386 (1969)

66 REEVE, J., HESP, R., WILLIAMS, S., HULME, P., KLENERMAN, L., ZANELLI, J. M., DARBY, A. J., TREGEAR, G. W. and PARSONS, J. A. Anabolic effect of low doses of a fragment of human parathyroid hormone on the skeleton in postmenopausal osteoporosis. *Lancet*, **1**, 1035–1038 (1976)

67 RUDE, R. K., OLDHAM, S. B. and SINGER, F. R. Functional hypoparathyroidism and parathyroid hormone end-organ resistance in human magnesium deficiency. *Clinical Endocrinology*, **5**, 209–224 (1976)

68 RUDE, R. K., SHARP, C. F., FREDERICKS, R. S., OLDHAM, S. B., ELBAUM, N., LINK, J., IRWIN, L. and SINGER, F. R. Urinary and nephrogenous adenosine 3',5'-monophosphate in the hypercalcaemia of malignancy. *Journal of Clinical Endocrinology and Metabolism*, **52**, 765–771 (1981)

69 SAMIY, A. H., HIRSCH, P. F. and RAMSAY, A. G. Localisation of the phosphaturia effect of parathyroid hormone in the nephron of the dog. *American Journal of Physiology*, **28**, 73–77 (1965)

70 SEGRE, G. V., BRINGHURST, R., PERKINS, A. S., LAUGHARN, J. A., REINER, B. L., JACOBS, J. W. and POTTS, J. T. Metabolism of parathyroid hormone by the liver. In *Hormonal Control of Calcium Metabolism*, edited by D. V. Cohn, R. V. Talmage and J. L. Matthews, pp. 70–73. Amsterdam, Excerpta Medica (1981)

71 SEGRE, G. V., NIALL, H. D., HABENER, J. F. and POTTS, J. T. Jr. Metabolism of parathyroid hormone. *American Journal of Medicine*, **56**, 774–784 (1974)

72 SEGRE, G. V., PERKINS, A. S., WITTERS, L. A. and POTTS, J. T. Metabolism of parathyroid hormone by isolated rat Kupffer cells and hepatocytes. *Journal of Clinical Investigation*, **67**, 449–457 (1981)

73 SHERWOOD, L. M., POTTS, J. T., Jr, CARE, A. D., MAYER, G. P. and AURBACH, G. D. Evaluation by radioimmunoassay of factors controlling the secretion of parathyroid hormone: intravenous infusions of calcium and ethylenediamine tetra acetic acid in the cow and goat. *Nature*, **209**, 52–55 (1966)

74 SPIEGEL, A. M., MARX, S. J., BRENNAN, M. F., BROWN, E. M., DOWNS, R. W., GARDNER, D. J. and ATTIE, M. F. Parathyroid function after parathyroidectomy: evaluation by measurement of urinary cAMP. *Clinical Endocrinology*, **15**, 66–73 (1981)

75 SPIEGEL, A. M., MARX, S. J., BRENNAN, M. F., BROWN, E. M., KOEHLER, J. O. and AURBACH, G. D. Urinary cyclic AMP excretion during surgery: an index of successful parathyroidectomy in patients with primary hyperparathyroidism. *Journal of Clinical Endocrinology and Metabolism*, **47**, 800–806 (1978)

76 STEWART, A. F., HORST, R., DEFTOS, L. J., CADMAN, E. C., LANG, R. and BROADUS, A. E. Biochemical evaluation of patients with cancer-associated hypercalcaemia: evidence for humoral and non-humoral groups. *New England Journal of Medicine*, **303**, 1377–1383 (1980)

77 TARGOVNIK, J. H., RODMAN, J. S. and SHERWOOD, L. M. Regulation of parathyroid hormone secretion in vitro: quantitative aspects of calcium and magnesium ion control. *Endocrinology*, **88**, 1477–1482 (1971)

78 VAES, G. The role of lysosomes and of the enzymes in the development of bone resorption induced by parathyroid hormone. In *Parathyroid Hormone and Thyrocalcitonin (Calcitonin)*, edited by R. V. Talmage and L. F. Belanger. pp. 318–328 Amsterdam, Excerpta Medica (1968)

79 WALKER, D. A., DAVIES, S. J., SIDDLE, K. and WOODHEAD, J. S. Control of renal tubular phosphate reabsorption by parathyroid hormone in man. *Clinical Science and Molecular Medicine*, **53**, 431–438 (1977)

80 WALTON, R. J. and BIJVOET, O. L. M. Nomogram for derivation of renal threshold phosphate concentration. *Lancet*, **2**, 309–310 (1975)

81 WATSON, L., MOXHAM, J. and FRASER, P. Hydrocortisone suppression test and discriminant analysis in differential diagnosis of hypercalcaemia. *Lancet*, **1**, 1320–1325 (1980)

82 WIDROW, S. H. and LEVINSKY, N. G. The effect of parathyroid extract on renal tubular calcium reabsorption in the dog. *Journal of Clinical Investigation*, **41**, 2151–2159 (1962)

83 WOODHEAD, J. S., ADDISON, G. M. and HALES, C. N. The immunoradiometric assay and related techniques. *British Medical Bulletin*, **30**, 44–49 (1974)

84 WOODHEAD, J. S., O'RIORDAN, J. L. H., KEUTMANN, H. T., STOLTZ, M. L., DAWSON, B. F., NIALL, H. D., ROBINSON, J. C. and POTTS, J. T. Jr. Isolation and chemical properties of porcine parathyroid hormone. *Biochemistry*, **10**, 2787–2792 (1971)

85 WOODHEAD, J. S., SIMPSON, J. S. A., DAVIES, S. J., FOSTER, H. and DAVIES, C. J. Accuracy and precision in automated immunoassay systems. In *Quality Control in Clinical Endocrinology*, edited by D. W. Wilson, S. Gaskell and K. Griffiths, pp. 117–125. Cardiff, Alpha Omega (1981)

86 WOODHEAD, J. S. and WALKER, D. A. Assay of parathyroid hormone in human serum and its uses. *Annals of Clinical Biochemistry*, **13**, 549–554 (1976)

5
Bisphosphonates
R. G. G. Russell

INTRODUCTION

Several bisphosphonates have been studied over the past 10 years for the treatment of a variety of disorders of calcium metabolism, including Paget's disease, dystrophic and metastatic calcification, renal calculi, hypercalcaemia and osteoporosis.

Bisphosphonates are analogues of pyrophosphate in which the labile phosphorus-oxygen bonds (P-O-P) are replaced by P-C-P bonds which are stable towards chemical and enzymatic degradation. Several 1,1 substituted bisphosphonates of this type inhibit both the growth and dissolution[23] of hydroxyapatite crystals *in vitro* and retard bone resorption and bone formation in experimental animals[24, 27, 45]. The recently recommended terminology described these compounds as bisphosphonates rather than as diphosphonates. Unfortunately this is likely to cause great confusion about nomenclature particularly since abbreviations now in common usage, for example EHDP, Cl_2MDP and APD, depend on the diphosphonate terminology. The history of development of the diphosphonates or bisphosphonates and their biochemistry and pharmacology has been reviewed elsewhere[25, 45] and there have been two recent symposia[12, 17]. This chapter will deal mainly with their clinical properties.

The effects of bisphosphonates in reducing bone resorption and bone turnover[8, 9, 31] have been demonstrated in a variety of tissue culture systems and in animal models. A major question still exists as to whether the effects on bone turnover, both in experimental animals and in man, can be accounted for by their known effects on crystal behaviour or whether they have direct inhibitory actions on cellular metabolism. Several recent papers indicate that high doses of some bisphosphonates can alter the metabolic properties of cells, particularly of skeletal origin[18–21, 33, 34]. They also have anti-inflammatory effects[26, 28].

Three bisphosphonates (*Figure 5.1*) have been used in clinical studies, namely EHDP (disodium etidronate, or disodium 1-hydroxy-ethylidene-1, 1- diphosphonate or bisphosphonate), Cl_2MDP (clodronate disodium, or dichloromethylene diphosphonate or bisphosphonate), and APD (3-amino, 1-hydroxypropylidene-1, 1-bisphosphonate). The first of these, disodium etidronate, is now licensed for distribution in several countries under the trade names of Didronel or Etidron. Both Cl_2MDP and APD are undergoing clinical trials but are unlikely to become generally available in the immediate future. A fourth bisphosphonate (6-aminohexane-1, 1-bisphosphonate) is undergoing preliminary clinical studies.

In both experimental animals and in man the intestinal absorption of the drugs is poor and variable, and to some extent dependent on the dose administered, but rarely exceeds 10%.

When given parenterally, the major fraction of absorbed bisphosphonates are taken up by bone, presumably reflecting their high affinity for bone mineral, and this is the basis for their use as bone scanning agents. EHDP is not metabolized and

	Common abbreviation	Name	Trade name

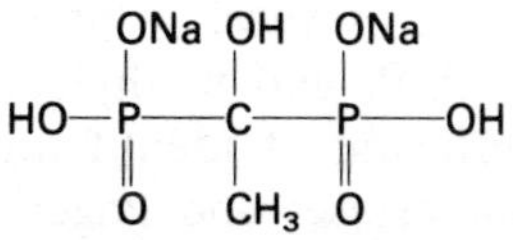

```
       ONa  OH  ONa
        |   |    |
HO—P———C———P———OH       EHDP              Etidronate disodium       Didronel
   ‖    |    ‖                                                      Etidron
   O   CH₃   O
```

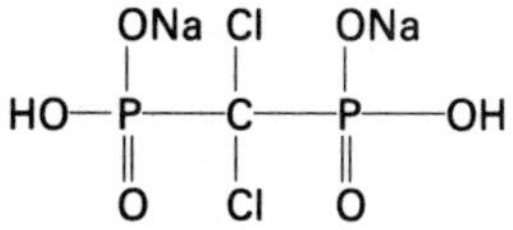

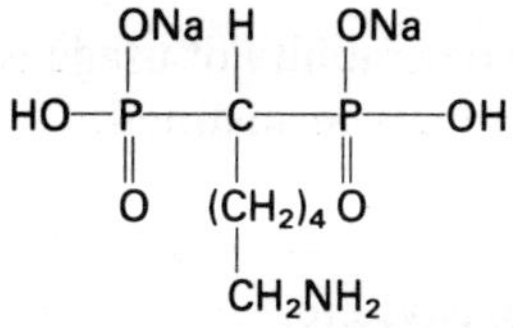

(1-hydroxyethylidene) bisphosphonic acid
Disodium salt

```
       ONa  Cl  ONa
        |   |    |
HO—P———C———P———OH       Cl₂MDP            Clodronate disodium
   ‖    |    ‖
   O   Cl    O
```

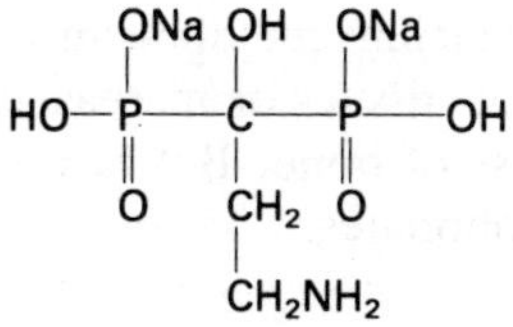

(Dichloromethylene) bisphosphonic acid
Disodium salt

```
       ONa  OH  ONa
        |   |    |
HO—P———C———P———OH       APD
   ‖    |    ‖
   O   CH₂   O
        |
       CH₂NH₂
```

(3-amino-1-hydroxypropylidene) bisphosphonic acid
Disodium salt

```
       ONa  H   ONa
        |   |    |
HO—P———C———P———OH
   ‖    |    ‖
   O  (CH₂)₄  O
        |
       CH₂NH₂
```

(6-aminohexylidene) bisphosphonic acid

Figure 5.1 Diphosphonates or bisphosphonates so far studied in man. Only EHDP (disodium etidronate) is licensed for use in Paget's disease and heterotopic ossification. There is some confusion about the correct nomenclature for the bisphosphonates or diphosphonates – bisphosphonate is the preferable term for 1,1 substituted phosphonates. The names given here are those used by IUPAC (1979)

about half the absorbed dose is excreted into the urine. The disappearance of bisphosphonates from blood is extremely rapid but the release of the drug taken up by the skeleton occurs slowly and presumably depends upon the rate of skeletal renewal as with other bone-seeking agents. In growing rats, the half-time of release is about 2–4 weeks, but the comparable figure in man is not known.

BONE SCANNING

The high affinity[7] of bisphosphonates for crystals of calcium phosphate has been exploited in bone scintigraphy. Bone scanning agents have been devised which utilize the well-recognized advantages of ^{99m}Tc as a γ-emitter and consists of a complex of ^{99m}Tc with a bisphosphonate in the presence of stannous ions. Like the corresponding pyrophosphate and polyphosphate compounds, several bisphosphonates, including methylene bisphosphonate (MDP), EHDP, and methylene hydroxy bisphosphonate (MHDP), appear to be highly efficient at identifying regions of increased skeletal turnover, particularly bone metastases and Paget's disease. The ^{99m}Tc polyphosphate or bisphosphonate compounds have distinct advantages over other bone scanning agents and are now the major class of agents used in clinical practice.

MEDICAL USES OF BISPHOSPHONATES

The experimental studies with bisphosphonates led naturally to the suggestion that they might be used in the therapy of various disorders of calcium metabolism in man, particularly where there is abnormal calcification in soft tissues or increased bone resorption leading to excess bone turnover or net loss of bone. Below are listed some of the potential clinical applications of bisphosphonates.

(1) Well established uses.
    (a) Bone scanning agents (e.g. ^{99m}Tc-Sn-EHDP).
    (b) Paget's disease of bone
(2) Indications for use of bisphosphonates where efficacy or desirability of usage is less well established but where use in selected instances may be justified.
    (a) *Ectopic calcification*
        Myositis ossificans progressiva
        Myositis of other types, such as paraplegia, arthroplasty, etc.
        Calcinosis, such as scleroderma, dermatomyositis, vascular calcification
        Dental calculus
    (b) *Excess bone loss*
        Acute osteoporosis (immobilization, for example after spinal cord injuries)
        High turnover osteoporosis
        Hypercalcaemia and osteolysis secondary to myeloma and cancer

(3) Other possible indications where efficacy is either not tested or not proven.
   (a) Bone dysplasias (to reduce high bone turnover)
   (b) Postmenopausal and senile osteoporosis (to prevent bone loss, possibly in combination with other drugs)
   (c) Renal osteodystrophy (to prevent high bone turnover, osteopenia and ectopic calcification)
   (d) Rheumatoid arthritis (as anti-inflammatory agents and to prevent bone erosion)
   (e) Ankylosing spondylitis (to prevent calcification and erosive changes)
   (f) Hyperlipidaemias[11].

Use of disodium etidronate (EHDP) in Paget's disease

There is more information available about the use of EHDP in Paget's disease than in the other conditions so far mentioned. Indeed, the past 10 years have witnessed a remarkable advance in the drug treatment of Paget's disease of bone[3, 35]. Three groups of agents, the calcitonins, bisphosphonates and mithramycin, have all been shown to produce impressive effects on the symptomatic, biochemical and histological features of the disease.

The doses of EHDP which have been used in Paget's disease range from 1–20 mg (4–80 μmol)/kg body weight/day. Between 5 and 20 mg/kg/day (20–80 μmol), there is a dose-dependent reduction in symptoms, and in the abnormal biochemical and histological findings[1, 2, 37, 46, 49].

The choice of dose poses some problem. The dose of 5 mg (20 μmol)/kg/day, which is most frequently recommended, takes longer to produce any given degree of suppression of disease activity than doses of 10 or 20 mg (40 or 80 μmol)/kg/day, but it is less frequently associated with the side-effects of hyperphosphataemia and impaired bone mineralization, and some investigators prefer this dose.

Disodium etidronate (EHDP) at a dose of 20 mg (80 μmol)/kg/day given by mouth is almost always effective in reducing bone turnover. Plasma alkaline phosphatase and urinary hydroxyproline can be suppressed into the normal range in about 70% of the patients.

The histological responses in bone biopsies from patients treated with 20 mg (80 μmol) of EHDP/kg/day also show uniform suppression of bone cellular activity with a diminution in the number of active osteoclasts and osteoblasts. Marrow fibrosis often disappears to be replaced by normal haematopoietic marrow. However, with high doses of EHDP, i.e. 10 mg (40 μmol)/kg/day, but only rarely with low doses and not with other compounds (such as Cl_2MDP and APD), there may be an impairment of bone mineralization leading to histological accumulation of unmineralized osteoid[39].

Biochemical and histological suppression of the disease may persist for a long time, even up to several years after cessation of treatment. The duration of remission is partly related to the dosage used and duration of treatment.

In double-blind studies to assess pain relief, EHDP has been shown to be more effective than placebo in reducing pain[2].

Other objective evidence for the effects of EHDP in Paget's disease include reduction of skin temperature, improvement of bone scans, and diminution of cardiac output. There have been claims for radiographic improvement, but these require further study.

A number of different dose regimes are presently being evaluated to combine maximum efficacy and safety. Until the results of these studies are available it is recommended that the majority of patients should be treated with a dose of 5 mg (20 μmol)/kg/day for an initial period not exceeding 6 months. If on stopping the drug there is a clinical relapse then a further course of therapy is given.

EHDP and myositis ossificans progressiva

Myositis ossificans progressiva (MOP) is a rare congenital disorder characterized by skeletal deformities and formation of ectopic bone in muscle. It usually leads to severe crippling and early death. Disodium etidronate (EHDP) has been given orally, usually in doses of 10–30 mg (40–120 μmol)/kg/day to prevent the mineralization of ectopic bone, particularly after surgery, and appears to be successful in many of the patients treated[32]. Unfortunately, because of the rarity of this condition, there have been no double-blind controlled studies of the effects of EHDP. However, as would be predicted on theoretical grounds, case studies suggest that EHDP is better at preventing progression at new sites of calcification than in reversing existing lesions.

EHDP and ectopic calcification

EHDP has been given to a small number of patients with ectopic calcification associated with scleroderma, dermatomyositis, or calcinosis universalis[32]. The published reports are difficult to interpret, particularly because it has been difficult to assess any benefit from EHDP when exacerbations and remissions occur spontaneously, and when only small numbers of patients have been studied in uncontrolled series.

EHDP and heterotopic ossification

In two double-blind studies by Bijvoet et al.[5] and Finerman et al.[22], EHDP was shown to inhibit the calcification of heterotopic bone around the hip after total hip replacement. There was evidence of recurrence of calcification when treatment with EHDP was stopped 3 months after surgery, which suggests that EHDP did not block the production of ectopic matrix but only its mineralization, as probably also happens in myositis ossificans progressiva. It is possible that if the matrix is prevented from mineralizing for a sufficient time, greater mobility may be achieved postoperatively, and there was some evidence that this happened.

EHDP and urolithiasis

Since EHDP inhibits the growth and aggregation of both calcium phosphate and calcium oxalate crystals *in vitro*, and prevents urolithiasis in animals[29], there has been some interest in using it to prevent calcium-containing stones in the urinary tract. When used in divided doses to produce adequate urinary concentrations, EHDP appears to be effective in reducing stone incidence in some patients[4]. However, EHDP is not a drug of first choice in urolithiasis because it suppresses normal skeletal turnover and mineralization at the doses necessary to prevent stone formation. Its use can only be justified in the rare but severe cases of recurrent stone formation resistant to other treatment. In theory, however, it might be possible to develop other bisphosphonates having similar physicochemical effects in urine but without effects on bone.

EHDP and osteoporosis

Several experimental studies in animals suggest that bisphosphonates might be used to diminish bone loss in osteoporosis. Several studies in man indicate that both EHDP and Cl_2MDP may be able to slow down bone loss during immobilization[38], especially after spinal injuries[42, 50]. There is interest in the possible use of bisphosphonates to prevent the loss of bone that occurs during immobilization in space flight.

In postmenopausal or senile osteoporosis, the results are less clear, partly because of the time required for changes in skeletal mass to become apparent. EHDP does reduce bone turnover, as measured by ^{45}Ca kinetics in osteoporotic women[47], but this will only be of value if it is associated with increased calcium retention or diminished calcium loss over a long period. In future experimental studies more emphasis may be placed on the possibility of using bisphosphonates on an intermittent basis in combination with drugs that increase bone turnover.

Adverse effects

Disodium etidronate (EHDP) has little toxicity in animal studies apart from its skeletal effects[41]. Its use in man is sometimes associated with diarrhoea which may disappear spontaneously or be managed by dividing the dose into a twice-daily rather than once daily regime. Disodium etidronate also produces a rise in plasma phosphate due to enhanced renal tubular reabsorption of phosphate[52]. This change in the renal handling of phosphate, which only occurs with doses above 10 mg (40 μmol)/kg/day, is not associated with any other detectable endocrine disturbance (in parathyroid, pituitary, adrenal or thyroid function), and has no detectable metabolic consequences.

In some patients with Paget's disease, perhaps 5% of those treated, severe pain has developed in involved bones during the first 1–2 months of treatment[10]. The incidence of this side-effect, which appears to be real, varies in different series. The reason for it is unknown but it may be more common in patients with severe osteolytic disease.

In some series an increased incidence of fracture has also been reported, particularly in patients treated for prolonged periods with high doses of the drug[36]. This is not surprising since fractures also occur in experimental animals given high doses of EHDP for prolonged periods. The fractures can presumably be ascribed to the diminution of bone turnover induced by the drug, which may make it more difficult for microfractures to heal. However, there is an increased incidence of fractures in untreated Paget's disease and there is no sound evidence at present that the incidence of fractures is increased when EHDP is used at the recommended doses of 5–20 mg (20–80 µmol)/kg/day for not longer than 3–6 months in any course of treatment.

Considerable attention has been paid to the development of mineralization defects in bone biopsies from patients treated with high doses of EHDP. These appear to occur most frequently at doses of 10 mg (40 µmol) and especially 20 mg (80 µmol)/kg/day, but may occur at any dose if the absorption of the drug is high enough (between 1–10% of EHDP administered by mouth is absorbed). This mineralization defect is largely reversible when treatment stops. Although anxiety has been expressed about these changes, many patients can show them without developing fractures and while showing good biochemical and symptomatic responses. Indeed, it may be more likely that bony complications would arise because of the suppressive effects of EHDP on normal bone turnover, rather than because of the mineralization defect *per se*.

In occasional patients, marked radiological changes occur during treatment[43]. This usually involves the loss of radiological density, particularly of cortical bone, and may be associated with rapid new bone formation which fails to mineralize under the influence of the drug. This appearance has been mistaken for the development of sarcoma, but probably constitutes an indication for withdrawing treatment. The radiolucent zones will usually rapidly mineralize when treatment is stopped.

There are no known interactions of EHDP with other drugs, although its absorption may be impaired by giving it with meals or with antacids such as magnesium trisilicate.

OTHER BISPHOSPHONATES

Dichloromethylene diphosphonate

Dichloromethylene diphosphonate (or clodronate disodium – Cl_2MDP) is one of the other bisphosphonates currently undergoing clinical trial and which may eventually become generally available for the treatment of Paget's disease and other disorders. In experimental studies, Cl_2MDP is an extremely potent inhibitor of bone resorption, but unlike EHDP does not impair bone mineralization except at very high doses. Preliminary studies in Paget's disease, using doses of 400 and 1600 mg (140 and 560 µmol)/day, show that there is a rapid suppression of raised plasma alkaline phosphatase and urinary hydroxyproline, and that histological suppression also occurs[14–16,40]. Cl$_2$MDP also inhibits osteolysis in myeloma and other hypercalcaemias of malignancy[13,15,48]. Further work is needed before its proper place in treatment can be evaluated.

3-Amino-1-hydroxypropylidene-1,1-bisphosphonate

Another new bisphosphonate which is a strong inhibitor of bone resorption[44] is 3-amino-1-hydroxypropylidene-1,1-bisphosphonate (ADP) and shares with Cl$_2$MDP a much weaker effect on inhibition of bone mineralization than EHDP. Preliminary studies indicate that APD is also rapidly effective in Paget's disease, at both a biochemical and hisotological level, and that it also suppresses symptoms[6,30]. It has also been successfully used to treat hypercalcaemia associated with myeloma and malignant disease[6,51]. APD has interesting effects on lymphocytes and monocytes which may be important in its mechanism of action, and preliminary results suggest that it may have potential anti-inflammatory effects in rheumatoid arthritis.

References

1 ALEXANDRE, C., MEUNIER, P. J., EDOUARD, C., KHAIRI, M. R. A. and JOHNSTON, C. C. Effects of ethane-1, hydroxy-1, 1 diphosphonate (5 mg/kg/day dose) on quantitative bone histology in Paget's disease of bone. *Metabolic Bone Disease and Related Research*. (In press)

2 ALTMAN, R., JOHNSTON, C. C., Jr., KHAIRI, M. R. A., WELLMAN, H., SERAFINI, A N. and SANKEY, R. R. Influence of disodium etidronate on clinical and laboratory manifestations of Paget's disease of bone (osteitis deformans). *New England Journal of Medicine*, **289**, 1279–1384 (1973)

3 ALTMAN, R. D. and SINGER, F. (eds.). Paget's disease of bone. In *Arthritis and Rheumatism* (Proceedings of the Kroc Foundation Conference), Volume 23 (1980)

4 BAUMANN, J. M., BISAZ, S., FLEISCH, H. and WACKER, M. Biochemical and clinical effects of ethane-1-hydroxy-1, 1-diphosphonate in calcium nephrolithiasis. *Clinical Science and Molecular Medicine*, **54**, 509–516 (1978)

5 BIJVOET, O. L. M., NOLLEN, A. J. G. SLOOF, T. J. J. H. and FEITH, R. Effect of a diphosphonate on para-articular ossification after total hip replacement. *Acta Orthopaedica Scandinavica*, **45**, 926–934 (1974)

6 BIJVOET, O. L. M., FRIJLINK, W. B., JIE, K., VAN DER LINDEN, H., MEIJER, C. J. L. M., MULDER, H., VAN PAASSEN, H. C., REITSMA, P. H., TE VELDE, J., DE VRIES, E. and VAN DER WEY, J. P. APD in Paget's disease of bone. Role of the mononuclear phagocyte system? *Arthritis and Rheumatism*, **23**, 1193–1204 (1980)

7 BISAZ, S., JUNG, A. and FLEISCH, H. Uptake of bone of pyrophosphate, diphosphonates and their technetium derivatives. *Clinical Science and Molecular Medicine*, **54**, 265–272 (1978)

8 BONJOUR, J.-P., RUSSELL, R. G. G., MORGAN, D. B. and FLEISCH, H. Intestinal calcium absorption, Ca-binding protein, and Ca-ATPase in diphosphonate-treated rats. *American Journal of Physiology*, **224**, 1011–1017 (1973)

9 BONJOUR, J.-P., TROHLER, U., PRESTON, C. and FLEISCH, H. Parathyroid hormone and renal handling of Pi: effect of dietary Pi and diphosphonates. *American Journal of Physiology*, **234**, F487–F505 (1978)

10 CANFIELD, R., ROSNER, W., SKINNER, J., McWHORTER, J., RESNICK, L., FELDMAN, F., KAMMER-MAN, S., RYAN, K., KUNIGONIS, M. and BOHNE, W. Diphosphonate therapy of Paget's disease of bone. *Journal of Clinical Endocrinology and Metabolism*, **44**, 96–106 (1977)

11 CANIGGIA, A. and GENNARI, C. Effect of ethane hydroxy diphosphonate (etidronate) on plasma cholesterol and total lipids in man. *Artery*, **3**, 188–192 (1977)

12 CANIGGIA, A. (ed.). *Proceedings of the First International Symposium on Diphosphonate in Therapy*. Italy, Istituto Gentili (1980)

13 CHAPUY, M. C., MEUNIER, P. J., ALEXANDRE, C. M. and VIGNON, E. P. Effects of disodium dichloromethylene diphosphonate on hypercalcaemia produced by bone metastases. *Journal of Clinical Investigation*, **65**, 1243–1247 (1980)

14 DELMAS, P. and MEUNIER, P. Le dichloromethylene diphosphonate (Cl₂MDP) en thérapeutique. *Thèse*, Lyon (1981)

15 DOUGLAS, D. L., RUSSELL, R. G. G., PRESTON, C. J., PRENTON, M. A., DUCKWORTH, T., KANIS, J. A., PRESTON, F. E., WOODHEAD, J. S. Effect of dichloromethylene diphosphonate in Paget's disease of bone and in hypercalcaemia due to primary hyperparathyroidism or maligant disease. *Lancet*, **1**, 1043 1047 (1980)

16 DOUGLAS, D. L., DUCKWORTH, T., KANIS, J. A., PRESTON, C., BEARD, D. J., SMITH, T. W. D., UNDERWOOD, I., WOODHEAD, J. S. and RUSSELL, R. G. G. Biochemical and clinical responses to dichloromethylene diphosphonate (Cl₂MDP) in Paget's disease of bone. *Arthritis and Rheumatism*, **23**, 1185–1192 (1980)

17 DONATH, A. (ed.). *CEMO Symposium on Diphosphonates*, Nyon, (in press)

18 FAST, D. K., FELIX, R., DOWSE, C., NEUMAN, W. F. and FLEISCH, H. The effects of diphosphonates on the growth and glycolysis of connective tissue cells in culture. *Biochemical Journal*, **172**, 97–107 (1978)

19 FELIX, R., RUSSELL, R. G. G. and FLEISCH, H. The effect of several diphosphonates on acid phosphohydrolases and other lysosomal enzymes. *Biochemica Biophysica Acta*, **429**, 429–438 (1976)

20 FELIX, R. and FLEISCH, H. Increase in alkaline phosphatase activity in calvaria cells cultured with diphosphonates. *Biochemical Journal*, **183**, 73–81 (1979)

21 FELIX, R. and FLEISCH, H. Increase in fatty acid oxidation in calvaria cells cultured with diphosphonates. *Biochemical Journal*, **196**, 237–245 (1981)

22 FINERMAN, G. A. M., KRENGEL, W. F., Jr., LOWELL, J. D., MURRAY, W. R., VOLZ, J. G., BOWERMAN, J. W. and GOLD, R. H. Role of diphosphonate (EHDP) in the prevention of heterotopic ossification after total hip arthroplasty: a preliminary report. In *The Hip* (Proceedings of the Fifth Open Scientific Meeting of the Hip Society, 1977), pp. 222–234. St Louis, C. V. Mosby (1977)

23 FLEISCH, H., RUSSELL, R. G. G. and FRANCIS, M. D. Diphosphonates inhibit hydroxyapatite dissolution *in vitro* and bone resorption in tissue culture and *in vivo*. *Science*, **165**, 1262–1264 (1969)

24 FLEISCH, H., RUSSELL, R. G. G., BISAZ, S., MUHLBAUER, R. C. and WILLIAMS, D. A. The inhibitory effect of phosphonates on the formation of calcium phosphate crystals *in vitro* and on aortic and kidney calcification *in vivo*. *European Journal of Clinical Investigation*, **1**, 12–18 (1970)

25 FLEISCH, H. Diphosphonates: history and mechanisms of action. *Metabolic Bone Disease and Related Research*. (in press)

26 FLORA, L. Comparative anti-inflammatory and bone protective effects of two diphosphonates in adjuvant arthritis. *Arthritis and Rheumatism*, **22**, 340–346 (1979)

27 FRANCIS, M. D., RUSSELL, R. G. G. and FLEISCH, H. Diphosphonates inhibit formation of calcium phosphate crystals *in vitro* and pathological calcification *in vivo*. *Science*, **165**, 1264–1266 (1969)

28 FRANCIS, M. D., FLORA, L. F. and KING, W. F. The effects of disodium ethane-1-hydroxy-1, 1-diphosphonate on adjuvant-induced arthritis in rats. *Calcified Tissue Research*, **9**, 109–121 (1972)

29 FRASER, D., RUSSELL, R. G. G. POHLER, O., ROBERTSON, W. G. and FLEISCH, H. The influence of disodium ethane-1-hydroxy-1, 1-diphosphonate (EHDP) on the development of experimentally induced urinary stones in rats. *Clinical Science*, **42**, 197–207 (1972)

30 FRIJLINK, W. B., BIJVOET, O. L. M., VELDE, J., HEYNEN, G. Treatment of Paget's disease with (3-amino-1-hydroxypropylidene)-1, 1-bisphosphonate (APD). *Lancet*, **1**, 799–802 (1979)

31 GASSER, A. B., MORGAN, D. B., FLEISCH, H. A. and RICHELLE, L. J. The influence of two diphosphonates on calcium metabolism in the rat. *Clinical Science*, **43**, 31–45 (1972)

32 GEHO, W. B. and WHITESIDE, J. A. Experience with disodium etidronate in diseases of ectopic calcification. In *Clinical Aspects of Metabolic Bone Disease*, edited by B. Frame, A. M. Parfitt and H. Duncan, pp. 506–511. Amsterdam, Excerpta Medica (1973)

33 GUENTHER, H. L., GUENTHER, H. E. and FLEISCH, H. Effects of 1-hydroxyethane-1, 1-diphosphonate and dichloromethane-diphosphonate on rabbit articular chondrocytes in culture. *Biochemical Journal*, **184**, 203–214 (1979)

34 GUENTHER, H. L., GUENTHER, H. E. and FLEISCH, H. The effects of 1-hydroxyethane-1, 1-diphosphonate and dichloromethane-diphosphonate on collagen synthesis by rabbit articular chondrocytes and rat bone cells. *Biochemical Journal*, **196**, 293–301 (1981)

35 HAMDY, R. C. *Paget's Disease of Bone: Assessment and Management*. New York, Praeger (1981)

36 KANTROWITZ, F. G., BYRNE, M. H., SCHILLER, A. L. and KRANE, S. Clinical and biochemical effects of diphosphonate in Paget's disease of bone. *Arthritis and Rheumatism*, **18**, 407 (1975)

37 KHAIRI, M. R. A., ALTMAN, R. D., DeROSA, G. P., ZIMMERMAN, J., SCHENK, R. K. and JOHNSTON, C. C. Sodium etidronate in the treatment of Paget's disease of bone. *Annals of Internal Medicine*, **87**, 656–663 (1977)

38 LOCKWOOD, D. R., VOGEL, J. M., SCHNEIDER, U. S. and HULLEY, S. B. Effect of the diphosphonate, EHDP, on bone mineral metabolism during prolonged bed rest. *Journal of Clinical Endocrinology and Metabolism*, **41**, 533–541 (1975)

39 MEUNIER, P., CHAPUY, M. C., COURPRON, P., VIGNON, E., EDOUARD, C. and BERNARD, J. Effects cliniques, biologiques et histologiques de l'ethane-1-hydroxy 1, 1-diphosphonate (EHDP) dans la maladie de Paget. *Revue du Rhumatisme*, **42**, 699–705 (1975)

40 MEUNIER, P. J., CHAPUY, M. C., ALEXANDRE, C., BRESSOT, C., EDOUARD, C., VIGNON, E., MATHIEU, L. and TRECHSEL, U. Effects of disodium dichloromethylene diphosphonate (Cl_2MDP) on Paget's disease of bone. *Lancet*, **2**, 489–492 (1979)

41 MICHAEL, W. R., KING, W. R. and WAKIM, J. M. Metablsm of disodium ethane-1-hydroxy-1, 1-diphosphonate (disodium etidronate) in the rat, rabbit, dog and monkey. *Toxicology and Applied Pharmacology*, **21**, 503–515 (1972)

42 MINAIRE, P., MEUNIER, P. J., BERARD, E., EDOUARD, C., GOEDERT, G. and PILONCHERY, G. Effects du dichloromethylene diphosphonate sur la perte osseuse précoce du paraplégique. *Annales de Médecine Physique*, **23**, 37–43 (1980)

43 NAGANT DE DEUXCHAISNES, C., MALDAGUE, B., MALGHEM, J., DEVOGELAER, J. P., HUAUX, J. P. and ROMBOUTS-LINEMANS, C. The action of the main therapeutic regimes on Paget's disease of bone, with a note on the effect of vitamin D deficiency. *Arthritis and Rheumatism*, **23**, 1215–1234 (1980)

44 REITSMA, P. H., BIJVOET, O. L. M., VERLINDEN-OOMS, H. AND VAN DER WEE-PALLS, L. J. A. Kinetic studies of bone and mineral metabolism during treatment with (3-amino-1-hydroxypropylidene)-1, 1-bisphosphonate (APD) in rats. *Calcified Tissue International*, **32**, 145–147 (1980)

45 RUSSELL, R. G. G. and FLEISCH, H. Pyrophosphate and diphosphonates. In *The Biochemistry and Physiology of Bone*, edited by G. Bourne, Volume IV, Chapter 2. New York, Academic Press (1976)

46 RUSSELL, R. G. G., SMITH, R., PRESTON, C., WALTON, R. J. and WOODS, C. G. Diphosphonates in Paget's disease. *Lancet*, **1**, 894–898 (1974)

47 SAVILLE, P. D. and HEANEY, R. Treatment of osteoporosis and diphosphonates. *Seminars in Drug Treatment*, **2**, 47–50 (1972)

48 SIRIS, E. S., SHERMAN, W. H., BAQUIRAN, D. C., SCHLATTERER, J. P., OSSERMAN, E. F. and CANFIELD, R. E. Effects of dichloromethylene diphosphonate on skeletal mobilisation of calcium in multiple myeloma. *New England Journal of Medicine*, **302**, 310–315 (1980)

49 SIRIS, E. S., CANFIELD, R. E., JACOBS, T. P. and BAQUIRAN, D. C. Long-term therapy of Paget's disease of bone with EHDP. *Arthritis and Rheumatism*, **23**, 1177–1184 (1980)

50 STOVER, S. L., HAHN, H. R. and MILLER, J. M. Disodium etidronate in the prevention of heterotopic ossification following spinal cord injury. *Paraplegia*, **14**, 146–156 (1976)

51 VAN BREUKELEN, F. J. M., BIJVOET, O. L. M. and VAN OOSTEROM, A. T. Inhibition of osteolytic bone lesions by 3-amino-1-hydroxypropylidene-1, 1-bisphosphonate (APD). *Lancet*, **1**, 803–805 (1979)

52 WALTON, R. J., RUSSELL, R. G. G. and SMITH, R. Changes in the renal handling of phosphate induced by disodium etidronate (EHDP) in man. *Clinical Science and Molecular Medicine*, **49**, 45–56 (1975)

6
Acquired disorders of vitamin D metabolism

M. G. Dunnigan, W. B. McIntosh, J. A. Ford and Iris Robertson

INTRODUCTION

The present chapter reviews the epidemiology of rickets and osteomalacia in the light of the classical model of these diseases as a product of either ultraviolet deprivation or of a lack of dietary vitamin D. Inconsistencies in the model are discussed which may necessitate its modification, particularly in the light of recent epidemiological and clinical observations on the occurrence of Asian rickets and osteomalacia in the United Kingdom. Possible interpretations of the observations are reviewed together with their implications for the prevention of vitamin D deficiency. In this chapter, the unqualified terms rickets and osteomalacia refer to the occurrence of these diseases in the absence of gastrointestinal, hepatobiliary, or renal disease where environmental influences are assumed to be dominant.

The view that rickets and osteomalacia result from an interaction of man with unfavourable aspects of his environment may recently have had less attention than it deserves. Just as the prevalence of ischaemic cardiovascular disease cannot be understood solely in terms of disordered lipid metabolism, so rickets and osteomalacia cannot be understood purely in terms of disordered vitamin D metabolism without reference to the environmental influences which have brought this about. In considering the latter, it should be remembered that an earlier period of fruitful research into the causes of rickets and osteomalacia began at the end of the First World War[6]. This earlier 'golden age' remains of great interest not only on historical grounds but because it provides information on the prevalence of these disorders when they were both commoner and existed in more florid forms than is the case today, at least in the developed world. The changing prevalence of rickets and osteomalacia in Europe and North America in the present century is of great importance to the understanding of the epidemiology of rickets and osteomalacia.

AETIOLOGICAL VIEWS OF RICKETS AND OSTEOMALACIA

For 250 years following the first clear description of rickets by Glisson, knowledge of the cause of the disease advanced scarcely at all though rickets was recognized as a major cause of disability and deformity in all the major cities of northern Europe. No real advance occurred until Mellanby and McCollum demonstrated an antirachitic fat-soluble substance in certain foods and Huldshinsky, followed by Hess and Unger, showed that rickets could be cured by the exposure of affected animals and children to ultraviolet light. The subsequent identification and chemical characterization of vitamin D_2, vitamin D_3 and its precursors transformed the understanding and treatment of rickets and osteomalacia.

It was assumed until recently that in northern latitudes vitamin D derived both from diet and sunlight contributed significantly to vitamin D intake although the proportions derived from each source were unknown. It was further assumed that lack of dietary vitamin D in foods such as eggs, butter, fat fish, milk and margarine could result in rickets and osteomalacia. The advent of sensitive assays for vitamin D metabolites, and particularly for serum 25-hydroxyvitamin D, has clarified this matter. It is now clear that more than 90% of circulating serum 25-hydroxyvitamin D is derived from synthesis in the skin in response to ultraviolet radiation. This finding was first reported by Haddad and Hahn in American subjects, and has been confirmed by Preece et al.[50] in British subjects with lower dietary intakes of vitamin D living in more northerly latitudes. The latter authors' ingenious demonstration of the inability of nuclear submariners subjected to prolonged ultraviolet deprivation to maintain serum 25-hydroxyvitamin D levels on a balanced western diet makes this point forcibly. Poskitt et al.[48] have obtained similar results in white subjects in Britain. The normal range of serum 25-hydroxyvitamin D in Britain is about 20–75 nmol/l (8–30 ng/ml) depending on seasonal variation and ultraviolet exposure. It now seems clear that not more than 2.5–5 nmol/l (1–2 ng/ml) of this is of dietary origin in subjects on a normal British diet of about 2.5 µg of vitamin D daily.

Similar conclusions have been drawn from vitamin D dose–response studies involving the administration of vitamin D supplements within and just above the range found in the normal western diet. A significant rise in serum 25-hydroxyvitamin D is not produced by adding less than the equivalent of 10 µg of vitamin D orally daily to the diets of Asian[16, 47] or elderly white subjects (*Figure 6.1*). This is four times the vitamin D found in the average British diet. Dietary vitamin D, even in northern industrialized countries, contributes little to total vitamin D intake and appears irrelevant to the maintenance of normal vitamin D status. Vitamin D can be viewed as a hormone synthesized in skin in response to ultraviolet radiation and Lawson's view[39] that dietary vitamin D can be discounted in considering the causes of vitamin D deficiency seems justifiable. The recent demonstration that 1,25-dihydroxyergocalciferol was not demonstrable in the serum of normal British subjects adds support to this view[29].

Preece et al.[49] confirmed directly that rickets and osteomalacia were due to vitamin D deficiency by demonstrating low or unrecordable levels of serum 25-hydroxyvitamin D in Asian subjects with these diseases. The central role of vitamin D in the aetiology of rickets and osteomalacia has been further clarified by the demonstration of low serum 24, 25; 25, 26; and 1,25-dihydroxycholecalciferols in Asian rickets and osteomalacia[45]. Treatment with 1,25-dihydroxycholecalciferol produced biochemical and radiological healing without any change in levels of

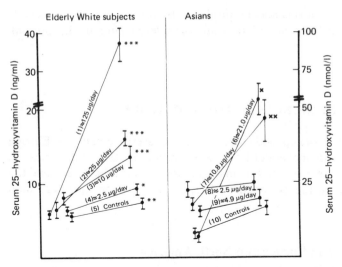

Figure 6.1 The response of serum 25-hydroxyvitamin D levels (with mean ± SEM) to varying oral intakes of vitamin D_2 (ergocalciferol) in Asian and elderly subjects in Glasgow[16, 47]. The additional vitamin D was provided as a weekly supplement (trials 1,2,3,7,9) or as butter fortified to a level of 90 μg/kg (trials 4,8) or 360 μg/kg (trial 6). Significance levels refer to paired differences for each group)*P<0.05; **P<0.01; ***P<0.001)

serum 25-hydroxyvitamin D, 24,25 or 25,26-dihydroxycholecalciferols. It therefore seems that 1,25-dihydroxycholecalciferol is the most important metabolite for the healing of vitamin D-deficiency osteomalacia and rickets, and the other hydroxy metabolites seem unimportant.

Although vitamin D deficiency is central to the causation of human rickets and osteomalacia, attention has also been devoted to the possible aetiological role of deficient mineral intake. In a series of investigations in puppy rickets Mellanby showed that an anticalcifying factor was present in wholemeal cereals. The identification of this factor as phytic acid suggested that high extraction and wholemeal cereals might be rachitogenic in man by binding dietary calcium. McCance and Widdowson confirmed that high intakes of dietary phytate might induce a negative calcium balance in human volunteers and this work led directly to the fortification of the British national loaf with calcium carbonate during the Second World War. A number of studies have cast doubt on the relevance of Mellanby's work to man by demonstrating that considerable adaptation can occur to wholemeal and high extraction cereals in respect of calcium absorption and that many populations on poor diets with low dietary calcium intakes show no evidence of rickets or osteomalacia.

In recent years, the possible rachitogenic role of dietary constituents other than vitamin D has again been raised by studies suggesting that unleavened bread[26, 51, 52, 64] and the habit of vegetarianism[23, 34] are involved in the aetiology of rickets and osteomalacia. It has recently been suggested that low calcium rickets with normal serum 25-hydroxyvitamin D levels may be produced by certain vegetarian diets[46]. These problems and their possible solution are considered later in the present chapter.

THE EPIDEMIOLOGY OF RICKETS AND OSTEOMALACIA

The present distribution of rickets and osteomalacia is described below in Europe and North America and in the underdeveloped nations of Asia and Africa. A comparison is made with their distribution in the comparatively recent past, and the risk factors associated with the occurrence of rickets and osteomalacia are then reviewed.

Rickets and osteomalacia in Europe and North America

At present, rickets and osteomalacia are rare in North America and uncommon in Europe with the exception of a proportion of the elderly, in immigrants from underdeveloped countries such as India, Pakistan and Turkey[14] and in a small number of white children in poor socioeconomic circumstances. Rickets has also occurred in a small number of food faddists living on lactovegetarian and macrobiotic diets in Europe[55] and North America[23], and a number of cases have been associated with the administration of anticonvulsant drugs. The prevalence of rickets and osteomalacia has been most extensively studied in recent years in the United Kingdom.

Infantile rickets in Britain

The introduction of dried milks and infant foods fortified with vitamin D and the ready availability of vitamin D supplements from child welfare clinics during the Second World War virtually eradicated infantile rickets from the United Kingdom. In the early 1960s infantile rickets was found in immigrant children in London who were not being provided with these sources of vitamin D. A similar situation was reported among white infants in Glasgow in 1963. A small number of cases have occurred since in white infants in Britain though recently the number of cases has been declining. Only 25 white infants were discharged from all Glasgow hospitals with mild rickets in the 11-year period 1968–78[16].

Infantile rickets continues to occur among Asian children in Britain and in a smaller proportion of West Indian children[30] (*Figure 6.2a*). This is due to lack of utilization of welfare foods to which the additional risk factors of skin pigmentation, prolonged breastfeeding and lactovegetarian diets in later infancy may be added. In recent years the hazard of macrobiotic cult diets has been associated with multiple nutritional deficiencies including rickets in a very small number of white infants[55].

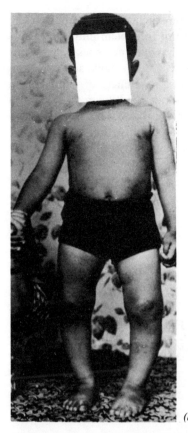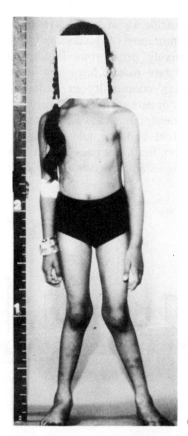

(a)   (b)

Figure 6.2(a) Typical infantile rickets in a 2-year-old Asian child showing bowing of both tibiae. (*b*) Severe late rickets in an 8-year-old Asian girl who required bilateral osteotomies

Neonatal hypocalcaemia was described among Asian infants in Birmingham associated with maternal vitamin D deficiency in 1972, and in 1973 neonatal rickets was described in Asian infants in Glasgow[27]. Several descriptions of this condition have appeared since. The prerequisite for fetal or neonatal rickets is latent or overt maternal osteomalacia and this is confined to the Asian population of the United Kingdom. Prevention of the condition depends upon the provision of vitamin D supplements for all Asian mothers in pregnancy.

Late rickets and osteomalacia in Britain

In the present century, rickets in the white population of the United Kingdom has been confined to the first 2 or 3 years of life. Active rickets after this age suggests underlying renal or gastrointestinal disease, vitamin D-resistant rickets or the ingestion of anticonvulsants. This situation also obtains for osteomalacia presenting in a white adult on a western diet under the age of 60 years.

In 1962 a high incidence of late rickets and osteomalacia was described in the Glasgow Asian community[17]. The disease differed from European infantile rickets in affecting relatively prosperous families and showing no social gradient. Osteomalacia and late rickets have now been described in many surveys from almost every Asian community in Britain[28]. The prevalence of biochemical evidence of rickets or osteomalacia has varied from about 30–40% in most surveys and radiological abnormalities have been reported in approximately 10% of Asian schoolchildren. Most children and adults are asymptomatic but a significant minority suffer from limb and back pain and a small minority progress to severe deformity requiring osteotomy (*see Figure 1.2b*).

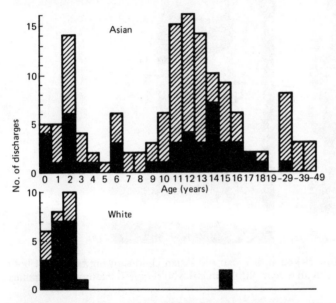

Figure 6.3 Numbers of white and Asian patients discharged from all Glasgow hospitals with nutritional rickets and osteomalacia between 1968 and 1978. Each case record was examined. (□, Female; ■, male) (After Dunnigan *et al.*[16], courtesy of the Editor and Publishers, *British Medical Journal*)

Figure 6.3 shows the age distribution of white and Asian children and adults discharged from Glasgow hospitals between 1968–78 with the diagnosis of rickets and osteomalacia. A bimodal distribution is evident in Asian children with peaks in late infancy and at the pubertal growth spurt. The sex distribution is equal until puberty with a female preponderance of approximately 2:1 in adolescence and an almost total female preponderance in adult life. From 1968–78, the probability of a Glasgow Asian schoolchild being admitted to hospital with rickets between 5 and 16 years of age was 1 in 29. A survey of all Asian families in a single practice in the city in 1979 showed that one child in eight (12%) had been referred to hospital with confirmed rickets. In this practice 44% of schoolchildren who were not taking vitamin D supplements had serum 25-hydroxyvitamin D levels of less than

12.5 nmol/l (5 ng/ml); 39% had abnormal routine biochemistry and 14% had radiological evidence of rickets[16].

The impact of osteomalacia on the Asian female population of London has recently been reviewed by Stamp *et al.*[62] who consider that the condition remains common and is a significant cause of disability among young and middle-aged Asian females. Studies have also confirmed the widespread prevalence of vitamin D deficiency among pregnant Asian women with its possible sequelae of neonatal hypocalcaemia and rickets[5, 11].

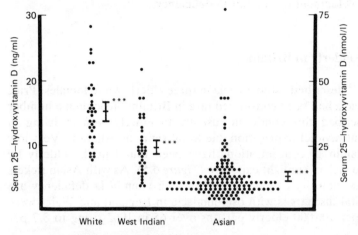

Figure 6.4 Serum 25-hydroxyvitamin D levels (with mean ± SEM) in white, West Indian and Asian children in Bradford. (After Ford *et al.*[28], courtesy of the Editor and Publishers, *Archives of Disease in Children*) Significance levels refer to differences between adjacent groups (***P<0.001)

The Asian community consitutes by far the greatest reservoir of vitamin D deficiency in Britain. This situation has no counterpart in the West Indian, Chinese or white populations outside infancy and old age (*Figure 6.4*). Hospital discharges with Asian rickets and osteomalacia in England and Wales were estimated to be 100 per 100 000 Asians *per annum* in 1962, falling gradually to 50 per 100 000 *per annum* in 1974 (J. Ablett, personal communication). Further analysis of the data shows that the trend is not uniform and that the incidence of rickets has fallen while that of osteomalacia has remained relatively constant. There has also been a tendency for the incidence of rickets and osteomalacia to rise following successive waves of immigration into the United Kingdom[13, 18]. Many patients with rickets and osteomalacia are now treated as outpatients and the true incidence of the more severe forms of the disease is likely to be appreciably greater than indicated by the hospital activity analysis data quoted above.

A suggestion that vitamin D deficiency might be widespread among white adolescents in Britain has not been confirmed[24]. In the 11-year period 1968–78 only two white adolescent boys were discharged from all Glasgow hospitals with a diagnosis of rickets unassociated with gastrointestinal, renal or hepatic disease[16]. In one the condition was asymptomatic, and in a second with mild limb pains and biochemical evidence of rickets, radiology was negative. It is of interest that this boy ate a diet unusually low in meat and meat products, resembling the lacto-vegetarian Asian diet.

Late rickets and osteomalacia are absent from the black West Indian immigrant population[14, 28]. Serum 25-hydroxyvitamin D levels in this group are intermediate in value between those of the Asian and white populations (*see Figure 6.4*) although overt biochemical and radiological evidence of rickets and osteomalacia are absent[28]. This supports the view that skin pigmentation may be a minor but definite risk factor for the development of vitamin D deficiency.

Osteomalacia in the elderly in Britain

In 1964, Gough *et al.*[31] described osteomalacia in three elderly white females. Prior to this time osteomalacia had been considered rare in Britain. Since then a number of studies have described this condition, usually in elderly woman living in conditions of severe ultraviolet deprivation due to infirmity or isolation. Very low serum 25-hydroxyvitamin D concentrations have been found in the elderly by Lawson *et al.*[40] due to lack of sunlight exposure (*Figure 6.5*). As with Asian rickets and osteomalacia, the majority of elderly women with vitamin D deficiency are asymptomatic. Hospital discharges with osteomalacia in England and Wales were estimated to be 0.7 per 100 000 elderly persons over 65 in 1962 rising to 5.7 per

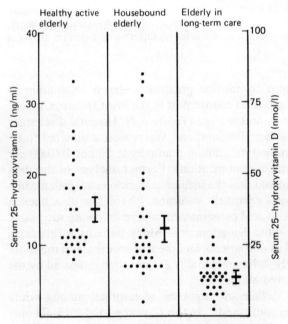

Figure 6.5 Serum 25-hydroxyvitamin D levels (with mean ± SEM) in elderly subjects in Glasgow showing the effect of severe ultraviolet deprivation on the 'long-term care' group. Significance level refers to differences between adjacent groups (**P*<0.01)

100 000 in 1974 (J. Ablett, personal communication). The reasons for this apparent rise remain speculative but an increased awareness of the diagnosis and more widespread use of automated biochemistry are likely to be important. Despite this rise, the incidence of clinically significant rickets and osteomalacia in the Asian population of the United Kingdom remains ten times that in the elderly white population.

Several studies in Britain have suggested that osteomalacia may be important in the aetiology of fractures in the elderly, particularly of the femoral neck. Aaron *et al.*[1] noted that 20–30% of women and 40% of a smaller group of men with fractured femoral necks in Leeds had histological evidence of osteomalacia. Faccini *et al.*[25] also noted an association between fracture of the femoral neck and an increase in the proportion of osteoid in addition to osteoporosis. The incidence of reported osteomalacia in elderly Asian and West Indian patients is so far low, but may be expected to rise as the immigrant population ages.

Rickets and osteomalacia in Asia and Africa

Rickets and osteomalacia remain prevalent in the tropical and subtropical countries of Africa and Asia where ultraviolet radiation is abundant. Rizvi *et al.*[54] regard rickets in India as a national problem. Rickets has been reported from Nigeria in children up to 4 years and in Jamaica in children between 3 and 8 years[13]. Rickets is common in Iran; in one hospital 15% of children admitted had X-ray evidence of the disease[59]. A feature of some reports of rickets in Iran is its occurrence in abundant sunshine in rural areas where ultraviolet deprivation is difficult to demonstrate[51]. In Israel[32] 16% of children under 2 had histological evidence of rickets at post mortem examination in hospital. A World Health Organization survey[13] demonstrated evidence of rickets in 3–18% of children from Algeria, Libya, Tunisia and Morocco. Rickets has been frequently described in non-European infants in South Africa and late rickets has been described in rural Bantu children subsisting on maize diets with abundant sunlight exposure and normal serum 25-hydroxyvitamin D levels[46].

Osteomalacia has been prevalent in northern India for many years. Vaishnava[63] reported on 593 cases of osteomalacia, mainly in women, living in urban slums in New Delhi on poor vegetarian diets. He comments that osteomalacia is the commonest metabolic disease seen in Delhi and possibly in northern India although it appears to be rare in southern India. Osteomalacia was extensively described in northern China[33]; recent reports on the prevalence of osteomalacia in China are lacking. Osteomalacia has been described among Bedouin women of the Negev desert who at the time of the study lived in conditions of almost total ultraviolet deprivation, living in tents and covered with black clothes when out of doors[13].

In summary, rickets and osteomalacia remain important health problems in many parts of Asia, the Middle East and Africa. The paradoxical situation that rickets and osteomalacia remain common in countries with relatively abundant sunshine, while they have virtually disappeared (with the exceptions noted above) from the relatively sunless countries of northern Europe and North America, has a bearing on the risk factors responsible for these diseases.

THE PREVALENCE OF RICKETS AND OSTEOMALACIA IN THE PAST

Descriptions of the prevalence of rickets and osteomalacia in India from earlier in the present century are similar to those reported recently[63], suggesting that the environmental factors responsible for these conditions have not greatly changed. This may also be true of other Afro-Asian countries although earlier accounts of prevalence are lacking. In contrast, the incidence of rickets in the industrialized countries of the northern hemisphere has fallen strikingly in the present century. In 1917 Hess and Unger reported that rickets affected 90% of black infants in New York, and Melvyn Howe[43] cites evidence that 50% of children in poor areas of Leeds in the north of England had marked rickets in Victorian times. Many reports agree on the high incidence and exceptional severity of rickets in Glasgow. Ferguson and Findlay, in a survey carried out in 1918 commented 'it was only with the greatest difficulty that Sister Elinor could find among the patients of the Dispensary of the Royal Hospital for Sick Children a sufficient number of non-rachitic families for the needs of the present research'. The British Paediatric Association reported in a multicentre survey that in 1943 13% of British children had clinical signs of rickets.

The measures leading to the virtual disappearance of infantile rickets in Britain and other western countries are well known and have been previously discussed. It is less well recognized that osteomalacia was endemic until the latter half of the 19th century in many European countries and contributed to the mortality statistics of Germany, Britain, Switzerland, France, Austria and Italy. A fuller discussion of the prevalence of osteomalacia in these countries and throughout the world is contained in Hess' classical monograph[33]. Particular areas of Europe seem to have been affected, for example, the Rhine valley, the Ergolz valley in Switzerland, Calabria in Italy and especially the city of Vienna. In France, Brittany seems to have been singled out by the disorder.

In the present century late rickets and osteomalacia made a dramatic reappearance in epidemic form in Austria and Germany at the end of the First World War and disappeared in 1921[6]. A striking rise in the incidence of rickets in late infancy and in preschool children occurred in Ireland during the Second World War associated with changes in the extraction rate of the national flour[36]. The implications of these changes in the prevalence of rickets and osteomalacia are discussed below.

RISK FACTORS FOR THE DEVELOPMENT OF RICKETS AND OSTEOMALACIA

Three stages may be recognized in elucidating the aetiology of a given disease. First, 'soft' epidemiological evidence provides tentative clues whose significance is often capable of differing interpretations. Second, the risk factors involved may be quantified and analysed by appropriate statistical techniques. This approach has been most highly developed in the field of ischaemic cardiovascular disease. Third, an aetiological mechanism, biochemical, toxic or infective is identified and the causal chain is completed. In the study of rickets and osteomalacia the first stage is well developed, a small number of studies have been undertaken in the second stage, while in the third, except for the establishment of the central importance of vitamin D deficiency, many postulated mechanisms remain speculative. Current evidence for the main risk factors associated with rickets and osteomalacia is reviewed below.

Ultraviolet deprivation

The demonstration that rickets could be healed by ultraviolet radiation provided a firm foundation for the crucial role of this narrow segment of the electromagnetic spectrum in the causation and prevention of vitamin D deficiency. Evidence that the greater part of circulating serum 25-hydroxyvitamin D is derived from synthesis in the skin in response to ultraviolet radiation even in industrialized northern cities has emphasized man's dependence on a limited supply of summer sunshine[48, 50]. This may provide only a marginally sufficient supply of vitamin D in northern latitudes which may be further compromised by slum conditions, habits of dress, atmospheric pollution and skin pigmentation.

Much evidence supports the view that urbanization is a risk factor for the development of rickets and osteomalacia. The widespread appearance of the disease in the 17th century coincided with overcrowding in the towns of Germany, the Low Countries and Britain. The demonstration of a marked urban–rural gradient in India is similarly convincing and the religious habit of female purdah provides an additional risk factor for the population of the subcontinent. In Britain, the overcrowded city of Glasgow with its high tenement buildings had a much higher incidence of rickets than other cities of Scotland. Serum alkaline phosphatase levels in white Glasgow schoolchildren were significantly higher than in schoolchildren living in a nearby small town[15]. Asian children living in the small town of Stornoway in the Outer Hebrides showed no biochemical evidence of rickets compared with a high incidence in their counterparts in Glasgow. Nevertheless, serum 25-hydroxyvitamin D levels were lower in Asian children in Stornoway than in white children in Glasgow[50].

The importance of ultraviolet deprivation in the aetiology of osteomalacia is strikingly seen in the housebound and institutionalized elderly. *Figure 6.5* (p. 132) shows serum 25-hydroxyvitamin D levels in healthy, housebound and institutionalized elderly subjects in Glasgow. Dietary intakes in all three groups were similar. The low levels of serum 25-hydroxyvitamin D in the long-term care group are due to almost total ultraviolet deprivation.

Despite much evidence that ultraviolet deprivation is a major risk factor for the development of rickets and osteomalacia, a number of studies have shown that absolute or moderately severe ultraviolet deprivation may not always be demonstrable in certain communities and individuals with rickets and osteomalacia.

Wilson[65] observed severe osteomalacia in the rural Kangra valley of Kashmir among field workers whose sunshine exposure was high. His observations are supported by those of Reinhold[51] who found rickets in older children in rural Iran whose exposure to strong sunlight outside infancy seemed adequate. The observations of Pettifor *et al.*[46] on late rickets in rural Bantu children exposed to strong sunshine have been previously noted (p. 133).

Evidence that severe ultraviolet deprivation may be lacking in the presence of widespread rickets or osteomalacia has also come from observations of the outdoor exposure habits of the British Asian population. Most Asian children in Glasgow have casual outdoor exposure similar to their white counterparts. Measurements of daylight exposure in both winter and summer showed no significant differences between 10 rachitic and 10 non-rachitic Asian children and 21 white children[14]. A more recent study of a larger sample of 84 Asian children has, however, demonstrated that rachitic children have significantly less outdoor exposure than non-rachitic children[57] (*see below*). Compston[7] observed Asian women in London with nutritional osteomalacia whose outdoor exposure seemed similar to their white counterparts. Some of her patients wore western dress and even sunbathed on occasion.

In summary, ultraviolet deprivation is a major risk factor for the development of rickets and osteomalacia, but these diseases can also develop in circumstances in which severe ultraviolet deprivation is not demonstrable. Additional factors appear to be required to produce rickets and osteomalacia in these circumstances.

Skin pigmentation

Hess and Unger observed that negro children living in New York were more prone to rickets than their white counterparts and suggested that skin pigmentation might impose a barrier to the passage of ultraviolet irradiation. Hess' observation that black rats require a more intense level of ultraviolet radiation to protect them from rickets than white rats supported this view[33]. Doubt has been cast on the role of skin pigmentation in the aetiology of vitamin D deficiency by observations that the British West Indian population is free of clinical rickets and osteomalacia outside infancy in contrast to the severely affected but less pigmented Asian community[14, 28]. Stamp[61] found no difference in serum 25-hydroxyvitamin D levels following ultraviolet radiation in white, Asian and West Indian subjects. This study is open to the objection that intense levels of ultraviolet radiation were employed which might have exceeded the barrier effect of skin pigment. Black skin transmits ultraviolet radiation less well than white skin, and two studies have shown that levels of serum 25-hydroxyvitamin D in the West Indian community are intermediate between levels in the Asian and white communities of Britain[24, 28]. The evidence thus suggests that skin pigmentation is a minor risk factor for the development of rickets and osteomalacia but may add significantly to the total risk if the other major risk factors are present.

Dietary factors

The discovery that vitamin D is present in certain foods such as milk, butter, fat fish and eggs suggested that the absence of these foodstuffs might produce rickets or osteomalacia. Evidence that at least 90% of circulating serum 25-hydroxyvitamin D is not of dietary origin and that 1,25-dihydroxyergocalciferol is not detectable in normal subjects makes this hypothesis difficult to accept[29, 48, 50]. In considering the role of diet in the causation of rickets and osteomalacia, a major problem is created by the presence in many studies of the coexisting risk factors of ultraviolet deprivation and skin pigmentation. The habit of vegetarianism is frequently associated with a habit of sun avoidance or of purdah in dark-skinned African or Asian communities. It is therefore useful to obtain evidence from populations in which these risk factors are absent. Alternatively, the significance of several risk factors may be analysed independently.

Diet and infantile rickets

Cows' milk contains little vitamin D even in summer and the use of 'doorstep', or condensed milks are well-known risk factors for the development of rickets when the infant is little exposed to the sun. Fortified dried milks and vitamin D supplements are essential in the first 2 years of life and their use has virtually eradicated rickets from western countries where they are readily available. Breast milk has been shown to contain more vitamin D in a water-soluble form than was previously thought[38]. Lackdawala and Widdowson[38] have stated, without citing any evidence, that breastfed children do not develop rickets and this statement has gained wide acceptance. There is good evidence, however, that prolonged breast-feeding associated with delayed weaning is a marked risk factor for infantile rickets. Both Chick *et al.*[6] and Hess[33] state unequivocally that breastfed children can develop severe rickets. More recent evidence of infantile rickets associated with prolonged breastfeeding has come from the Tower Hamlets study of the nutrition of Asian children in London (R. J. Harris, personal communication). Similar evidence has come from a resurgence of infantile rickets associated with maternal vegetarianism and breastfeeding in the United States among the Black Muslim community[23]. Recent studies by Leerbeck and Søndergaard[41] have suggested that the water-soluble vitamin D in breast milk is not antirachitic in the rat and may therefore be metabolically inactive in man also. There is a need to re-emphasize that breastfeeding does not protect against rickets and that vitamin D supplements remain essential to the breastfed infant. This is particularly true if breastfeeding is prolonged beyond 2 or 3 months and if the milk is derived from a vitamin D-deficient mother.

Diet and late rickets and osteomalacia

Hess, in his detailed review of osteomalacia in Europe and Asia[33] stated that cereals formed the staple diet of the population wherever the disease occurred in endemic form. In northern India the staple cereal was wheat and in northern China millet; more detailed accounts of these dietaries are found in the original monograph. The truth of this general statement is attested to by much supporting evidence. Recent studies of rickets and osteomalacia in India indicate that the conditions are associated with poor vegetarian and cereal-based diets although interpretation of this evidence is made difficult by the possible presence of coexisting ultraviolet deprivation associated with slum conditions, female seclusion and skin pigmentation[63]. The occurrence of endemic osteomalacia in European countries such as France in the 19th century becomes understandable when the diet of the population is considered[66]. Until almost the end of the 19th century the French peasant diet consisted largely of vegetables, bread and a porridge obtained by boiling maize or wheat; meat was an expensive luxury. This diet resembled that of the present-day Indian or Chinese peasant, but was not associated with the confounding variables of skin pigmentation or sun-avoidance on cultural or religious grounds.

Osteomalacia and late rickets appeared in Austria and Germany at the end of the First World War in epidemic form[6]. The outbreak was associated with reversion to a vegetarian diet consisting almost entirely of bread and vegetables. The disease subsided as the population returned to a more normal western diet in 1921. Skin pigmentation and ultraviolet deprivation were also not confounding variables in this cruel nutritional 'experiment' produced by war which clearly illustrates the role of vegetarianism in the aetiology of rickets and osteomalacia. Chick *et al.*[6] observed that osteomalacia in Vienna in 1919 and 1920 showed a seasonal variation identical to that of rickets and responded promptly to the administration of cod liver oil. These observations strongly suggest that a vegetarian diet mediates rickets and osteomalacia through vitamin D deficiency. A less severe recurrence of osteomalacia occurred in Holland at the end of the Second World War in association with similar famine conditions and responded well to treatment with vitamin D.

Although Ireland was not involved in the Second World War a marked rise in the incidence of rickets in older infants and preschool children was noted in 1941 when the extraction rate of the national flour was raised from 70% to 100%. The Irish National Nutrition Survey observed the incidence of rickets in Dublin between 1942–48 and concluded that the increase was due to a change from white to wholemeal flour[36]. The incidence of rickets subsided as the extraction rate was reduced. We have re-examined the evidence of this survey together with data on national food consumption at the time and in the light of recent vitamin D dose–response studies[56]. The only significant variable over the years of the survey was the changing extraction rate of the national flour. Intakes of dietary vitamin D, dairy foods, vegetable foods, meat and meat products did not vary significantly. Ultraviolet exposure was constant. This unwitting nutritional 'experiment' thus supports the view that high extraction cereals are rachitogenic and operate independently of other dietary variables, skin pigmentation or ultraviolet deprivation.

Dietary studies of Asian rickets in Britain

Dunnigan and Smith[19] found that the dietary vitamin D intakes of Glasgow Asian schoolchildren with and without rickets did not differ from those of white schoolchildren. Subsequent studies have confirmed these findings which add weight to other evidence that dietary vitamin D in the amounts present in the normal western diet is irrelevant to the aetiology of rickets and osteomalacia[28]. Two studies have shown that the serum 25-hydroxyvitamin D levels of vegetarian Asian women in pregnancy are lower than those of non-vegetarian women[5,11], but interpretation of the role of diet in these studies is made difficult by the presence in some Asian women of the habit of sun-avoidance and purdah.

Reinhold observed late rickets in rural Iranian children with adequate sunshine exposure who consumed large quantities of unleavened bread as *tanok*[51] and suggested that the consumption of unleavened bread as chupatty might be equally rachitogenic in the British Asian community[52]. Two uncontrolled studies suggested biochemical improvement in children with Asian rickets when chupatties were withdrawn[26,44] but a subsequent study found no short-term changes in calcium balance when chupatties were added to the diet[12].

Review of a previous 7-day weighed dietary study carried out in Glasgow showed that the chupatty intakes of 11 Asian children with rickets, most with moderate to severe clinical disease, were greater than those of 14 non-rachitic Asian children. Furthermore, in the group as a whole the chupatty intake was highly correlated with the serum alkaline phosphatase level[14]. An extension of this analysis by multiple regression techniques has shown that the relationship between chupatty and alkaline phosphatase levels is independent of age, caloric intake and other food classes.

In a 7-day weighed dietary study of 82 Ugandan Asians in London, Hunt *et al.*[35] examined differences in dietary patterns and outdoor exposure between various religious groups. A subsequent multiple regression analysis suggested that, in descending order of magnitude, intakes of chupatty and animal protein, outdoor exposure and dietary vitamin D were significantly related to serum 25-hydroxy-vitamin D levels in Asians[34]. Two weighed dietary studies carried out on 16 asymptomatic Asian children in Coventry and 21 asymptomatic Asian children in Birmingham showed no significant differences between the diets of children with and without biochemical evidence of rickets[24,44].

THE ROLE OF DIETARY FACTORS AND DAYLIGHT OUTDOOR EXPOSURE IN THE AETIOLOGY OF ASIAN RICKETS

We have recently completed a 7-day weighed dietary survey with measurements of daylight outdoor exposure in 84 Glasgow Asian schoolchildren between 8 and 16 years of age. The results have further clarified the relative roles of diet and ultraviolet deprivation in the aetiology of late rickets in Asian children.

Moderate to severe clinical rickets was found in 16 children with deformity (six children), difficulty in walking or running, and biochemical and X-ray evidence of disease. These formed a group with 'clinical rickets'. There were 28 children without symptoms who showed milder biochemical evidence of rickets and formed a second group with 'asymptomatic rickets', 40 children with normal routine biochemistry (serum calcium, inorganic phosphorus and alkaline phosphatase), and no symptoms of rickets formed a third 'non-rachitic' group.

More detailed results of the study will be published in due course[57]; the main conclusions are given here. The diets of children with 'clinical rickets' contained much less meat, meat products and fish than the diets of 'non-rachitic' children. Intakes of eggs and dairy foods (milk, butter and margarine) were also less and intakes of chupatty were greater. Ultraviolet exposure was less in children with 'clinical rickets' than in their 'non-rachitic' counterparts. The diets of children with 'asymptomatic rickets' showed less marked differences from the diets of 'non-rachitic' children. Intakes of meat, meat products and fish were lower, intakes of

Table 6.1 Significant relative risks for Asian children with 'clinical rickets' compared with 'non-rachitic' children

Variable	Relative risk	P*
Meat†	0.2	0.008
Chupatty	3.3	0.04
Fibre	6.8	0.004
Phytic acid	3.1	0.05
Phosphorus	0.2	0.02
Outdoor exposure	0.2	0.04
Age	3.8	0.03

*Fisher's exact probability
†Includes meat, meat products and fish

Table 6.2 Significant relative risks for Asian children with 'asymptomatic rickets' compared with 'non-rachitic' children

Variable	Relative risk	P*
Pulses	4.9	0.007
Calcium	2.4	0.04
Outdoor exposure	0.2	0.007
Age	3.2	0.03

*Fisher's exact probability

dairy foods, pulses and chupatty were higher. Ultraviolet exposure was less in children with 'asymptomatic rickets' than in 'non-rachitic' children. The general trend of the diets in the three groups of children was thus to progressively severe lactovegetarianism with increasing severity of rickets.

The components of the diet of each of the 84 children (comprising the three rachitic groups) were then examined in detail and the food classes contributing to the significant components were identified. In the initial analysis, the distribution of each dietary component and food class was studied for the entire group and each subject was classified as having a 'high' or 'low' exposure to that component or food class relative to this particular group. The relative risk of high exposure to each component and food was calculated for both the 'asymptomatic rickets' and the 'clinical rickets' groups relative to the 'non-rachitic' group. The significant relative risks are shown in *Tables 6.1* and *6.2*. Relative risks greater than one suggest that a high level of the factor is associated with rickets, whereas a relative risk less than one suggests that a low level of the factor is associated with rickets. In this context 'high' and 'low' exposure are used relative to the whole group and not as absolute terms. 'High' levels of fibre, chupatty and age and 'low' levels of phosphorus, meat and outdoor exposure are associated with 'clinical rickets', whereas 'high' levels of pulses and calcium (associated with higher milk consumption) and 'low' levels of outdoor exposure are associated with 'asymptomatic rickets'.

In the examination of these relative risks, there is no indication of the extent, if any, of the overlap of these factors in their contribution to the increased risk. To take account of this problem, a stepwise logistic regression model of rachitic category on dietary components, age, and outdoor exposure was fitted to the results. The analysis of dietary components gave, in a stepwise manner, the independent and non-overlapping contributions to the logistic model. The results for the 'clinical rickets' and 'asymptomatic rickets' groups are shown, relative to the 'non-rachitic' group, in *Table 1.3* with factors listed in order of importance in the model.

Table 6.3 Independent factors in logistic model of dietary components, age and outdoor exposure, standardized for caloric intake, in order of importance. The main food classes contributing to component factors are given in parentheses

	Boys	Girls
Asymptomatic rickets	Outdoor exposure Fibre (pulses) Phosphorus (meat, pulses) Age	Outdoor exposure Fibre (chupatty, pulses) Vitamin D (milk)
Clinical rickets	Fibre (chupatty, pulses, fruit) Phosphorus (meat, dairy foods) Age	Outdoor exposure Fibre (chupatty, pulses) Phosphorus (fish, chupatty, pulses) Carbohydrate (chupatty, fruit)

Important differences in the dietary patterns of the boys and girls, due mainly to higher meat intakes in the boys, were evident in all groups. The results are therefore listed separately for boys and girls. Overall, although the order of importance of the component factors varies from group to group, the principal factors common to all groups are outdoor exposure, fibre and phosphorus. In the analysis reported in *Table 6.3*, all factors have been standardized for caloric intake so that these independent factors do not simply reflect differences in the amount of food eaten.

An examination of the major food classes from which these important components arise shows that the differences in fibre intake arise from chupatty, pulses and fruit and the differences in phosphorus intake come from meat, fish, pulses and dairy foods. The phosphorus sources are somewhat different in the boys and girls, with meat predominating in the boys and fish in the girls.

The detailed logistic regression model thus supports the view that the lacto-vegetarian diet is rachitogenic independent of outdoor exposure. Dietary fibre derived from high extraction wheat cereal as chupatty, fruit and pulses is the most important rachitogenic factor and meat and fish are the most important protective foods. Dairy foods appear mildly protective, possibly by 'diluting' more rachitogenic components. Dietary vitamin D is unimportant. The emergence of vitamin D as an independent component in girls with 'asymptomatic rickets' reflects higher milk (and vitamin D) intakes in this group compared with 'non-rachitic' girls. The dietary risk factors operate in a context of moderate ultraviolet deprivation; this may be little more than that imposed by residence in an urban industrial environment at high latitude.

ENDOGENOUS RISK FACTORS FOR THE DEVELOPMENT OF RICKETS AND OSTEOMALACIA

The influence of age on the incidence of rickets is a function of growth velocity in the first 2 years of life and at puberty, and in the osteomalacia of old age reflects ultraviolet deprivation. The reasons for the female propensity to rickets and osteomalacia are unknown and are independent of environmental factors such as ultraviolet exposure and diet. Serum 25-hydroxyvitamin D levels in Asian males and females are similar[28] and in adolescents at least outdoor exposure does not differ between boys and girls[14] although girls have a much higher incidence of late rickets. The suggestion that there is a racial predisposition to vitamin D deficiency among Asians has not been confirmed[24] and overall, with the exception of age and sex, environmental factors seem overwhelmingly dominant in the aetiology of rickets and osteomalacia.

POSSIBLE MECHANISMS INVOLVED IN THE AETIOLOGY OF RICKETS AND OSTEOMALACIA

The evidence presented above suggests that both ultraviolet deprivation and lactovegetarianism are major risk factors for the development of rickets and osteomalacia. Lack of dietary vitamin D does not appear to be a risk factor. More detailed studies suggest that high intakes of fibre and low intakes of meat, meat products and fish are the main dietary risk factors for the development of vitamin D deficiency. Since the final common path for almost all human rickets and osteomalacia is vitamin D deficiency, low calcium and phosphorus, intakes, dietary phytate and phytate-derived polyphosphate esters seem unlikely to be involved in the aetiology of human rickets and osteomalacia other than in extreme circumstances of severe calcium or phosphorus deprivation. Low phosphorus osteomalacia has been reported in patients taking large quantities of aluminium hydroxide as an antacid[4] and, as noted above, low calcium intakes have been incriminated in the aetiology of late rickets in Bantu children in South Africa[46].

The tentative model which emerges from the epidemiological evidence is of an interaction of diet and ultraviolet exposure in which dietary factors modulate aspects of the vitamin D pathway and increase effective vitamin D requirement. There is now evidence for an enterohepatic circulation of metabolites of vitamin D and this may provide a mechanism for such interactions[2]. Interruption of such a functionally important enterohepatic circulation by constituents of high extraction cereals may be important to the aetiology of vitamin D deficiency. Lignin, a component of wheat fibre, combines with bile acids and increases their excretion[21]. Reinhold[53] has suggested that should vitamin D or a metabolite of vitamin D become attached to the fibre–bile-acid complex, which is chemically likely, it may be transported through the gut. Vegetarian diets and diets rich in wholemeal and high extraction cereal may thus lead to enough wastage of vitamin D and of vitamin D metabolites derived from ultraviolet radiation to lead to rickets and osteomalacia.

An alternative reason for the protective role of animal foods such as meat and eggs may be that these foods contain more vitamin D than is currently believed from standard analyses. Poultry, cattle and pigs often receive diets heavily fortified with vitamin D. Further analyses of the vitamin D content of these foods may, as with milk, reveal a greater content of vitamin D or of vitamin D metabolites than is currently believed.

THE RELATIONSHIP OF GASTROINTESTINAL DISEASE TO VITAMIN D DEFICIENCY

The occurrence of rickets and osteomalacia in diseases of the gastrointestinal tract and hepatobiliary system raises similar issues to those posed by vitamin D deficiency associated with the dietary risk factors discussed above. Since the dietary contribution to total vitamin D status is small, it is at first sight difficult to understand why serum 25-hydroxyvitamin D levels should be low in many patients after gastric surgery[22], jejunoileal bypass, coeliac[8] and Crohn's disease[3]. Ultraviolet exposure is frequently normal in such patients and it seems necessary to postulate an interaction between endogenously synthesized vitamin D and the pathological processes concerned with malabsorption to explain these findings.

There is now evidence that circulating isotopically labelled vitamin D appears in bile in the form of water-soluble polar metabolites. In the rat 8–40% of tritiated vitamin D or 25-hydroxyvitamin D appeared in bile within 2 hours of injection as water-soluble glucuronide conjugates which were reabsorbed in the proximal and distal intestines and re-excreted in bile[60]. Evidence for a conservative enterohepatic circulation of 25-hydroxyvitamin D in man[2] suggests that as much as 85% of labelled metabolites of 25-hydroxyvitamin D entering the duodenum may be reabsorbed. Recent evidence has also suggested a conservative enterohepatic circulation for 1,25-dihydroxycholecalciferol in the rat[37]. It has been reported that cholestyramine is effective in the treatment of experimental vitamin D intoxication in the rat, presumably by interrupting the enterohepatic circulation of vitamin D and its metabolites[58]. This may be a useful illustration of the functional importance of a conservative enterohepatic circulation for vitamin D; interruption of such an enterohepatic circulation by intestinal malabsorptive disease may lead to enough wastage of vitamin D metabolites to produce rickets or osteomalacia.

Not all the bone disease associated with gastrointestinal and hepatobiliary disease is due to vitamin D deficiency. Osteoporosis has been reported after gastric surgery, in Crohn's disease and in primary biliary cirrhosis, and secondary hyperparathyroidism may also be present. Deficient mineral absorption may also contribute to the overall picture, which is more complex than in simple vitamin D deficiency rickets and osteomalacia, and much higher doses of vitamin D are required to produce healing. Nevertheless, the view that the requirement of endogenously derived vitamin D is increased by certain alimentary diseases and dietary factors provides an intelligible explanation for the occurrence of rickets and osteomalacia associated with alimentary malabsorption and vegetarianism.

THE TREATMENT OF RICKETS AND OSTEOMALACIA

Rickets and osteomalacia associated with ultraviolet deprivation, a vegetarian diet or the taking of anticonvulsants responds rapidly to an oral dose of 100 μg (4000 i.u.) of vitamin D daily given for 2 or 3 months. The dose may then be reduced to a supplement of 10 μg (400 i.u.) daily. Calcium supplements are unnecessary. In patients who may not receive regular oral medication a single injection of 10 mg (400 000 i.u.) of vitamin D is effective and no further treatment is usually needed although an oral supplement of 10 μg of vitamin D should be recommended to prevent recurrence in future years.

The osteomalacia associated with gastric surgery also responds readily to vitamin D; this is best given parenterally and most patients respond well to a single intramuscular dose of 10 mg of vitamin D. The osteomalacia of coeliac disease is initially resistant to large oral and parenteral doses of vitamin D and doses of as much as 1 mg orally or 0.25 mg daily by injection may be required for healing. The bone disease heals well with a gluten-free diet and vitamin D can usually be discontinued after 2 or 3 months.

Osteomalacia associated with other forms of malabsorption such as small bowel resection or Crohn's disease may require large doses of parenteral vitamin D for healing of the order of 1 mg intramuscularly once weekly. The newer vitamin D metabolites should normally be reserved for the treatment of renal osteodystrophy, vitamin D-resistant rickets and hypoparathyroidism. However, a recent report of the healing of osteomalacia associated with small bowel resection with oral

1α-hydroxyvitamin D_3 (1α-OHD$_3$) where large doses of parenteral vitamin D had been only partially effective suggests a possible role for this metabolite in certain patients with osteomalacia associated with malabsorption[9]. The response of a patient with primary biliary cirrhosis to 1,25-dihydroxycholecalciferol where vitamin D and 1α-hydroxyvitamin D_3 had been ineffective also illustrates the possible use of this metabolite in certain cases of osteomalacia associated with severe hepatobiliary disease where the further hydroxylation step required to convert 1α-hydroxyvitamin D_3 to the active metabolite 1,25 hydroxyvitamin D_3 may be defective (I.T. Boyle, personal communication).

THE PREVENTION OF RICKETS AND OSTEOMALACIA

Although aspects of the aetiology of rickets and osteomalacia require clarification, prevention of these diseases is, in principle, straightforward. This can be achieved by the consumption of not more than an additional 10 µg (400 i.u.) of vitamin D daily to the normal diet. Vitamin D dose–response studies have shown that this will produce a satisfactory rise in serum 25-hydroxyvitamin D levels[16, 47]. Calciferol (vitamin D_2) is cheap and effective and the newer vitamin D metabolites such as 1α-hydroxyvitamin D are unnecessary for routine prophylaxis. The fortification of foodstuffs such as milk and chupatty[47] flour has been rejected as a vehicle for providing the extra vitamin D required to at-risk groups in the United Kingdom. A preventive policy based on the ready availability of vitamin D supplements backed by appropriate health education measures to reach community health service personnel and the Asian community has increased supplement uptake eight-fold in Asian children in Glasgow over a 2-year period[16]. The incidence of hospital admissions for Asian rickets has fallen in this time although longer-term evaluation of the programme is required. Similar policies are required on a national scale to reach not only the at-risk Asian community but the housebound and institutionalized elderly.

The taking of 10 µg (400 i.u.) of vitamin D daily to prevent rickets and osteomalacia carries no risk of vitamin D intoxication even in susceptible individuals. In older children and adults this rarely occurs with daily vitamin D intakes of less than 1 mg (40 000 i.u.) daily over a prolonged period of time. The mild form of infantile hypercalcaemia[42] found in the United Kingdom in the years following the Second World War was associated with the consumption of between 50 µg (2000 i.u.) and 875 µg (35 000 i.u.) of vitamin D daily due to the overfortification of infant foods. Even the lower level of dosage associated with this disorder is five times greater than the quantity of vitamin D required for the effective prophylaxis of simple vitamin D deficiency.

CONCLUSION

The present western diet, characterized by the consumption of refined carbohydrate and high intakes of animal products such as meat, meat products and eggs appears highly protective against rickets and osteomalacia. In the longer term a degree of adaptation of the Asian community in Britain to such a diet should bring about a corresponding reduction in their incidence of rickets and osteomalacia. Evidence that the incidence of rickets in the Asian community has fallen by approximately half over a period of 16 years, while the incidence of osteomalacia has remained relatively constant, is consistent with this hypothesis[18]. Personal observation suggests that second-generation Asian children in Britain are partially adapting to western diets while first-generation Asian adults retain their traditional dietary habits. The changing incidence of Asian rickets in Britain supports the view that both marginal ultraviolet exposure and dietary factors determine the prevalance of vitamin D deficiency in a given community or country. It seems likely that the present western diet, as characterized above, has been the major factor in producing a rapid decline in the incidence of endemic late rickets and osteomalacia in the present century in Europe. The current occurrence of small pockets of vitamin D deficiency in certain communities in Europe and North America is associated with habits of vegetarianism or lactovegetarianism[23].

The prescient comments of Chick *et al.*[6], based on observations in Vienna between 1919 and 1922, aptly summarize our views of the probable relationship of ultraviolet exposure and diet in the aetiology of rickets and osteomalacia, whatever the ultimate mechanism of their interaction proves to be: 'The adherents of both the dietetic and hygienic theories have urged the sufficiency of their particular view of the matter. It is now abundantly clear, however, that in the prevention of rickets both diet and sunlight play a part and that, in so far as it is not exclusive, each theory resumes a measure of truth.'

Acknowledgements

The serum 25-hydroxyvitamin D assays carried out in Stobhill Hospital were made possible by a grant from the Medical Research Council. We are most grateful for helpful comments and information provided by Dr J. G. Ablett of the Nutrition Section, Department of Health and Social Security, London. The most recent dietary study was made possible by a grant from the Biomedical Research Committee of the Scottish Home and Health Department; the study was carried out by Mrs Janette B. Henderson.

References

1 AARON, J. E., GALLAGHER, J. C., ANDERSON, J., STASIAK, L., LONGTON, E. B., NORDIN, B. E. C. and NICHOLSON, M. Frequency of osteomalacia and osteoporosis in fractures of the proximal femur. *Lancet*, **1**, 229–233 (1974)

2 ARNAUD, S. B., GOLDSMITH, R. S., LAMBERT, P. N. and GO, V. L. W. 25-hydroxyvitamin D_3: evidence of an enterohepatic circulation in man. *Proceedings of the Society for Experimental Biology and Medicine*, **149**, 570–572 (1975)

3 ARNAUD, S. B., NEWCOMER, A. D., HODGSON, S. F., JOWSEY, J. O and GO, V. L. W. Serum 25-hydroxyvitamin D (25-OHD) and the pathogenesis of osteomalacia in patients with non-typical sprue. *Gastroenterology*, **72**, 1025 (1977)

4 BAKER, L. R. I. Iatrogenic osteomalacia and myopathy due to phosphate depletion. *British Medical Journal*, **3**, 150–152 (1974)

5 BROOKE, O. G., BROWN, I. R. F., BONE, C. D. M., CARTER, N. D., CLEEVE, H. J. W., MAXWELL, J. D., ROBINSON, V. P. and WINDER, S. M. Vitamin D supplements in pregnant Asian women: effects on calcium status and fetal growth. *British Medical Journal*, **1**, 751–754 (1980)

6 CHICK, H., DALYELL, E. J., HUME, E. M., MACKAY, H. M. M. and HENDERSON SMITH, H. Studies of rickets in Vienna, 1919–1922: report of the Accessory Food Factors Committee. *Medical Research Council Special Report Series No. 77*. London, HMSO (1923)

7 COMPSTON, J. E. Rickets in Asian immigrants. *British Medical Journal*, **2**, 612 (1979)

8 COMPSTON, J. E. and CREAMER, B. Plasma levels and intestinal absorption of 25-hydroxyvitamin D in patients with small intestinal resection. *Gut*, **18**, 171–175 (1977)

9 COMPSTON, J. E., HORTON, L. W. L. and TIGHE, J. R. Oral 1α-hydroxyvitamin D$_3$ in the treatment of osteomalacia associated with malabsorption. *Clinical Endocrinology*, **7**, 245S–246S (1977)

10 COOKE, W. T., SWAN, C. H. J., ASQUITH, P., MELIKIAN, V. and McFEELY, W. E. Serum alkaline phosphatase and rickets in urban schoolchildren. *British Medical Journal*, **1**, 324–327 (1973)

11 DENT, C. E. and GUPTA, M. M. Plasma 25-hydroxyvitamin-D levels during pregnancy in Caucasians and in vegetarians and non-vegetarian Asians. *Lancet*, **2**, 1057–1060 (1975)

12 DENT, C. E., ROUND, J. M., ROWE, D. J. F. and STAMP, T. C. B. Effect of chapattis and ultraviolet irradiation on nutritional rickets in an Indian immigrant. *Lancet*, **1**, 1282–1284 (1973)

13 DEPARTMENT OF HEALTH AND SOCIAL SECURITY. *Report on Health and Social Subjects, 19*. Rickets and osteomalacia. London, HMSO (1980)

14 DUNNIGAN, M. G. Asian rickets and osteomalacia in Britain. In *Child Nutrition and its relation to Mental and Physical Development*, Stretford, Manchester, Kellogg Company of Great Britain. pp. 43–70 (1977)

15 DUNNIGAN, M. G. and GARDNER, M. O. Serum alkaline phosphatase in urban and semi-rural Scottish children. *Scottish Medical Journal*, **10**, 325–327 (1965)

16 DUNNIGAN, M. G., McINTOSH, W. B., SUTHERLAND, G. R., GARDEE, R., GLEKIN, B., FORD, J. A. and ROBERTSON, I. Policy for prevention of Asian rickets in Britain: a preliminary assessment of the Glasgow rickets campaign. *British Medical Journal*, **282**, 357–360 (1981)

17 DUNNIGAN, M. G., PATON, J. P. J., HAASE, S., McNICOL, G. W., GARDNER, M. D. and SMITH, C. M. Late rickets and osteomalacia in the Pakistani Community in Glasgow. *Scottish Medical Journal*, **7**, 159–167 (1962)

18 DUNNIGAN, M. G. and ROBERTSON, I. Residence in Britain as a risk factor for Asian rickets and osteomalacia. *Lancet*, **1**, 770 (1980)

19 DUNNIGAN, M. G. and SMITH, C. M. The aetiology of late rickets in Pakistani children in Glasgow. Report of a diet survey. *Scottish Medical Journal*, **10**, 1–9 (1965)

20 DRISCOLL, R. H., MEREDITH, S., WAGONFELD, J. W. and ROSENBERG, I. H. Bone histology and vitamin D status in Crohn's disease: assessment of vitamin D therapy. *Gastroenterology*, **72**, 1051 (1977)

21 EASTWOOD, M. A. and HAMILTON, D. Studies on the absorption of bile salts to non-absorbed components of diet. *Biochemica Biophysica Acta*, **152**, 165–173 (1968)

22 EDDY, R. L. Metabolic bone disease after gastrectomy. *American Journal of Medicine*, **50**, 442–449 (1971)

23 EDIDIN, D., LEVITSKY, L. L., SCHEY, W., DUMBOVIC, R. and CAMPOS, A. Resurgence of nutritional rickets associated with breast feeding and special dietary practices. *Pediatrics*, **62**, 232–235 (1980)

24 ELLIS, G., WOODHEAD, J. S. and COOKE, W. T. Serum 25-hydroxyvitamin-D concentrations in adolescent boys. *Lancet*, **1**, 825–828 (1977)

25 FACCINI, J. M., EXTON-SMITH, A. N. and BOYDE, A. Disorders of bone and fracture of the femoral neck. *Lancet*, **1**, 1089–1092 (1976)

26 FORD, J. A., COLHOUN, E. M., McINTOSH, W. B. and DUNNIGAN, M. G. Biochemical response of late rickets and osteomalacia to a chupatty-free diet. *British Medical Journal*, **3**, 446–447 (1972)

27 FORD, J. A., DAVIDSON, D. C., McINTOSH, W. B., FYFE, W. M. and DUNNIGAN, M. G. Neonatal rickets in Asian immigrant population. *British Medical Journal*, **3**, 211–212 (1973)

28 FORD, J. A., McINTOSH, W. B., BUTTERFIELD, R., PREECE, M. A., PIETREK, J., ARROWSMITH, W. A., ARTHURTON, M. W., TURNER, W., O'RIORDAN, J. L. H. and DUNNIGAN, M. G. Clinical and subclinical vitamin D deficiency in Bradford children. *Archives of Disease in Childhood*, **51**, 939–943 (1976)

29 FRAHER, L. J., JONES, G., CLEMENS, T. L., ADAMI, S. and O'RIORDAN, J. L. H. Radio-assays of vitamin D_2 and D_3 metabolites. *Acta Endocrinologica*, **97** Supplementum 243, Advance abstracts of papers, XIIIth Acta Endocrinologica Congress, Cambridge, August (1981)

30 GERTNER, J. M. and LAWRIE, B. Preventing nutritional rickets. *Lancet*, **1**, 257 (1977)

31 GOUGH, K. R., LLOYD, O. C. and WILLIS, M. R. Nutritional osteomalacia. *Lancet*, **2**, 1261–1264 (1964)

32 GRIFFEL, B. and WINTER, S. T. The prevalence of rickets at autopsy in a subtropical climate. *Journal of Tropical Pediatrics and Environmental Child Health*, **4**, 13–16 (1958)

33 HESS, A. F. *Rickets including Osteomalacia and Tetany*. London, Henry Kimpton (1930)

34 HUNT, S. P., NASH, A. H., WATSON, R. and TRUSWELL, A. S. Vitamin D status in different subgroups of British Asians. *British Medical Journal*, **1**, 641 (1977)

35 HUNT, S. P., O'RIORDAN, J. L. H., WINDO, J. and TRUSWELL, A. S. Vitamin D status in different subgroups of British Asians. *British Medical Journal*, **2**, 1351–1354 (1976)

36 JESSOP, W. H. E. Results of rickets surveys in Dublin. *British Journal of Nutrition*, **4**, 289–295 (1950)

37 KUMAR, R., NAGUBANDI, S., MATTOX, U. R. and LONDOWSKI, J. M. Enterohepatic physiology of 1,25-dihydroxyvitamin D_3. *Journal of Clinical Investigation*, **65**, 277–284 (1980)

38 LAKDAWALA, D. R. and WIDDOWSON, E. M. Vitamin D in human milk. *Lancet*, **1**, 167–168 (1977)

39 LAWSON, D. E. M. Dietary vitamin D. *Lancet*, **2**, 1021 (1979)

40 LAWSON, D. E. M., PAUL, A. A., BLACK, A. E., COLE, T. J., MANDAL, A. R. and DAVIE, M. Relative contributions of diet and sunlight to vitamin D status in the elderly. *British Medical Journal*, **2**, 303–305 (1979)

41 LEERBECK, E. and SØNDERGAARD, H. The total content of vitamin D in human milk and cows' milk. *British Journal of Nutrition*, **44**, 7–12 (1980)

42 LIGHTWOOD, R. Idiopathic hypercalcaemia in infants with failure to thrive. *Archives of Disease in Childhood*, **27**, 302–303 (1952)

43 MELVYN HOWE, G. *Man, Environment and Disease in Britain*. Harmondsworth, Penguin Books Ltd., p. 207 (1976)

44 O'HARA-MAY, J. and WIDDOWSON, E. M. Diets and living conditions of Asian boys in Coventry with and without signs of rickets. *British Journal of Nutrition*, **36**, 23–36 (1976)

45 PAPAPOULOS, S. E., CLEMENS, T. L., FRAHER, L. J., GLEED, J. and O'RIORDAN, J. L. H. Metabolites of vitamin D in human vitamin D deficiency; effect of vitamin D or 1,25 dihydroxycholecalciferol. *Lancet*, **2**, 612–615 (1980)

46 PETTIFOR, J. M., ROSS, P., WANG, J., MOODLEY, G. and COUPER-SMITH, J. Rickets in children of rural origin in South Africa: is low dietary calcium a factor? *Journal of Pediatrics*, **92**, 320–324 (1978)

47 PIETREK, J., WINDO, J., PREECE, M. A., O'RIORDAN, J. L. H., DUNNIGAN, M. G., McINTOSH, W. B. and FORD, J. A. Prevention of vitamin-D deficiency in Asians. *Lancet*, **1**, 1145–1148 (1976)

48 POSKITT, E. M. E., COLE, T. J. and LAWSON, D. E. M. Diet, sunlight and 25-hydroxy-vitamin D in healthy children and adults. *British Medical Journal*, **1**, 221–223 (1979)

49 PREECE, M. A., FORD, J. A., McINTOSH, W. B., DUNNIGAN, M. G., TOMLINSON, S. and O'RIORDAN, J. L. H. Vitamin D deficiency among Asian immigrants to Britain. *Lancet*, **1**, 907–910 (1973)

50 PREECE, M. A., TOMLINSON, S., RIBOT, C. A., PIETREK, J., KORN, H. T., DAVIES, D. M., FORD, J. A., DUNNIGAN, M. G. and O'RIORDAN, J. L. H. Studies of vitamin D deficiency in man. *Quarterly Journal of Medicine*, **44**, 575–589 (1975)

51 REINHOLD, J. G. High phytate content of rural Iranian bread: a possible cause of human zinc deficiency. *American Journal of Clinical Nutrition*, **24**, 1204–1206 (1971)

52 REINHOLD, J. G. Nutritional osteomalacia in immigrants in an urban community. *Lancet*, **1**, 386 (1972)

53 REINHOLD, J. G. Rickets in Asian immigrants. *Lancet*, **2**, 1132 (1976)

54 RIZVI, S. N. A., CHAWLA, S. C, SINHA, S., MALHOTRA, P., GULATI, P. D. and VAISHNAVA, H. Some observations on the prevalence of vitamin D deficiency rickets amongst families of osteomalacics. *Journal of the Association of Physicians of India*, **24**, 833–838 (1976)

55 ROBERTS, I. F., WEST, R. J., OGILVIE, D. and DILLON, M. J. Malnutrition in infants receiving cult diets; a form of child abuse. *British Medical Journal*, **1**, 296–298 (1979)

56 ROBERTSON, I., FORD, J. A., McINTOSH, W. B. and DUNNIGAN, M. G. The role of cereals in the aetiology of nutritional rickets: the lesson of the Irish National Nutrition Survey 1943–8. *British Journal of Nutrition*, **45**, 17–22 (1981)

57 ROBERTSON, I., GLEKIN, B. M., HENDERSON, J. G., McINTOSH, W. B., LAKHANI, A. and DUNNIGAN, M. G. Nutritional deficiencies among ethnic minorities in the United Kingdom. *Proceedings of the Nutrition Society*. In press

58 ROSENBERG, I. H., SITRIN, M. D. and BOLT, M. J. G. The enterohepatic circulation of vitamin D: potential clinical implications. In *Vitamin D. Basic Research and Its Clinical Application* (Proceedings of the Fourth Workshop on vitamin D). Berlin, Walter de Gruyter and Co., pp. 487–492 (1979)

59 SALIMPOUR, R. Rickets in Tehran: study of 200 cases. *Archives of Disease in Childhood*, **50**, 63–66 (1975)

60 SITRIN, M., BOLT, M. and ROSENBERG, I. H. Characterisation and quantitative analysis of the biliary excretion products of vitamin D and 25-OH vitamin D. *Clinical Research*, **26**, 285A (1978)

61 STAMP, T. C. B. Factors in human vitamin D nutrition and in the production and cure of classical rickets. *Proceedings of the Nutrition Society*, **34**, 119–130 (1975)

62 STAMP, T. C. B., WALKER, P. G., PERRY, W. and JENKINS, M. V. Nutritional osteomalacia and late rickets in Greater London 1974–79: clinical and metabolic studies in 45 patients. *Clinics in Endocrinology and Metabolism*, **9**, 81–105 (1980)

63 VAISHNAVA, H. Vitamin D deficiency in Northern India. *Journal of the Association of Physicians of India*, **23**, 477–484 (1975)

64 WILLS, M. R., DAY, R. C., PHILLIPS, J. B. and BATEMAN, E. C. Phytic acid and nutritional rickets in immigrants. *Lancet*, **1**, 771–773 (1972)

65 WILSON, D. C. Incidence of osteomalacia and late rickets in Northern India. *Lancet*, **2**, 10–12 (1931)

66 ZELDIN, T. *France 1848–1949. Volume Two: Intellect, Taste and Anxiety*. Oxford, Clarendon Press, p. 725 (1977)

7

Renal osteodystrophy

Burt A. Liebross and Jack W. Coburn

INTRODUCTION

When the life of a patient with advanced renal failure is prolonged, either through conservative therapy or renal 'replacement' with dialysis, renal osteodystrophy may arise as a formidable consequence. We shall use the term renal osteodystrophy to include several skeletal syndromes and the alterations of divalent ion metabolism that occur when kidney function is reduced. The kidneys are known to play an important role in the regulation of calcium, phosphorus, and magnesium metabolism through control of their urinary excretion and by the generation of 1,25-dihydroxyvitamin D_3 (1,25 $(OH)_2D_3$); also they are major organs responsible for the degradation of parathyroid hormone (PTH). As the kidneys fail, various homeostatic mechanisms are activated in an apparent attempt to adjust for disturbances in divalent ion metabolism. These homeostatic processes themselves may have certain adverse effects; thus, the increased secretion of parathyroid hormone, which occurs in renal insufficiency, is a major factor leading to altered skeletal structure and may even contribute to other uremic symptoms.

SKELETAL PATHOLOGY IN RENAL OSTEODYSTROPHY

Several forms of skeletal pathology occur with advanced renal failure. The type of bone disease may depend upon a number of factors, including the relative prominence of certain specific pathogenic processes described below, the presence of uremic toxins, the age of the patient, the rate of skeletal turnover, the duration and rate of progression of renal insufficiency, differences in dietary intake, the nature of pharmacological intervention, and the duration and adequacy of dialysis. The skeletal pathology varies from patient to patient, but the most common form in uremic adults is that of osteitis fibrosa (fibro-osteoclasia) which arises due to the action of excess PTH. Osteomalacia, or impaired mineralization of bone, is also common; it is usually accompanied by a variable degree of osteitis fibrosa. These forms of skeletal pathology are described below.

Osteitis fibrosa (fibro-osteoclasia)

Osteitis fibrosa is characterized by augmented numbers of both osteoclasts and osteoblasts and an increase in marrow fibrosis which is localized along peritrabecular surfaces. The activation of osteoclasts is mediated by high concentrations of PTH; this results in increased resorption of both mineral and matrix along the surfaces of trabecular bone and within the Haversian canals of cortical bone[71]. Rows of osteoblasts lay down wide seams of newly synthesized, unmineralized osteoid along the surfaces of trabecular bone and within the sites of earlier resorptive cavities or Howships lacunae. This excess of unmineralized osteoid develops in osteitis fibrosa as a consequence of more rapid synthesis of matrix rather than because there is impaired mineralization. Another feature of osteitis fibrosa is the presence of 'woven' osteoid with the layers of collagen arranged in a haphazard, irregular fashion; this contrasts with the orderly, lamellar arrangement of the collagen fibrils in normal bone. A pattern of woven bone also occurs in other conditions characterized by increased bone turnover, such as Paget's disease, hyperthyroidism, and acromegaly. Another feature of woven bone is the deposition of calcium as amorphous calcium phosphate, instead of as hydroxyapatite which is deposited in normal, lamellar bone. It has been proposed that a greater quantity of woven than lamellar bone may be needed to produce a similar degree of mechanical strength[71]. Thus, the appearance of osteosclerosis, which is a common feature of secondary hyperparathyroidism, may represent an increased mineralization with amorphous calcium phosphate deposited in woven bone in an attempt to maintain mechanical stability.

Osteomalacia

The term osteomalacia is used to describe defective mineralization of bone. However, the histological criteria used for the diagnosis of osteomalacia vary between laboratories. Osteomalacia is most commonly identified by the finding of wide osteoid seams; however, the presence of widened osteoid seams does not, in itself, indicate the presence of osteomalacia. As noted in the discussion of osteitis fibrosa, the seams are widened when skeletal mineralization does not keep pace with an increased rate of matrix synthesis. Other 'static' features of osteomalacia include the finding of an increased number of unmineralized osteoid lamellae and an increase in the fraction of trabecular surface that is covered with osteoid. The best method of identification of defective mineralization involves the use of tetracycline which is incorporated into newly forming bone. With the administration of tetracycline on two separate occasions, separated by a known time interval, the apposition rate or bone formation rate can be calculated, permitting a dynamic approach to bone histomorphometry. Such measurements disclose a reduced rate of bone formation in osteomalacia. In most patients with osteomalacia, there coexists a variable degree of secondary hyperparathyroidism and the bone shows concomitant features of osteitis fibrosa; that is, increased resorption and peritrabecular fibrosis. These lesions have been classified as showing 'mixed' features of both osteitis fibrosa and osteomalacia[23, 76].

Another subset of patients with advanced renal failure show isolated or 'pure' osteomalacia and totally lack the features of secondary hyperparathyroidism[1, 38]. Most of these patients have been treated with hemodialysis for a substantial period, and the pathogenesis of this variety of osteomalacia, which is discussed below, may differ from that leading to osteitis fibrosa or the mixed lesion of osteomalacia combined with osteitis fibrosa.

PATHOPHYSIOLOGY OF ALTERED CALCIUM HOMEOSTASIS

Under normal circumstances, the kidneys play a vital role in mineral homeostasis. Thus, they act to maintain the external balance for calcium, phosphorus and magnesium; they are the principal tissues responsible for hydroxylating 25-hydroxyvitamin D to 1,25-dihydroxyvitamin D and 24,25-dihydroxyvitamin D; also, they are responsible for certain aspects of the degradation of parathyroid hormone. With the loss of certain of these functions with renal insufficiency, it is not surprising that mineral homeostasis is deranged. There is generally an orderly sequence of disturbances that occur with the reduction in functioning nephron population with chronic renal failure; however, certain selective renal disorders may have a preponderance of one pathophysiological alteration. For example, patients with Fanconi's syndrome may have hypophosphatemia and inappropriate activation of vitamin D to $1,25(OH)_2D_3$, while patients with the nephrotic syndrome often have excessive urinary losses of 25-hydroxyvitamin D, which is excreted in the urine bound to the vitamin D-binding protein of plasma.

Hypocalcemia and secondary hyperparathyroidism

When the glomerular filtration rate falls below 50–75 ml/min, an early and persistent abnormality is an elevation in the serum level of immunoreactive parathyroid hormone (iPTH)[70]. This increase in serum iPTH occurs because PTH secretion is increased, but it also arises, in part, due to reduced metabolic clearance of iPTH. Many immunoassay procedures detect primarily the carboxyl (C–) terminal fragments of the PTH molecule. These C-terminal fragments which are biologically inactive are normally cleared from the circulation entirely by glomerular filtration[42]; with progressive renal insufficiency, their metabolic clearance rate is greatly reduced, leading to a major increase in their blood levels. Thus, the presence of modestly increased blood levels of C-terminal PTH fragments in patients with renal insufficiency may not necessarily indicate the existence of biological hyperparathyroidism. Nonetheless, bone biopsies done on patients with mild renal insufficiency generally show some evidence of increased parathyroid action[49]. As renal failure progresses and glomerular filtration rate (GFR) falls below 30 ml/min, evidence of secondary hyperparathyroidism becomes more marked as do morphological findings of hyperparathyroidism in bone[10]. There are several factors responsible for the production of hypocalcemia and secondary hyperparathyroidism in renal failure; these include phosphate retention, an altered calcemic response to the action of parathyroid hormone, and abnormal vitamin D metabolism.

Phosphate retention

An increase in plasma inorganic phosphorus is associated with a reciprocal fall in plasma calcium. Retention of phosphate due to a drop in GFR early in the course of renal insufficiency may cause a fall in blood ionized calcium and initiate the increased secretion of PTH. The increase in level of PTH would cause phosphaturia, lower serum phosphorus levels to normal, and restore serum calcium, but only at the expense of a higher serum level of PTH. Bricker, Slatopolsky *et al.*[74, 79] have shown the fundamental importance of dietary phosphate in the development of secondary hyperparathyroidism in animals with experimental renal failure. Thus, it has been shown that a decrease in dietary phosphate intake in proportion to the degree of reduction in GFR can result in normal serum levels of calcium and phosphorus and only a moderate increase in levels of iPTH. In contrast, azotemic dogs fed constant, normal amounts of phosphate developed substantial secondary hyperparathyroidism.

The mechanism whereby minimal phosphate retention stimulates the secretion of PTH is not certain; serum phosphorus levels have usually been normal or even slightly decreased in patients with mild renal insufficiency[48]. Also, it has been shown that the excretion of an increased fraction of filtered phosphate, a uniform feature of renal failure and thought to arise primarily because of the high PTH levels, can also occur in the absence of the parathyroid glands[86]. Moreover, it is possible that phosphate retention could inhibit the generation of 1,25-dihydroxyvitamin D_3, and thereby lead to reduced calcium absorption, hypocalcemia, and parathyroid hypersecretion. Overt hyperphosphatemia does not generally appear in patients with renal failure until their renal function decreases to below 25% of normal. When it occurs, the overt hyperphosphatemia can clearly contribute to the hypocalcemia and consequent secondary hyperparathyroidism.

Skeletal resistance to the calcemic action of parathyroid hormone

Another factor which contributes to hypocalcemia and the degree of secondary hyperparathyroidism in renal failure is skeletal resistance to the calcemic action of PTH. Thus, a higher concentration of PTH may be needed to maintain serum calcium at normal levels. In patients with advanced renal failure and in those treated with dialysis, the administration of exogenous parathyroid extract fails to produce a normal increment of serum calcium[52, 53]. Moreover, patients with mild renal insufficiency exhibit delayed recovery from the hypocalcemia induced by the infusion of ethylenediamine tetracetic acid (EDTA) despite a greater than normal increment in serum iPTH[46]. The factors responsible for this skeletal resistance to the calcemic action of PTH may include decreased generation of 1,25-dihydroxyvitamin D_3[55] and/or 24,25 $(OH)_2D_3$,[83] phosphate retention[84], and the presence of certain 'uremic toxins'[92]. It is possible that the rate of bone resorption may be maximal in uremia so that a further increase in PTH can produce little enhanced skeletal action[53]; alternatively, the activity of each osteoclast or osteocyte may be decreased in uremia.

Abnormalities of vitamin D production

The kidney is the major organ which generates 1,25-dihydroxyvitamin D_3 $(1,25(OH)_2D_3)$, the active hormonal form of vitamin D. The blood level of this sterol is normally maintained under close metabolic control. Thus, under normal circumstances, the generation of $1,25(OH)_2D_3$ from $25(OH)D_3$ is stimulated by hypocalcemia, presumably via the effect of parathyroid hormone, and by phosphate deprivation or a fall in serum phosphate level; the effect of phosphate is believed to act directly on the enzyme. Conversely, hyperphosphatemia or calcium loading may depress the generation of $1,25(OH)_2D_3$. The activity of the $25(OH)D_3-1\alpha$-hydroxylase, the enzyme responsible for generating $1-25(OH)_2D_3$, can also be inhibited by its product $1,25(OH)_2D_3$ or by acidosis.

Inability of the diseased kidney to produce $1,25(OH)_2D_3$ plays an important role in the pathogenesis of altered calcium homeostasis in renal insufficiency[18]. In patients with advanced renal failure, the intestinal absorption of calcium is impaired and the plasma levels of $1,25(OH)_2D$ are uniformly depressed[13, 25]. Moreover, the administration of modest doses of $1,25(OH)_2D_3$ can restore the intestinal absorption of calcium to normal in uremic patients[12].

These observations provide strong evidence that vitamin D metabolism is abnormal in advanced renal failure. However, it is not clear when in the course of renal insufficiency these abnormalities of vitamin D metabolism develop, nor is it known whether they contribute to the pathogenesis of altered calcium homeostasis in the early course of renal insufficiency. Most patients with mild-to-moderate renal insufficiency (that is, serum creatinine levels below 225 µmol/l (2.5 mg/dl) or creatinine clearance rates greater than 50 ml/min) exhibit normal intestinal calcium absorption[19, 51], and preliminary data in adults with moderate insufficiency suggest that plasma levels of $1,25(OH)_2D$ may be normal[80]. It should be noted that these findings in early renal failure may not represent the normal response of the tubular cells to the high levels of PTH, which should lead to increased generation of $1,25(OH)_2D_3$. Preliminary observations in children with mild renal disease due to tubulointerstitial disorders have revealed low serum levels of $1,25(OH)_2D$[67], an observation suggesting that the 'pathway' to secondary hyperparathyroidism may differ from patient to patient.

The kidney is also the organ which is primarily responsible for generation of 24,25 dihydroxyvitamin D_3 $(24,25(OH)_2D_3)$, a sterol of uncertain physiological role[41]. This sterol probably does not stimulate intestinal calcium absorption without being converted by the kidney to 1,24,25 trihydroxyvitamin D_3; however,

24,25$(OH)_2D_3$ may have effects different from 1,25$(OH)_2D_3$[47]. Whether the reduced levels of 24,25$(OH)_2D_3$ in uremia play a role in the pathogenesis of bone disease is uncertain.

Factors causing defective mineralization (osteomalacia)

The pathogenesis of osteomalacia or the defective mineralization seen in patients with advanced renal failure is less certain than are the factors leading to secondary hyperparathyroidism and osteitis fibrosa; some of the factors that are believed to contribute are shown in *Table 7.1*. Because of the deranged vitamin D metabolism

Table 7.1 Factors which may contribute to osteomalacia in renal failure

(1) Altered vitamin D status
    (a) Nutritional vitamin D deficiency (25(OH)D low)
    (b) Intestinal malabsorption of vitamin D_2 or D_3*
    (c) Reduced 25$(OH)D_3$ due to nephrotic syndrome or anticonvulsant therapy
    (d) Reduced 1,25$(OH)_2D_3$ arising through renal disease
    (e) End-organ unresponsiveness to 1,25$(OH)_2D_3$*

(2) Accumulation of toxic substances which may impair bone mineralization
    (a) Aluminum
    (b) Fluoride
    (c) Strontium*
    (d) Cadmium*
    (e) Lead*

(3) Phosphate deficiency or depletion (*see also* 5d)

(4) Altered quantities of normal skeletal constituents
    (a) Excess bone pyrophosphate*
    (b) Excess bone magnesium*†
    (c) Depletion of bone carbonate*†

(5) Therapeutic intervention
    (a) Administration of heparin*†
    (b) Treatment with anticonvulsants
    (c) Adrenal steroid therapy†
    (d) Excessive intake of Al$(OH)_3$ gels

* Theoretical causes of reduced mineralization, not proven.
† Probably contributory, not actual cause of osteomalacia.

in renal insufficiency, it is tempting to conclude that osteomalacia arises due to the altered vitamin D metabolism. Although the alterations in vitamin D metabolism may contribute to the osteomalacia, there is little evidence that patients with osteomalacia have alterations in plasma levels of vitamin D that differ from those seen in uremic patients who lack this skeletal lesion. Thus, anephric patients, who cannot generate 1,25$(OH)_2D_3$, do not invariably develop histological features of osteomalacia[11]. Also the blood levels of 24,25$(OH)_2D_3$ are reduced or absent in anephric patients; however, it is not certain whether this vitamin D sterol is needed for skeletal homeostasis[41, 88]. The role of these alterations in vitamin D metabolism in causing osteomalacia in uremia is poorly understood because there is uncertainty about how vitamin D leads to mineralization of bone in normals. Thus, it is uncertain whether vitamin D and its metabolites have a direct effect on mineralization of the skeleton or whether they act merely by elevating the calcium and phosphorus levels in the extracellular fluid which bathes the skeletal matrix. In occasional uremic patients, the plasma levels of 25(OH)D may be low providing evidence for the concomitant existence of a nutritional deficiency of vitamin D[24]. Such cases are unusual, and most uremic patients with osteomalacia seen in the United States have normal levels of 25(OH)D[38].

Epidemiological evidence and case reports suggest possible roles of aluminum accumulation, phosphate depletion or hypophosphatemia, and treatment with certain drugs, such as phenobarbital, diphenylhydantoin or glutethimide in the pathogenesis of osteomalacia. Acidosis and treatment with heparin may inhibit bone formation[32]. Alternations in collagen synthesis or in crystal maturation may contribute to osteomalacia or be an integral component of this skeletal abnormality[3]. Also, the bone of a uremic patient may contain differing amounts of normal constituents, including the accumulation of magnesium or pyrophosphate and the loss of carbonate; such alterations may also contribute to defective mineralization.

A number of reports have shown a strong association between the use of untreated water for the preparation of dialysate and the prevalence of osteomalacia and encephalopathy[64, 65, 91]. Moreover, osteomalacia is uncommon in uremic patients who have not been treated with dialysis. Other clinical observations indicate that osteitis fibrosa may progress or change to osteomalacia. Aluminum could also accumulate by intestinal absorption during therapy with aluminum carbonate or aluminum hydroxide. The kidney is the only route for the excretion of aluminum that enters the body, and it is not surprising that aluminum may accumulate in patients with renal failure. Moreover, studies in experimental animals suggest that the parenteral administration of aluminum can impair the mineralization of epiphyseal cartilage[26]. Although the association between osteomalacia and aluminum accumulation is strong, such epidemiological observations do not prove a 'cause and effect'. Thus, aluminum could be present merely as an 'innocent bystander', or it could be a marker for the presence of another trace substance. The observations that osteomalacic bone disease is less common following the initiation of appropriate water treatment[65, 91] provide the most compelling evidence that aluminum or some other constituent of the water can cause osteomalacia in certain patients. Some patients may develop osteomalacic bone disease despite the use of water that has been 'appropriately treated', suggesting another cause or the entry of aluminum into the body through the enteric route[44, 69].

Data derived during the use of fluoride-containing water for the preparation of dialysate must be considered with the knowledge that such water may also have excessive quantities of other potentially toxic compounds, such as aluminum. The purification of tap-water with removal of the fluoride could have led to removal of aluminum and other trace compounds. Thus, such observations do not prove the cause of the abnormal bone formation.

In occasional patients, the intake of a low phosphate diet or the overzealous use of phosphate-binders can produce phosphate depletion or hypophosphatemia, which can impair bone mineralization[45]. Such hypophosphatemia is probably the cause of osteomalacic bone disease in only a small number of uremic patients. Similarly, the number of cases that arise as a consequence of treatment with phenobarbital, phenytoin, or glutethimide must be relatively small.

Other factors in patients with advanced renal failure lead to alterations in skeletal mineralization. These include magnesium accumulation, chronic acidosis, an increase in skeletal pyrophosphate, regular treatment with heparin, and reduced bone bicarbonate. Each of these pathophysiological features, in themselves, might lead to certain alteration in skeletal homeostasis. On the other hand, there are no data to indicate that these factors are altered to a greater degree in the uremic patients who develop osteomalacia than in other patients who lack osteomalacia.

Another factor which has been implicated as a possible contributor to the development of 'pure' osteomalacia and the low rate of bone turnover is the presence of low levels of parathyroid hormone (PTH)[28, 38, 89]. Total parathyroidectomy has been implicated as predisposing to this syndrome[89], and preliminary observations suggest there may be impaired release of PTH in response to hypocalcemia in uremic patients with osteomalacia, even in those who have not undergone parathyroid surgery[46].

A unified concept to explain the osteomalacia that develops in a small fraction of patients with end-stage uremia is not possible. Indeed, certain pathogenic factors, such as reduced serum levels of both $1,25(OH)_2D$ and $24,25(OH)_2D$ and the skeletal accumulation of aluminum, exist in most patients with advanced renal failure. Thus, it is surprising that osteomalacia is not seen uniformly in uremic patients; and the search for the factor or factors which prevent the development of osteomalacia in uremic patients might be profitable. No candidates are obvious, but it should be remembered that many forms of osteomalacia, such as with vitamin D deficiency, with mesenchymal tumors, and with sex-linked hypophosphatemic rickets, have hypophosphatemia as a prominent feature. On the other hand, patients with end-stage uremia usually have normal or elevated serum phosphorus levels. Thus, the lack of hypophosphatemia could be a factor that prevents the development of osteomalacia in many uremic patients.

CLINICAL FEATURES OF RENAL OSTEODYSTROPHY

Certain signs, symptoms, and clinical features which are associated with altered divalent ion metabolism in renal failure are shown in *Table 7.2*. Some clinical features can arise in patients with advanced renal failure specifically from the alterations of mineral metabolism; these include bone pain, fractures, skeletal deformities, and in children, growth failure. On the other hand, certain signs and symptoms may be due to the uremic state, *per se*. Thus, pruritus can show substantial amelioration following parathyroidectomy in some patients, while it

Table 7.2   Features associated with renal osteodystrophy

---

(1) Musculoskeletal system
   (a) Bone pain
   (b) Fractures
   (c) Acute pseudogout
   (d) Calcific periarthritis
   (e) Skeletal deformities
   (f) Proximal myopathy
   (g) Spontaneous tendon rupture
   (h) Growth retardation
   (i) Slipped epiphyses
   (j) Tumoral calcification

(2) Cardiopulmonary system
   (a) Myocardial calcification, heart block, heart failure
   (b) Pulmonary vascular calcification
   (c) Hypertension (?)

(3) Dermatological features
   (a) Pruritus
   (b) Cutaneous calcification

(4) Ophthalmological features
   (a) Corneal calcification (band keratopathy)
   (b) Conjunction calcification (i.e., with 'red eye' or 'white eye')

(5) Metabolic and endocrine features
   (a) Insulin resistance
   (b) Hypertriglyceridemia
   (c) Impotence
   (d) Menstrual abnormalities and/or sterility

(6) Hematological features
   (a) Anemia
   (b) Pancytopenia

(7) Neurological features
   (a) Dialysis encephalopathy
   (b) Peripheral neuropathy (?)
   (c) Altered cognitive function
   (d) Abnormal EEG (?)

---

exists in other uremic patients who have little or no evidence of secondary hyperparathyroidism. Also, profound myopathy may show an impressive response to treatment with active vitamin D sterols, while in other cases the course of this problem seems totally unaltered by therapy directed to the altered calcium metabolism. It is apparent that uremia, *per se*, represents a complex biochemical milieu, and it would not be surprising if more than one causal factor is responsible for many specific clinical features.

As noted above under 'skeletal pathology', patients with uremia may exhibit osteitis fibrosa, a feature of secondary hyperparathyroidism, osteomalacia, or combinations of the two. Although there is considerable overlap of the signs and symptoms present in patients with the differing types of skeletal pathology, certain clinical patterns are more common with a given pathological feature. When this seems to occur, these differences will be mentioned. In general, when clinical symptoms are present there is usually far-advanced renal insufficiency. Certain symptoms may occur with moderate renal failure, in other words, when renal function is reduced to 15–20% of normal, particularly in children who are still growing or with a renal disease which causes slow progression of the renal insufficiency.

Bone pain

The bone pain of renal osteodystrophy is extremely variable; very severe pain usually appears insidiously with findings of either osteomalacia or with osteitis fibrosa, and the pain is often dismissed as neurotic or due to 'muscular strain'. The presence of severe bone pain may be associated with marked radiographic findings in some patients; however, other patients exhibit severe debility or pain with little or no X-ray abnormalities. This is particularly true in patients with osteomalacia. At times, the bone pain is related to the presence of a fracture, such as a crush fracture of a vertebral body or of one or more ribs. The pain is often described as deep-seated, and it is aggravated by weight-bearing or muscular effort. Often the pain is totally relieved when the effect of gravity is removed by immersing the patient in water. Pain most commonly occurs about the lower back, the hips or the rib cage, and less frequently about the knees, ankles and/or feet. Usually the pain is poorly localized.

Physical findings are usually lacking, although some patients occasionally exhibit localized bony tenderness. Warmth, redness and swelling are usually absent. The resolution of severe bone pain upon treatment with active forms of vitamin D or following parathyroidectomy may provide the most convincing evidence that such symptoms were due to renal osteodystrophy.

Skeletal deformities

Skeletal deformities most commonly develop during periods of active bone remodeling or growth. Deformities can be marked in children, but can also occur in adults, either as a consequence of fractures or associated with bone remodeling. A cause of substantial skeletal deformity of children, and usually involving the wrists and hips, is a slipped epiphysis; these usually arise as a consequence of osteitis fibrosa affecting the epiphyseal growth plate[60]. Genu valgum or 'knock-knee' is a feature almost limited to patients with uremia during late childhood and adolescence. Substantial deformities of the thoracic spine, with profound loss of height and a 'pigeon' chest, arise due to recurrent rib fractures in adults; such deformities may be more common in patients with osteomalacia[62]. Occasionally, skeletal abnormalities of the jaw and maxilla may be profound; this may be associated with loosening, drifting and loss of teeth.

Fractures

Spontaneous fractures most commonly affect the axial skeleton where they involve the vertebral bodies, ribs, and hips. Such fractures are most commonly associated with osteomalacia and are a prominent feature of the syndrome of dialysis osteomalacia (*see below*). Fractures often occur with minimal trauma. Thus, crush vertebral fractures may occur spontaneously, rib fractures can occur during a sneeze or cough, and hip fractures may occur with minor trauma, such as when a patient steps off a curb. Less frequently fractures involve the long bones. Spontaneous rib fractures are frequently multiple, and little displacement may be seen on X-ray; hence, they may be more easily identified with a bone scintiscan, where they may be indistinguishable from stress fractures or pseudofractures.

Myopathy

Proximal myopathy of varying severity and affecting the muscles of the shoulder and pelvic girdles can appear in patients with end-stage uremia. The muscle weakness appears insidiously, with the patients noting difficulty in arising from a low chair, in climbing stairs or in holding objects above their head. Such patients frequently exhibit a characteristic waddling or 'penguin' gait.

A similar clinical syndrome is seen in patients with rickets or osteomalacia due to nutritional vitamin D deficiency, and such myopathy often responds dramatically to treatment with vitamin D sterols. Secondary hyperparathyroidism is usually present, and the myopathy has been attributed to the high levels of PTH[49]. Myopathy is more common in vitamin D deficiency than in hyperparathyroidism, providing further evidence for a special role of vitamin D in the myopathy[81]. The serum levels of muscle enzymes, that is, creatinine phosphokinase and aldolase, are generally normal in uremic patients with proximal myopathy.

The mechanism of proximal myopathy remains obscure. A cytosolic receptor for $1,25(OH)_2D_3$ similar to that identified in other target tissues has not been identified in muscle, an observation that has been used as evidence against $1,25(OH)_2D_3$ having a direct effect on muscle. However, there is impaired uptake of radio-calcium by the endoplasmic reticulum from muscle of vitamin D-deficient animals: this abnormality can be corrected by vitamin D or $1,25(OH)_2D_3$[56]. Also, the muscles from vitamin D-deficient animals exhibit a prolonged relaxation phase. Cytosolic binding of 25-hydroxyvitamin D have been shown in muscle[7], but the relationship between this finding and altered muscle function in uremia is uncertain since the plasma levels of 25(OH)D are generally normal[38].

Both motor and sensory neuropathy may occur in patients with chronic renal failure, and distal muscle weakness may occur as a consequence of neuropathy which may be totally unrelated to calcium metabolism. Clinically, it may be difficult to separate the weakness of peripheral neuropathy from that occurring due to proximal myopathy, *per se*. Also, bone pain and myopathy frequently coexist, and it may be difficult to separate them clinically; patients with overt bone disease and muscle weakness might have muscular weakness arising as a consequence of marked inactivity because of bone pain. Thus, it was surprising to observe substantial remission of pain and improved muscular strength while there was little or no change in the osteomalacic skeletal lesion[38].

Pseudogout and periarthritis

In uremia, episodes of acute arthritis or pseudogout sometimes occur; this clinically resembles gout but is associated with deposition of crystals of calcium pyrophosphate. More commonly, there is acute periarthritis with periarticular inflammation. This syndrome is frequently associated with extraskeletal calcification and presumably arises due to the deposition of calcium hydroxyapatite. The latter syndrome is more common in patients with marked hyperphosphatemia and high serum PTH levels. The symptoms respond to treatment with phenylbutazone or another non-steroidal anti-inflammatory agent, and they usually do not recur when there is adequate control of the serum phosphorus levels.

Spontaneous tendon rupture

The spontaneous rupture of a major tendon, usually the Achilles tendon, quadriceps tendon, or tendons of the fingers, can occur in patients with uremia. Such patients invariably have evidence of overt or marked secondary hyperparathyroidism. The lesions heal normally following surgical therapy, and reports of tendon rupture in patients with primary hyperparathyroidism suggest that excess PTH somehow plays a role. This may be due to alterations in the structure of collagen in the tendon, similar to those seen in uremic bone[3].

Growth retardation

Growth retardation is common in uremic children. Such children show impaired growth and delayed maturation of the skeleton. The mechanisms for the abnormalities of growth and skeletal maturation remain obscure. They may be related to the abnormal protein metabolism of uremia, reduced caloric intake[77], to the secondary hyperparathyroidism, and to the alterations of vitamin D metabolism. Observations that the rate of bone maturations and growth can improve substantially after treatment with an active vitamin D sterol[15, 43], provide support for a role of vitamin D.

Pruritus

Pruritus is a troublesome symptom in many patients with advanced renal failure. Although the pruritus often improves following the initiation of regular dialysis, it is sometimes persistent or even progressive. The observation that 'uremic' pruritis may improve within a few days after subtotal parathyroidectomy for secondary hyperparathyroidism suggests that it is in some way related to the level of calcium or phosphate in the extracellular fluid[33, 54]. The improvement of the pruritis usually occurs before there is any change in the calcium content of the skin[54]. The development of pruritis during hypercalcemia that is induced by vitamin D therapy after parathyroidectomy suggests that pruritus is related to blood calcium level rather than to parathyroid hormone, *per se*; nonetheless, its mechanism remains obscure. With better management and prevention of severe secondary hyperparathyroidism the occurrence of pruritus due to secondary hyperparathyroidism is less common than it was a few years ago.

Calciphylaxis

Calciphylaxis is an unusual yet devastating syndrome that can appear in patients with advanced stable renal failure, in those undergoing hemodialysis, and after successful renal transplantation. The syndrome is characterized by progressive ischemic ulcers of the extremities, the buttocks or thighs. There is usually extreme pain, often with Raynaud's phenomenon, and the lesions may progress with necrosis of the digits, fat or muscles. Extensive arterial calcification involving the media of the medium and large arteries is often seen radiographically, and most patients exhibit subperiosteal resorption and secondary hyperparathyroidism. Many of the patients have had a period of substantial hyperphosphatemia at some time in the past; however, the lesions can appear and progress in successful renal transplant recipients at a time when serum phosphorus levels are normal or even subnormal. Mild hypercalcemia is often present.

The pathogenesis of this lesion is obscure; a similar syndrome has been produced in animals with uremia fed a diet high in phosphate; treatment with glucocorticoids can predispose the animals to the lesion. Thus, it is possible that treatment with prednisone may predispose to the development of such a lesion following renal transplantation. Under most circumstances, mild hypercalcemia is present. In many patients, there is a prompt reversal of the ischemic lesions following parathyroidectomy with the consequent fall in serum levels of calcium and phosphorus. Such observations have suggested a relationship between this syndrome and altered divalent ion metabolism and secondary hyperparathyroidism. The very prompt improvement that may occur after parathyroid surgery suggests a role of vasoconstriction in causing the ischemic lesions rather than their arising as a consequence of the vascular calcification. This condition can be very severe and in some cases fatal[30]. Parathyroid surgery should be considered promptly when one encounters such an unfortunate patient.

Extraskeletal calcification

Extraskeletal calcification may arise in several forms. Large tumoral calcified masses can appear about the joints; these may develop in the same periarticular

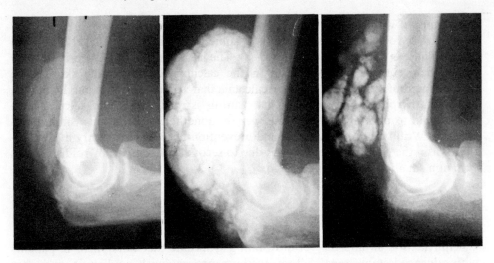

Figure 7.1   The development and partial resolution of a large, tumoral calcification about the right elbow of a patient with end-stage uremia. At the time of the first photograph (*left*), hemodialysis was initiated preceded by uncontrolled hyperphosphatemia for several months. Over the next 13 months, the patient was non-compliant with regard to phosphate-binding antacids. The mass increased in size, causing decreased mobility of the elbow (*center*). The patient then followed his prescribed phosphate binders and hyperphosphatemia was controlled; there was slow resolution of the calcification over the next 7 months (*right*)

sites as do the dystrophic calcifications seen in patients with normal kidney function. These lesions are associated with high calcium and phosphorus products in the serum, and the appropriate control of hyperphosphatemia with the use of aluminum hydroxide or aluminum carbonate is usually associated with their resolution (*Figure 7.1*). Although a role of calcium and phosphate, *per se*, has been implicated, observations that vascular calcifications may regress during vitamin D treatment as serum phosphorus is controlled[90] raise the possibility that high levels of parathyroid hormone may also play a pathogenic role.

An important factor affecting the incidence of such non-visceral calcifications is the age of the patient. Thus, calcifications of any kind are very rare in uremic children and infants despite the existence of high calcium and phosphorus products, while vascular calcifications are very common in adults over 40 years of age[72]. The mechanisms for such 'protection' in the young age-groups is unknown. Soft tissue calcifications may be extensive in the lungs, when they can lead to abnormal pulmonary function with decreased diffusion capacity, hypoxemia, and reduced vital capacity[21]. Vascular calcification may at times be quite extensive in skeletal muscle, leading to ischemic myopathy with muscle pain and weakness[31]. Cardiac calcifications may be asymptomatic or they may be associated with abnormalities of the conducting system with complete heart block[75]; extensive calcification of the myocardium can lead to congestive heart failure.

Calcification of the eye, a common finding in patients with advanced renal failure, may involve the bulbar conjunctiva and the cornea, where it causes band keratopathy. When the deposition of calcium is acute it may lead to an acute inflammatory response producing the so-called 'red-eye' syndrome[5].

Visceral calcification, which involves the lungs, muscle, or myocardium, is largely comprised of amorphous calcium phosphate; this differs from the more typical vascular and periarticular calcifications, which are made up of hydroxy-apatite. There seems to be little or no relationship between serum calcium and phosphorus products and the development of visceral calcification; a high serum magnesium may play an etiological role.

'Dialysis osteomalacia'

This is a syndrome characterized by recurrent fractures, bone pain, proximal myopathy, and the development of skeletal deformities which include lumbar and/ or thoracic scoliosis (*Figure 7.2*), the frequent development of hypercalcemia during treatment with small doses of vitamin D, and serum iPTH levels that are normal or lower than those in other dialysis patients. A high incidence of this syndrome has been reported in certain geographical areas, and aluminum or other contaminants in the water utilized for the preparation of dialysate have been implicated[64]. In other instances, the cases are sporadic, appearing in a small fraction of dialysis patients who utilize water treated with appropriate methods for water purification[38]. On bone biopsy, these patients usually exhibit only osteomala-cia with little or no evidence of hyperparathyroidism. The failure of the osteoid to mineralize despite the maintenance of serum calcium and phosphorus levels at or above normal levels and during treatment with $1,25(OH)_2D_3$ provide evidence that this defect of bone mineralization arises independent of serum levels of calcium, phosphorus or $1,25(OH)_2D$.

The pathogenesis of this lesion is obscure. It has been attributed to total parathyroidectomy in certain cases[28, 89]. The patients do show reduced rates of bone turnover, and reduced secretion of parathyroid hormone could be a factor leading to low turnover of bone. Another feature has been the high concentrations of aluminum in the bone; substantially more than occurs in the bone of uremic patients with other types of bone disease, such as osteitis fibrosa[38]. Also, there has been close correlation between the volume of unmineralized osteoid and the aluminum content[39]. Histochemical studies show the aluminum to be localized largely along the 'calcification front' of newly forming bone, a finding which is compatible with aluminum acting to inhibit mineralization. Studies in experimental animals have shown that large doses of parenteral aluminum can impair the mineralization of epiphyseal cartilage of rats given intraperitoneal aluminum[26]. The presence of a high content of aluminum in the tap-water used for preparing dialysate has been implicated as a source, and epidemiological studies suggest that the incidence of such lesions falls markedly after the initiation of appropriate water treatment. A role of oral aluminum carbonate and aluminum hydroxide in leading to the accumulation of aluminum is uncertain. This disorder may occur in occasional uremic patients who have not been treated with dialysis, and it may occur in dialysis patients who have used appropriate water treatment; thus, there must be other sources of aluminum. It is known that small quantities of oral aluminum may be absorbed[44, 69], and it is not surprising that uremic patients show a total body accumulation of aluminum because of the absence of the mechanism for its excretion.

There is a strong association between 'dialysis osteomalacia' and the syndrome of 'dialysis encephalopathy'[64], which has been attributed to the accumulation of aluminum in the brain. The hallmarks of this encephalopathy include stuttering speech, myoclonus, and a seizure disorder. In a substantial number of cases, the

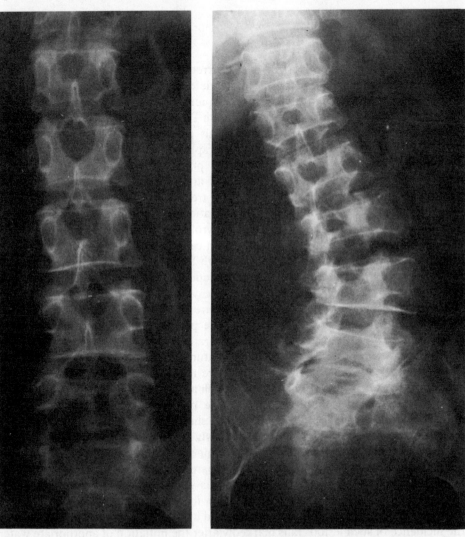

Figure 7.2 X-rays of the lumbar spine in a patient with 'dialysis osteomalacia'. This 40-year-old woman was treated with dialysis for 24 months (*left*) when she developed progressive bone pain. There was progressive shortening of her height and the development of marked lumbar scoliosis over the next 3 years (*right*). Bone biopsy disclosed severe osteomalacia with no evidence of secondary hyperparathyroidism

course has been progressive leading to the death of the patient. The electroencephalogram may be characteristic, with bilateral synchronous slow, sharp, triphasic waves and prominent spikes. Cerebrospinal fluid is generally normal, except for increased protein content in some cases. The initiation of appropriate water treatment has resulted in the disappearance of this lesion.

BIOCHEMICAL FEATURES OF RENAL OSTEODYSTROPHY

Serum phosphorus

Serum phosphorus levels are generally normal in early renal insufficiency, but as glomerular filtration rate (GFR) decreases to less than 25% of normal, serum phosphorus levels are often above normal. At this degree of renal insufficiency, changes in dietary phosphate intake can contribute to the degree of hyperphosphatemia. Some degree of dietary phosphate restriction is useful, and it is usually necessary to treat such patients with aluminum carbonate or aluminum hydroxide gels; compounds which bind phosphate in the gastrointestinal tract. Hemodialysis can provide for the removal of substantial phosphate, but the continued use of aluminium-containing phosphate binders is required in 85–95% of patients undergoing treatment with dialysis.

The efficiency of intestinal absorption of phosphorus is probably normal in most patients with renal failure. Treatment with an active vitamin D sterol can stimulate the absorption of both phosphate and calcium and thus may aggravate the hyperphosphatemia. It is common to think of parathyroid hormone as having an effect to lower serum phosphorus because of its phosphaturic action; however, this effect is quantitatively of little or no importance when renal function is markedly decreased. Thus, a patient with a glomerular filtration rate (GFR) below 10 ml/min invariably exhibits minimal tubular reabsorption of phosphate (in other words, the % tubular reabsorption of phosphate (TRP) approaches zero). Under such circumstances, an increase in PTH-induced bone resorption would augment the release of both calcium and phosphate into extracellular fluid; this would aggravate hyperphosphatemia. Under acute catabolic stress, hyperphosphatemia may become marked.

Occasionally, serum phosphorus levels may be subnormal in patients with renal failure. This may occur because of the overzealous use of phosphate binders and of severe restriction of dietary phosphate intake. It may also occur in rare uremic patients with reduced intestinal absorption of phosphate or during a period of protein anabolism, such as following recovery from marked malnutrition or a catabolic illness.

Serum calcium

The average serum calcium level of patients with advanced renal failure is lower than that seen in a control population; however, there is marked individual variation. The causes of hypocalcemia, which have been reviewed above, are of considerable interest. Patients with advanced chronic uremia often show a slight increase in the complexed fraction of plasma calcium; such calcium is presumably complexed to citrate, phosphate, and other organic anions. This results in a slightly lower level of ionized blood calcium for any given total serum calcium concentration. Upon initiation of regular hemodialysis, serum calcium levels increase toward normal in most patients with uremia; occasionally mild hypercalcemia is seen. Hypercalcemia can occur in patients with advanced renal failure due to marked secondary hyperparathyroidism ('tertiary' hyperparathyroidism); it may be associated with excess intake of oral calcium and treatment with various vitamin D sterols; and it is not uncommon in patients with the syndrome of 'dialysis osteomalacia'. Hypercalcemia can also arise in patients with renal failure due to other causes, such as sarcoidosis, malignancy, etc.

During treatment with regular dialysis, the use of dialysate with calcium levels of 1.5–1.75 mmol/l (3.0–3.5 mEq/l) results in postdialysis serum calcium levels which exceed normal. By the time of the next dialysis, the serum calcium levels have decreased to normal; however, the continued use of a dialysate calcium of 2.0 mmol/l (4.0 mEq/l) has led to persistent hypercalcemia in some patients[61].

Serum magnesium levels

As is the case for serum phosphorus, the levels of serum magnesium tend to increase as the glomerular filtration rate falls below 20–25% of normal. Indeed, acute hypermagnesemia may occur in uremic patients following an increase in dietary magnesium intake and in those ingesting magnesium-containing antacids. When dialysate magnesium concentration is lowered below 0.25–0.4 mmol/l (0.5 –0.8 mEq/l), serum magnesium may fall to normal. Intestinal magnesium absorption is usually normal in uremic patients; however, in uremic patients with a diarrheal disorder, severe hypomagnesemia and hypocalcemia can develop[29]. Decrease in the secretion of parathyroid hormone and development of skeletal unresponsiveness to the action of PTH[2,27] both contribute to the hypocalcemia of magnesium depletion.

Alkaline phosphatase

The total serum alkaline phosphatase reflects enzyme activities arising from hepatic, intestinal and skeletal sources. Despite this non-specific nature of alkaline phosphatase, a slow, progressive increase in serum level in a patient with end-stage renal failure may be the only clue to the development of overt bone disease. The skeletal alkaline phosphatase arises largely from osteoblasts, and a correlation between skeletal alkaline phosphatase and bone biopsy findings of osteitis fibrosa has been observed[66]. In uremic patients with osteomalacia, it has been suggested that the alkaline phosphatase may be normal[1], although others have noted no differences between various subgroups[38]. In a study with the measurement of specific skeletal isoenzymes of alkaline phosphatase, a good correlation between plasma skeletal alkaline phosphatase levels and the response to treatment with an active vitamin D metabolite was observed[66]. Other plasma markers of increased bone activity may include plasma hydroxyproline[34] and GLA protein[68]; but these measurements are not in wide use.

Serum immunoreactive parathyroid hormone

Serum levels of immunoreactive parathyroid hormone (iPTH) are almost invariably increased in patients with advanced renal failure. However, the degree of elevation above normal and the fraction of uremic patients showing markedly elevated levels vary consideraly with the region-specificity of the assay used. With an assay directed toward the amino terminus of the PTH molecule (N-terminal) and which would presumably detect intact PTH as well as amino-terminal fragments, serum iPTH levels may be only mildly elevated in uremia[35]. On the other hand, measurements sensitive to the carboxyl or C-terminal fragments, which are biologically inactive, reveal marked elevations in uremic patients, principally because these fragments of the PTH molecule are largely cleared by glomerular filtration[42].

RADIOGRAPHIC FEATURES OF RENAL OSTEODYSTROPHY

Techniques

In many hospitals, the techniques employed in obtaining bone radiographs result in poor quality films that are very insensitive to the changes of metabolic bone disease. Thus, a standard 'bone survey' is often done to identify metastatic lesions

Table 7.3   Radiographic features of osteodystrophy

Feature	Osteitis fibrosa	Osteomalacia
Demineralization	0 to +	+ +
Subperiosteal resorption	+ + +	0
Osteosclerosis	+ +	0 or +
Fractures	0 to +	+ + +
Looser's zone	0	0 to + +
Vascular calcification	0 to + +	0 to +
Periosteal neostosis	0 to + +	0
Brown tumors	0 to + + +	0
Cortical striation	+	0 to +
Protrusio acetabuli	0 to +	0 to +
Scintiscan	diffuse symmetrical uptake	pseudofractures

0, rare; + to + + + indicates varying prevalence and/or severity.

or bone fractures rather than to detect fine details of skeletal architecture. The use of precise and careful radiographic techniques can improve substantially the sensitivity and precision of the X-ray examination in both detecting and identifying metabolic bone disease[14] (*Table 7.3*).

Standard radiographic techniques and film are generally utilized for X-rays of the spine, pelvis, chest and shoulder girdle, due to the energy of X-rays and exposure time employed. There are, however, several techniques which can greatly enhance the sensitivity and accuracy of X-rays of the hands. Meema *et al.*[58] routinely utilize fine-grain film (Kodak, Type M film) for radiographs of the hand; these films, which are hand-developed by the hospital dental department, are then magnified 6 to 7-fold with a hand lens. Direct magnification X-rays, with enlargement by 3.5 to 4-fold, are recommended by others[14, 85], although special equipment is needed. Another technique is to utilize a fine-grain film, such as mammography film, which can be developed by automatic processing, and the X-rays viewed with visual enlargement with a hand lens.

There is disagreement about the sensitivity of these methods; thus investigators who utilize the direct magnification technique, report that this method is more sensitive than is the magnification of standard mammography films using a hand lens. On the other hand, Meema and Shatz[59] have reported a high sensitivity utilizing the hand lens enlargements of films obtained using fine-grain film. The technique of xeroradiography[82] appears to add little to these techniques.

Using hand X-rays without magnification, Meema and Schatz[59] detected subperiosteal resorption in only 8% of uremic patients, while 29% displayed resorption after hand lens magnification. Using mammography film with no magnification, Carr *et al.*[14] found superiosteal reabsorption in only 6%, compared to 56% showing abnormalities with the magnification films; there was a similar increase in the identification of intracortical striations.

X-ray features of osteitis fibrosa

A principal feature of secondary hyperparathyroidism on X-ray is subperiosteal erosion. Hand X-rays, evaluated by one of the sensitive methods described above, provide the most sensitive method to detect this feature (*Figure 7.3*). There is some disagreement about the appropriate site for evaluation; thus, Meema *et al.*[58] and Ritz *et al.*[73] emphasized the specificity of subperiosteal erosions on the radial surfaces of the phalanges of the first, second and third fingers. Such superiosteal resorptions correlated well with serum iPTH levels and also with histological features of osteitis fibrosa. Sandaram *et al.*[85] reported that the terminal phalangeal tuft revealed abnormalities more frequently than did the periosteal surfaces of the phalanges. They noted 'loss of the cortical margin of the tuft' which was often accompanied by a fine fraying or spiculated appearance at the end of the phalanx. Ritz *et al.*[73] concluded that the change in the tuft, termed 'acro-osteolysis', was less specific, and correlated less well with bone histological features of osteitis fibrosa than did resorptive changes in the phalanges.

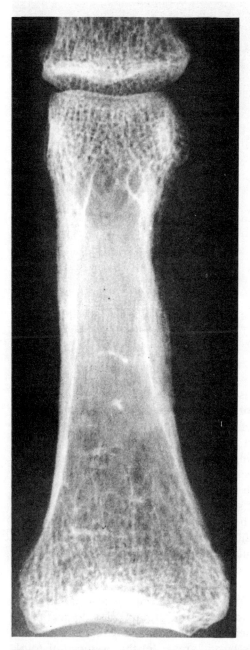

Figure 7.3 Middle phalanx of the second digit of the left hand of a patient treated with hemodialysis for 30 months. There is a marked subperiosteal resorption, seen along the radial surface of the distal third and proximal fifth of the third phalanx. The ulnar surface shows slight irregularity of the periosteal surface over the distal third of the phalanx

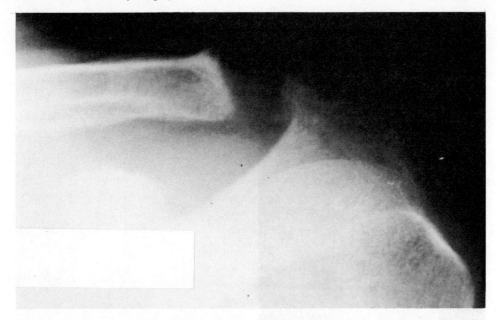

Figure 7.4   Substantial loss of the distal end of the left clavicle of the patient with secondary hyperparathyroidism whose hands are shown in *Figure 7.3*. Radiographs obtained 1 year earlier disclosed no recognizable abnormality of the clavicle

Subperiosteal resorption may occur elsewhere in the skeleton, including the distal clavicles (*Figures 7.4*), the surface of the ischium and pubis, and the surface of the long bones at the junction of the metaphysis and diaphysis. Erosions can sometimes create problems in differential diagnosis; thus, intra-articular erosions of the humeral head may simulate findings of erosive arthritis[8]. Other skeletal features of hyperparathyroidism include cortical striations, cystic abnormalities (brown tumors), and periosteal new bone formation[57].

General correlations exist between the severity of subperiosteal resorption and the degree of osteitis fibrosa detected on bone biopsy. A small fraction of patients who lack histological features of osteitis fibrosa may exhibit subperiosteal resorption. This may reflect the fact that trabecular bone, with a higher rate of turnover, is evaluated on bone biopsy, while X-ray features of erosion reflect changes in the cortical bone, with its slower rate of turnover.

The radiographic abnormalities of the skull, which occur in association with secondary hyperparathyroidism, include (a) a diffuse 'ground glass' appearance; (b) a generalized mottled or granular appearance which probably represents areas of increased resorption alternating with sclerotic areas; (c) the presence of focal radiolucent defects; and (d) focal areas of sclerosis. Dental X-rays may reveal the loss of lamina dura, although such a finding is non-specific. Slowly developing deformities of the pelvis can occur in patients with secondary hyperparathyroidism (*Figure 7.5*); these deformities are presumably brought about because of rapid bone remodeling in a part of the skeleton subject to weight-bearing.

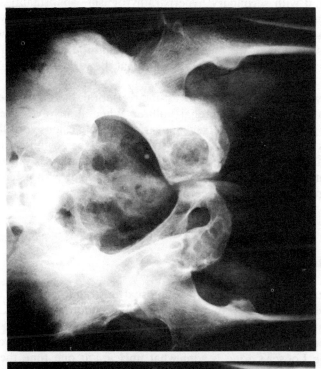

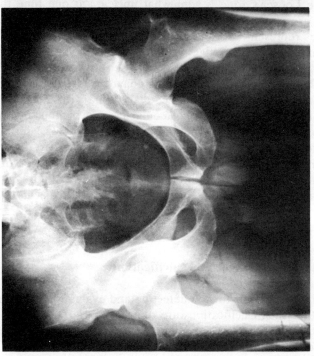

Figure 7.5 Profound radiographic features of secondary hyperparathyroidism developed in the pelvis of a man with advanced renal failure. This man, who had no symptoms related to his skeleton, developed a progressive deformity of the pelvis with cystic changes and patchy osteosclerosis (*right*) over 3 years after the initial X-ray (*left*); most of this developed before his renal failure had progressed to a degree at which dialysis was required. The skeletal lesions showed substantial improvement following subtotal parathyroidectomy

In uremic children with secondary hyperparathyroidism, abnormalities of the growth zone are common. The radiographic distinction between secondary hyperparathyroidism arising due to uremia from true 'rickets' may be difficult; with the former there is no widening of the metaphyseal zone, and the metaphyseal lucent zone, which blends into the subperiosteal resorption at the surface of the cortex, is very irregular[60].

Osteosclerosis, which commonly involves the vertebral bodies or pelvis, is common in patients with advanced renal failure. When it involves the spine, osteosclerosis may give the 'rugger jersey' appearance. Such lesions correlate best with other features of osteitis fibrosa[93]. An association between osteosclerosis and osteomalacia has also been reported[78], although the explanation is uncertain; it seems possible that the presence of osteosclerosis in a patient with osteomalacia could represent a remnant of prior hyperparathyroidism.

Radiographic features of osteomalacia

Specific X-ray features of osteomalacia are unusual in uremic patients, even in those with extensive osteomalacia. In our experience, pseudofractures or Looser's zones, which appear as wide, straight radiolucent bands abutting upon the cortex of bone and usually perpendicular to the long axis of the bone, are uncommon. The pathogenesis of the Looser's zone is somewhat unclear; at one time they were thought to arise as areas of erosion around nutrient arteries. Recent data suggest that pseudofractures represent undisplaced, 'stress' fractures, with resorption and slow healing around the fracture edge. A scintiscan of bone with technetium-labeled (^{99m}Tc) diphosphonate may be the most sensitive means for detecting pseudofractures. The other X-ray features of osteomalacia are non-specific. Some degree of rarefaction, particularly of the medullary bone with increased cortical striation, is commonly seen. Patients with osteomalacia may demonstrate profound generalized demineralization, but this finding is non-specific. The term 'dialysis osteopenia' is indeterminant as to the nature of the skeletal disorder; it seems likely that such patients may have had some degree of osteomalacia. The occurrence of fractures, particularly of the ribs, vertebral bodies, and hips, is more common in those with osteomalacia than in uremic patients lacking osteomalacia[78].

Radiographic features of extraskeletal calcification

Serial X-rays are the best means for the detection and evaluation of extraskeletal calcifications, whether such calcifications are tumoral, periarticular, or vascular. Profound calcifications of the small vessels of the lung may be detected by scintiscan at a time when they are not visible on X-ray[22]. The clinical features associated with such calcifications obviously vary with their site and their extent.

Quantitation of bone mass from radiographic measurement

Various techniques, utilizing measurements on radiographs, have been employed to evaluate bone mass. Measurements of the thickness of the cortex of the metacarpals and the cortical/total width ratios have been employed. These show a progressive decrease in 'bone mass' over time in patients with uremia. This loss of cortical bone mass may not correlate with either the type of extent of bone disease as identified by iliac crest bone biopsy[37]. In a longitudinal study of patients undergoing treatment with hemodialysis, a low-order correlation was seen between the quantity of heparin given and the rate of decrease in metacarpal cortical bone width in the male patients. Other observations suggest that rate of loss of cortical bone mass may depend upon the concentration of calcium utilized in dialysate[9].

Bone scintiscan

Scintiscans of bone, which utilize technetium-labeled diphosphonate, are of value in detecting and following the course of skeletal disease in patients with renal osteodystrophy. They may be useful in estimating the degree of secondary hyperparathyroidism or osteitis fibrosa; this is usually manifested by a symmetrical increase in uptake of the diphosphonate both by the axial skeleton and around the epiphyseal areas of the long bones[63]. The scintiscan may be of value in osteomalacia, with the identification of pseudofractures that are not visible on X-ray. Also, the scintiscan may be of value in the detection of ectopic calcification, particularly in the lungs and other soft tissues.

MANAGEMENT OF RENAL OSTEODYSTROPHY

Control of hyperphosphatemia

One essential goal in the management of patients with advanced renal failure (*Table 7.4*) is the prevention of hyperphosphatemia. The data indicating that phosphate retention plays a major role in the pathogenesis of renal osteodystrophy are quite convincing. Also, there is a direct contribution of hyperphosphatemia to extraskeletal calcification in uremia. Patients undergoing hemodialysis exhibit a 'saw tooth' pattern in their serum phosphorus levels, with a substantial fall during each dialysis; under these conditions a predialysis serum phosphorus level of 1.21–1.72 mmol/l (3.5–5.0 mg/dl) may be ideal. Two therapeutic procedures are generally needed to achieve appropriate levels of serum phosphorus: (a) a modest degree of phosphate restriction with total dietary phosphate intake to 27–35 mmol/day (800–1000 mg/day); and (b) the regular ingestion of aluminum-containing phosphate binders. The compounds employed, aluminum carbonate or aluminum hydroxide, render phosphate non-absorbable, both the phosphate ingested in the diet and the endogenous phosphate secreted into the intestinal lumen. The dosage of phosphate binders that is required varies widely from patient to patient and may vary from four to six capsules per day to as many as 30 to 40 capsules per day. A small number, perhaps less then 5–10% of dialysis patients, have normal serum phosphorus levels without the need for phosphate binders. This variability may depend on the intake of phosphate in the diet and differing phosphate absorption in individual patients

Table 7.4 Outline of management of renal osteodystrophy (*see text*) (modified from Coburn and Slatopolsky[20])

(1) Control serum phosphorus (i.e. 1.21–1.72 mmol/l, 3.5–5.0 mg/dl)
    (a) Restrict dietary phosphorus intake (27–35 mmol/day, 0.8–1.0 g/day)
    (b) Phosphate-binding antacids: aluminum hydroxide or carbonate – dosage adjusted on individual basis
    (c) Avoid hypophosphatemia

(2) Adequate calcium intake (when serum phosphorus is controlled)
    (a) Oral calcium supplements to provide 25 mmol/day, 1 g/day
    (b) Appropriate dialysate calcium (i.e. 1.5–1.625 mmol/l, 6.0–6.5 mg/dl)

(3) Vitamin D sterols – there should be adequate control of serum phosphorus
    Indications for treatment
    (a) Hypocalcemia (less than 2.25 mmol/l, 9.0 mg/dl)
    (b) Overt 2° hyperparathyroidism (high iPTH and bone erosions) with serum calcium less than 2.75 mmol/l, 11.0 mg/dl
    (c) Osteomalacia with 2° hyperparathyroidism
    (d) Most children with chronic renal failure
    (e) Renal failure with concomitant anticonvulsant therapy
    (f) Proximal myopathy
    (g) ? Prophylaxis in dialysis patients or chronic renal failure
    Approximate daily doses of various sterols (individualized)
    (a) Vitamin D_2 or D_3: 10 000–200 000 iu/day (0.25–5 mg/day)
    (b) Dihydrotachysterol: 0.25–2.0 mg/day
    (c) 25-hydroxyvitamin D_3 (calcifediol): 25–100 µg/day
    (d) 1,25-dihydroxyvitamin D_3 (calcitriol): 0.25–1.0 µg/day
    (e) 1α-hydroxyvitamin D_3: 0.5–2.0 µg/day

(4) Parathyroidectomy: indications – evidence of secondary hyperparathyroidism, such as bone erosions and significantly increased iPTH *plus* any of the following:
    (a) Persistent hypercalcemia (serum calcium more than 2.88–3.0 mmol/l, 11.5–12.0 mg/dl)
    (b) Progressive or symptomatic extraskeletal calcification*
    (c) Persistently elevated serum (calcium and phosphorus products)*
    (d) Pruritus not responding to other treatment
    (e) Calciphylaxis (ischemic ulcers and necrosis)
    (f) Symptomatic hypercalcemia after renal transplantation

(5) Other considerations:
    (a) Appropriate dialysate magnesium (i.e. 0.6–1.0 mg/dl, 0.25–0.35 mmol/l (0.5–0.7 mEq/l)
    (b) Appropriate water treatment for preparing dialysate (to remove fluoride, aluminum, sulfate, calcium and magnesium)
    (c) Avoid unnecessary treatment with barbiturates, phenytoin or glutethimide
    (d) Normalize acid–base status

* Hyperparathyroidism may recur if hyperphosphatemia is not prevented postoperatively.

The association between the excessive accumulation of aluminum and the occurrence of dialysis encephalopathy and the syndrome of 'fracturing osteomalacia' raises a question about the assumed safety of aluminum-containing phosphate binders. The 'outbreaks' of these syndromes have occurred with the probable source of the aluminum being the water used for preparing dialysate; however, there are other cases with aluminum accumulation that may occur via the intestinal absorption of aluminum present in phosphate binders. In considering the risks of phosphate binders, almost all patients with end-stage uremia will develop severe secondary hyperparathyroidism or extraskeletal calcifications if hyperphosphatemia is not prevented. On the other hand, severe aluminum accumulation may occur in only a small fraction of uremic patients; thus, the therapeutic choice of using these aluminum-containing compounds seems fairly obvious until other types of phosphate-binding compounds are developed.

Adequate calcium in both diet and dialysate

Calcium deficiency should be avoided by maintaining both adequate dietary intake of calcium and the use of an appropriate concentration of calcium in the dialysate. Because of restriction of dairy products in the diet, the intake of calcium is below normal in most patients with renal insufficiency[19]. It would seem advisable to increase the dietary intake of calcium to 37.5 mmol/day (1500 mg/day) or more which will generally result in a neutral or positive calcium balance in most patients with advanced renal failure; and a dietary supplement of calcium, 25 mmol/day (1.0 g/day), has been recommended[17, 20].

There may be both practical and theoretical problems with the prescriptions of oral calcium supplements. First, hypercalcemia may be seen in uremic patients given oral calcium supplements, particularly when the patients also receive active forms of vitamin D. When one gives an active vitamin D sterol to enhance the efficiency of calcium absorption by a dialysis patient, such a patient has no mechanism for adjusting the renal excretion of calcium; also, he undergoes dialysis against a dialysate calcium level that often exceeds the diffusible calcium level in the blood. Thus, it is not surprising that hypercalcemia may occur unless the rate of bone accretion exceeds the rate of its resorption. When the skeleton is not acting as a sump for calcium deposition, hypercalcemia may ensue during therapy with calcium even with doses of $1,25(OH)_2D_3$ that fail to lead to physiological blood levels of $1,25(OH)_2D_3$. Thus, there is a theoretical argument that calcium supplementation should not be given to patients who are receiving treatment with an active vitamin D sterol. Unfortunately, controlled data are not available to support or refute this recommendation.

The dialysate calcium level should be at a concentration that does not produce a negative balance for calcium during the dialysis procedure, and dialysate calcium levels of 1.5–1.75 mmol/l (3.0–3.5 mEq/l) are probably optimal. With dialysate concentrations above 1.75 mmol/l (3.5 mEq/l), there is little evidence for a beneficial effect on bone and there may be a chance of persistent hypercalcemia, with the possibility of detrimental effects.

Prevention of hypermagnesemia

Since the kidney is the major route for the excretion of magnesium it is not surprising that hypermagnesemia can occur in a renal failure patient following an increase in magnesium intake. This most commonly occurs following the ingestion of a laxative containing magnesium (that is, magnesium oxide, cascara segrada, etc.) or an antacid which contains magnesium. A dialysate magnesium of 0.6–1.0 mg/dl (0.25–0.35 mmol/l, 0.5–0.7 mEq/l) will usually result in predialysis serum magnesium levels that are slightly above normal; and significant hypomagnesemia during the postdialysis period can be prevented. The use of a dialysate magnesium of 0.75 mmol/l (1.5 mEq/l) leads to moderate hypermagnesemia in dialysis patients. A suggestion that a high level of magnesium in dialysate might be used to suppress secretion of PTH has not been substantiated by long-term studies.

With intestinal disorders that impair the intestinal absorption of magnesium, hypomagnesemia and magnesium depletion can develop in patients with renal insufficiency[29]. This may be associated with decreased secretion of PTH and reduced responsiveness of the skeleton to PTH with the appearance of marked hypocalcemia.

Treatment with vitamin D sterols

With knowledge that the kidney is the major organ responsible for the generation of 1,25-dihydroxyvitamin D_3 (calcitriol), the most active known hormonal form of vitamin D, it is apparent that therapy with this sterol should be considered. Presently, there are no firm data on when in the course of renal insufficiency, treatment with an active vitamin D sterol should be initiated. Also, there are no clear guidelines concerning the appropriate dosage. In a study of three patients with moderate renal insufficiency (creatinine clearance of 32–51 ml/min), treatment with calcitriol, 1.0 µg/day, for 6 months was associated with a slight increase in serum calcium, a fall in serum iPTH, and improvement in mild bone disease. Urinary calcium excretion increased moderately in two patients and markedly in the third. Thus, these observations suggest that calcitriol was safe and could produce a beneficial effect[36]. Other studies carried out in patients with more advanced renal failure suggested that a reversible deterioration of renal function occurred during treatment with $1,25(OH)_2D_3$[16]. The latter investigators did not prevent hypercalcemia or an increase in serum phosphorus during such treatment. Thus, it is possible that treatment with a vitamin D sterol might enhance the absorption of calcium and phosphorus, aggravate the hyperphosphatemia, and be a factor which contributes to an increased calcium content of the kidney; together, these processes might lead to more rapid deterioration of renal function. On the other hand, if there was suppression of PTH secretion, treatment with calcitriol might have a beneficial effect, particularly as PTH may be a factor which contributes to the progressive decrease in renal function.

In patients with advanced renal insufficiency and those undergoing hemodialysis, the lesions of secondary hyperparathyroidism are those which show the most

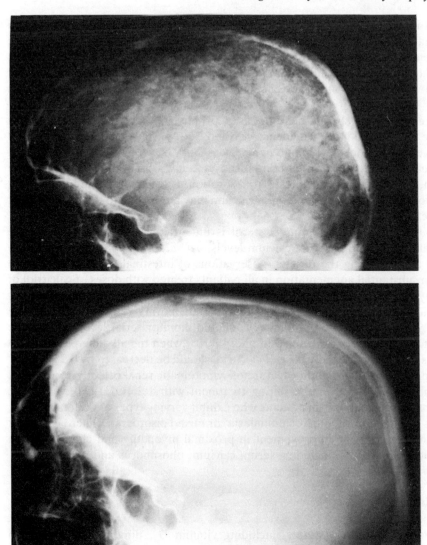

Figure 7.6 Features of secondary hyperparathyroidism affecting the skull of a renal failure patient undergoing regular hemodialysis (*above*). There are areas of lucency interspersed with mottled sclerosis; 6 months after initiation of treatment with calcitriol $(1,25(OH)_2D_3)$, the skull X-ray had returned to normal (*below*)

improvement during treatment with calcitriol. Thus, features of secondary hyperparathyroidism, such as markedly elevated serum iPTH, and elevated alkaline phosphatase, skeletal X-ray findings of subperiosteal resorption, and a bone biopsy showing osteitis fibrosa, generally improve with calcitriol therapy (*Figure 7.6*). In patients with features of secondary hyperparathyroidism and pretreatment hypercalcemia (that is, serum calcium levels of more than 2.7 mmol/l, 10.8 mg/dl) there is frequently a rapid worsening of hypercalcemia, probably due to the extensive parathyroid hyperplasia. In patients whose skeletal lesions show features of both osteomalacia and osteitis fibrosa, an improvement in both the osteomalacic component and the lesion of osteitis fibrosa is usual. Patients whose bone biopsies show isolated osteomalcia and little or no evidence of secondary hyperparathyroidism often show little or no improvement of the skeletal disease during therapy with calcitriol[38, 76].

Whether calcitriol should be used as a prophylactic agent in patients with end-stage uremia and lacking evidence of osteodystrophy is uncertain. Preliminary data suggest that patients with mild bone disease may be prone to the development of hypercalcemia[4, 6]. Thus, when bone turnover is low with a limited rate of bone accretion, the stimulation of intestinal absorption of calcium in a uremic patient with no route for the renal excretion of calcium may predispose to the development of hypercalcemia.

When therapy with a vitamin D sterol is undertaken, the dosage should be individualized. Although serum calcium levels, *per se*, have been suggested as the criterion for increasing the dosage, observations of intestinal calcium absorption indicate a substantial augmentation in all patients treated with doses of calcitriol of $0.5 \, \mu g/day$ or above; moreover, patients are prone to develop hypercalcemia after the serum alkaline phosphatase had decreased to the normal range. Thus, a dosage of $0.5–0.75 \, \mu g/day$ may be optimal. One should monitor serial levels of alkaline phosphatase as well as of calcium and phosphorus; when the alkaline phosphatase decreases to normal, the daily dose of calcitriol should be decreased by $0.25 \, \mu g/day$.

Proximal myopathy is another feature of symptomatic renal osteodystrophy that shows substantial improvement during treatment with $1,25(OH)_2D_3$. Moreover, the myopathy may improve in patients who exhibit varying types of skeletal lesions, including osteitis fibrosa, pure osteomalacia, or mixed disorders[38]. There is little or no relationship between improvement in proximal myopathy and changes in the biochemical parameters, including serum calcium, phosphorus and iPTH.

Other vitamin D sterols

Several other vitamin D sterols, including vitamin D_2, dihydrotachysterol and 25-hydroxycholecalciferol (calcifediol) have been utilized in uremic patients: 1α-hydroxyvitamin D_3 has undergone extensive usage in Europe; available data suggest that 1α-hydroxyvitamin D_3 is converted to and has actions similar to those of $1,25(OH)_2D_3$. Dihydrotachysterol (DHT), when given in doses of 0.2–2.0 mg/day, has been associated with improvement of uremic secondary hyperparathyroidism. Dihydrotachysterol presumably acts in patients with end-stage uremia because of the chemical structure of the A-ring of the sterol. The A-ring of DHT has a 3-hydroxyl group that is rotated 180°, so this 3-hydroxyl radical lies in a 'pseudo 1α-hydroxyl' position. This is presumably why DHT can act without 1α-hydroxylation by the kidney. Calcifediol (25-hydroxycholecalciferol) has been studied in a series of uremic patients studied with serial bone biopsies. Dosages of calciferol which elevated the plasma 25(OH)D to values above normal were associated with a reversal of features of secondary hyperparathyroidism; in some instances, there was improved mineralization. The failure to see an effect until the serum levels of 25(OH)D were above normal may suggest that the $25(OH)D_3$ exerts its action only when present in pharmacological quantities and with blood levels similar to those seen with vitamin D toxicity.

Another sterol which is being investigated is $24,25(OH)_2D_3$. This sterol, generated largely in the kidney, is found in reduced quantities in the serum of patients with advanced renal insufficiency. Short-term studies carried out in patients with nutritional vitamin D deficiency provide evidence that 24,25-dihydroxyvitamin D_3 may have effects that are qualitatively dissimilar from those of $1,25(OH)_2D_3$ alone. Thus, serum calcium levels fell and alkaline phosphatase levels increased in dialysis patients given $24,25(OH)_2D_3$[47]; moreover, there was evidence for improved mineralization in patients given $24,25(OH)_2D_3$ compared to those receiving $1,25(OH)_2D_3$ alone[40]. Although such data suggest that $24,25(OH)_2D_3$ may have different effects from those of $1,25(OH)_2D_3$, results in experimental animals provide little confirmation of a necessary action for this sterol[87]. Further physiological or pharmacological studies are needed to verify a possible role of $24,25(OH)_2D_3$.

Parathyroid surgery

A reduction of the magnitude of secondary hyperparathyroidism and improvement of osteitis fibrosa often occur with appropriate medical therapy described above. Under certain circumstances, however, surgical removal of hyperplastic parathyroid tissue may be indicated. With overt secondary hyperparathyroidism, characterized by a combination of X-ray evidence of bone erosions or histological features of osteitis fibrosa plus markedly elevated serum iPTH levels, parathyroid surgery may be indicated with any of the following *additional* features:

(1) persistent elevation of serum calcium to above 11.5 mg/dl;
(2) an increase in serum calcium and phosphorus products to 6.5–6.9 mmol/l × mmol/l (75–80 mg/dl × mg/dl), or above combined with progressive soft tissue calcification despite vigorous efforts at phosphate restriction;
(3) progressive skeletal lesions of secondary hyperparathyroidism with debilitating symptoms when a very prompt clinical response to surgery is highly desirable;
(4) intractable pruritis which is recalcitrant to standard medical therapy;
(5) calciphylaxis; perhaps the most imperative.

One important consideration is the availability of a surgeon who is highly experienced with parathyroid surgery. It is imperative that four parathyroid glands be identified, since the presence of a single parathyroid adenoma in a patient with chronic renal failure is exceedingly uncommon. The favored surgical approach should be removal of 3½ to 3¾ glands. Total parathyroidectomy with transplantation of some parathyroid tissue to the forearm is favored by some, but this seems to carry an increased risk of hypoparathyroidism and adds unnecessary surgery. During the postoperative period marked hypocalcemia, hypophosphatemia, and hypomagnesemia may occur with their severity depending on the extent of abnormality of the bone preoperatively. Pretreatment with calcitriol may aid in the management of hypocalcemia. Tetanic seizures, which lead to fractures, can occur after parathyroid surgery; of interest, such seizures are likely to occur during or immediately after hemodialysis. Therapy with supplemental calcium and an active vitamin D sterol may be needed for weeks or months. A return of plasma alkaline phosphatase to normal may be an indication that such treatment can be reduced or even discontinued. Efforts to prevent hyperphosphatemia after surgery are imperative to prevent a recurrence of secondary hyperparathyroidism.

References

1 ALVAREZ-UDE, F., FEEST, R. G., WARD, M. K., PIERIDES, A. M., ELLISE H. A., PEART, K. M., SIMPSON, W., WEIGHTMAN, D. and KERR, D. S. Hemodialysis bone disease: correlation between clinical, histologic and other findings. *Kidney International*, **14**, 68–73 (1978)

2 ANAST, O. A., MOHS, J. M., KAPLAN, S. L. and BURNS, T. W. Evidence for parathyroid failure in magnesium deficiency. *Science*, **177**, 606–608 (1972)

3 AVIOLI, L. V. Collagen metabolism, uremia and bone. *Kidney International*, **4**, 105–115 (1973)

4 BAKER, L. R. I., MUIR, J. W., CATELL, W. R., TUCKER, K. A., SHARMAN, L. V., GOODWIN, J. F., MARSH, P. F., HATEL, W., MORGAN, A. G. and CHAPUT de SAINTONGE, D. M. Use of 1,25(OH)$_2$-vitamin D$_3$ in prevention of renal osteodystrophy: preliminary observations. *Contributions to Nephrology*, **18**, 147–151 (1979)

5 BERLYNE, G. M. and SHAW, A. G. Red eyes in renal failure. *Lancet*, **1**, 4–7 (1967)

6 BINSWANGER, U., FISCHER, J. A., ISELIN, H., OSWALD, N., FREI, D. and WILLIMANN, P. 1,25-dihydroxycholecalciferol treatment of clinically asymptomatic renal osteodystrophy. *Mineral and Electrolyte Metabolism*, **2**, 103–115 (1979)

7 BIRGE, S. J. and HADDAD, J. G. 25-hydroxycholecalciferol stimulation of muscle metabolism. *Journal of Clinical Investigation*, **56**, 1100–1107 (1975)

8 BONAVITA, J. A. and DALINKA, M. K. Shoulder erosions in renal osteodystrophy. *Skeletal Radiology*, **5**, 105–108 (1980)

9 BONE, J. M., DAVISON, A. M. and ROBSON, J. S. Role of dialysate calcium concentration in osteoporosis in patients on hemodialysis. *Lancet*, **1**, 1047–1049 (1972)

10 BORDIER, P. J., ARNAUD, C., HAWKER, C., TUN-CHOT, S. and HIOCO, D. Relationship between serum immunoreactive parathyroid hormone. Osteoclastic and osteocytic bone resorption and serum calcium in primary hyperparathyroidism and osteomalacia. In *Clinical Aspects of Bone Diseases*, edited by B. Frame, A. N. Parfitt and H. H. Dunach, pp. 222–228, Amsterdam, Excerpta Medica (1973)

11 BORDIER, P. J., TUN-CHOT, S., EASTWOOD, J. B., FOURNIER, A. and DE WARDNER, H. E. Lack of histological evidence of vitamin D abnormality in the bones of anephric patients. *Clinical Science*, **44**, 33–41 (1973)

12 BRICKMAN, A. S., COBURN, J. W., MASSRY, S. G. and NORMAN, A. W. 1,25-dihydroxyvitamin D$_3$ in normal man and patients with renal failure. *Annals of Internal Medicine*, **80**, 161–168 (1974)

13 BRUMBAUGH, P. F., HAUSSLER, D. H., BRESSLER, R. and HAUSSLER, M. R. Radioreceptor assay for 1α,25-dihydroxyvitamin D₃. *Science*, **183**, 1089–1091 (1974)

14 CARR, D., DAVIDSON, J. K., McMILLAN, M. and DAVIDSON, J., Renal osteodystrophy: an underdiagnosed condition. *Clinical Radiology*, **31**, 55–59 (1980)

15 CHESNEY, R. W., MOORTHY, A. V., EISMAN, J. A., JAX, D. K., MAZESS, R. B. and DeLUCA, H. F. Increased growth after long-term and 1α,25-dihydroxyvitamin D₃ in childhood renal osteodystrophy. *New England Journal of Medicine*, **298**, 238–242 (1978)

16 CHRISTIANSEN, C., RØDBRO, P., CHRISTENSEN, M. S., HARTNACK, B. and TRANSBØL, I.Deterioration of renal function during treatment of chronic renal failure with 1,25-dihydroxycholecalciferol. *Lancet*, **2**, 700–703 (1978)

17 CLARKSON, E. M., EASTWOOD, J. B., KOUTSAIMANIS K. G. and DE WARDNER, H. E. Net intestinal absorption of calcium in patients with chronic renal failure. *Kidney International*, **3**, 258–263 (1973)

18 COBURN, J. W., HARTENBOWER, D. L. and BRICKMAN, A. S. Advances in vitamin D metabolism as they pertain to chronic renal disease. *American Journal of Clinical Nutrition*, **29**, 1283–1299 (1976)

19 COBURN, J. W., KOPPLE, M. H., BRICKMAN, A. S. and MASSRY, S. G. Study of intestinal absorption of calcium in patients with renal failure. *Kidney International*, **3**, 264–273 (1973)

20 COBURN, J. W. and SLATOPOLSKY, E. Vitamin D, parathyroid hormone, and renal osteodystrophy. In *The Kidney*, edited by B. M. Brenner and F. Rector, pp. 2213–2305, Philadelphia, Saunders (1981)

21 CONGER, J. D., HAMMOND, W. S., ALFREY, A. C., CONTIGUGLIA, S. R., STANFORD, R. E. and HUFFER, W. E. Pulmonary calcification in chronic dialysis patients. Clinical and pathologic studies. *Annals of Internal Medicine*, **83**, 330–336 (1975)

22 DAVIS, B. A., POULOSE, K. P. and REBA, R. C. Letter: Scanning for uremic pulmonary calcifications. *Annals of Internal Medicine*, **85**, 132 (1976)

23 DELLING, G., LÜHMANN, H., BULLA, M., FUCHS, C., HENNING, H. V., JANSEN, J. L. J., KOHNLE, W. and SCHULZ, W. The action of 1,25(OH)₂D₃ on turnover kinetic, remodelling surfaces and structure of trabecular bone in chronic renal failure. *Contributions to Nephrology*, **18**, 105–121 (1979)

24 EASTWOOD, J. B., HARRIS, E., STAMP, T. C. B. and DE WARDENER, H. E. Vitamin D-deficiency in the osteomalacia of chronic renal failure. *Lancet*, **2**, 1209–1211 (1976)

25 EISMAN, J. A., HAMSTRA, A. J., KREAM, B. E. and DE LUCA, H. F. 1,25-dihydroxyvitamin D in biological fluids: a simplified and sensitive assay. *Science*, **193**, 1021–1023 (1976)

26 ELLIS, H. A., McCARTHY, J. H. and HERRINGTON, J. Bone aluminum in haemodialysed patients and in rats injected with aluminum chloride; relationship to impaired bone mineralization. *Journal of Clinical Pathology*, **32**, 832–844 (1979)

27 ESTEP, H., SHAW, W., WATLINGTON, C. O., HOBE, C., HOLLAND, W. and TUCKER, H. ST. G. Hypocalcemia due to reversible hypomagnesemia and parathyroid hormone unresponsiveness. *Journal of Clinical Endocrinology*, **29**, 842–848 (1969)

28 FELSENFELD, A. J., HARRELSON, J. M., WELLS, S. A. and GUTMAN, R. A. Severe osteomalacia with hypercalcemia following subtotal parathyroidectomy. *Kidney International*, **16**, 952 (1979)

29 FREITAG, J., MARTIN, K. J., HRUSKA, K. A., ANDERSON, D., CONTRADES, M., LANDENSON, J., KLAHR, S. and SLATOPOLSKY, E. Impaired parathyroid hormone metabolism in patients with chronic renal failure. *New England Journal of Medicine*, **298,** 29–32 (1978)

30 GIPSTEIN, R. H., COBURN, J. W., ADAMS, D. A., LEE, D. B. N., PARSA, K. P., SELLERS, A., SUKI, W. N. and MASSRY, S. G. Calciphylaxis in man: a syndrome of tissue necrosis and vascular calcification in 11 patients with chronic renal disease. *Archives of Internal Medicine*, **136,** 1273–1280 (1976)

31 GOODHUE, W. W., DAVIS, J. N. and PORRI, R. S. Ischemic myopathy in uremic hyperparathyroidism. *Journal of the American Medical Association*, **221,** 911–912 (1972)

32 GRIFFITH, G. C., NICHOLS, G. Jr., ASHER, J. D. and FLANAGAN, B. Heparin osteoporosis. *Journal of the American Medical Association*, **193,** 85–94 (1965)

33 HAMPERS, C. L., KATZ, A. J., WILSON, R. E. and MERRILL, J. P. Disappearance of 'uremic' itching after subtotal parathyroidectomy. *New England Journal of Medicine*, **279,** 695–697 (1968)

34 HART, W., DUURSMA, S. A., VISSER, W. J. and NJIO, L. K. F. The hydroxyproline content of plasma of patients with impaired renal function. *Clinical Nephrology*, **4,** 104–108 (1975)

35 HAWKER, C. D. and DI BELLA, F. P. Parathyroid hormone in chronic renal failure: studies with two different parathyroid hormone immunoassays. *Contributions to Nephrology*, **20,** 2137 (1980)

36 HEALY, M. D., MALLUCHE, H. H., GOLDSTEIN, D. A., SINGER, F. R. and MASSRY, S. G. Effects of long-term therapy with calcitriol in patients with moderate renal failure. *Archives of Internal Medicine*, **140,** 1030–1033 (1980)

37 HENDERSON, R. G., RUSSELL, R. G. G., EARNSHAW, M. J., LEDINGHAM, J. G. G., OLIVER, D. O. and WOODS, C. G. Loss of metacarpal and iliac bone in chronic renal failure: influence of haemodialysis, parathyroid activity, type of renal disease, physical activity and heparin consumption. *Clinical Science*, **56,** 317–324 (1979)

38 HODSMAN, A. B., SHERRARD, D. J., WONG, E. G. C., BRICKMAN, A. S., LEE, D. B. N., ALFREY, A. C., SINGER, F. R., NORMAN, A. W. and COBURN, J. W. Vitamin D-resistant osteomalacia in hemodialysis patients lacking secondary hyperparathyroidism. *Annals of Internal Medicine*, **94,** 629–637 (1981)

39 HODSMAN, A. B., SHERRARD, D. J., BRICKMAN, A. S., ALFREY, A. C., GOODMAN, W. G., MALONEY, N., LEE, D. B. N. and COBURN, J. W. Bone aluminum in osteomalacic renal osteodystrophy correlation with excess osteoid. *Kidney International*, **19,** 127 (1981)

40 HODSMAN, A. B., WONG, E. G. C., SHERRARD, D. J., BRICKMAN, A. S., LEE, D. B. N., SINGER, F. R., NORMAN, A. W. and COBURN, J. W. Use of 24,25-dihydroxyvitamin D_3 in dialysis osteomalacia: preliminary results. In *Hormonal Control of Calcium Metabolism*, edited by D. V. Cohn, R. V. Talmage and J. L. Matthews, p. 460. Amsterdam, Excerpta Medica (1981)

41 HORST, R. L., LITTLEDIKE, E. T., GRAY, R. W. and NAPOLI, J. L. Impaired 24,25-dihydroxyvitamin D production in anephric human and pig. *Journal of Clinical Investigation*, **67,** 274–280 (1981)

42 HRUSKA, K. A., KOPELMAN, R., RUTHERFORD, W. E., KLAHR, S. and SLATOPOLSKY, E. Metabolism of immunoreactive parathyroid hormone in the dog: the role of the kidney and the effects of chronic renal disease. *Journal of Clinical Investigation*, **56**, 39–48 (1975)

43 JOHANNSEN, A., NIELSEN, H. E. and HANSEN, H. E. Bone maturation in children with chronic renal failure. Effect of 1α-hydroxyvitamin D_3 and renal transplantation. *Acta Radiologica Diagnosis*, **20**, 193–199 (1979)

44 KAEHNY, W. D., HEGG, A. P. and ALFREY, A. C. Gastrointestinal absorption of aluminum from aluminum-containing antacids. *New England Journal of Medicine*, **296**, 1389–1390 (1977)

45 KANIS, J. A., ADAMS, N. D., EARNSHAW, M., HEYNEN, G., LEDINGHAM, J. G. G., OLIVER, D. O., RUSSELL, R. G. G. and WOODS, C. G. Vitamin D, osteomalacia and chronic renal failure. In *Vitamin D: Biochemical, Chemical and Clinical Aspects Related to Calcium Metabolism*, edited by A. W. Norman, K. Schaefer, J. W. Coburn, H. F. DeLuca, D. Fraser, H. G. Grigoleit and D. v. Herrath, pp. 671–677. New York, Walter de Gruyter (1977)

46 KRAUT, J. A., SHINABERGER, J., SINGER, F. R., SHERRARD, D. J., SAXTON, J., HODSMAN, A. B., MILLER, J. H., KUROKAWA, K. and COBURN, J. W. Reduced parathyroid response to acute hypocalcemia in dialysis osteomalacia. *Clinical Research*, **29**, 102A (1981)

47 LLACH, F., BRICKMAN, A. S., SINGER, F. R. and COBURN, J. W. 24,25-dihydroxycholecalciferol, a vitamin D sterol with qualitatively unique effects in uremic man. *Metabolism of Bone Diseases and Related Research*, **2**, 11–15 (1979)

48 LLACH, F., MASSRY, S. G., SINGER, F. R., KUROKAWA, K., KAYE, J. H. and COBURN, J. W. Skeletal resistance of endogenous parathyroid hormone in patients with early renal failure: a possible cause for secondary hyperparathyroidism. *Journal of Clinical Endocrinology and Metabolism*, **41**, 338–345 (1975)

49 MALLETTE, L. E., PATTEN, B. M. and ENGEL, W. K. Neuromuscular disease in secondary hyperparathyroidism. *Annals of Internal Medicine*, **82**, 474–483 (1975)

50 MALLUCHE, H. H., RITZ, E. and LANGE, H. P. Bone histology in incipient and advanced renal failure. *Kidney International*, **9**, 355–362 (1976)

51 MALLUCHE, H. H., WERNER, E. and RITZ, E. Intestinal absorption of calcium and whole body calcium retention in incipient and advanced renal failure. *Mineral and Electrolyte Metabolism*, **1**, 263–270 (1978)

52 MASSRY, S. G., COBURN, J. W., LEE, D. B. N., JOWSEY, J. and KLEEMAN, C. R. Skeletal resistance to parathyroid hormone in renal failure: study in 105 human subjects. *Annals of Internal Medicine*, **78**, 357–264 (1973)

53 MASSRY, S. G., COBURN, J. W., LEE, D. B. N. and KLEEMAN, C. R. Effect of the infusion of parathyroid extract on serum calcium in patients with renal failure. In *Clinical Aspects of Metabolic Bone Disease*, edited by B. Frame, A. M. Parfitt and H. Duncan, pp. 578–581, Amsterdam, Excerpta Medica (1973)

54 MASSRY, S. G., POPOVTZER, M. M., COBURN, J. W., MAKOFF, D. L., MAXWELL, M. H. and KLEEMAN, C. R. Intractable pruritus as a manifestation of 2° hyperparathyroidism in uremia. Disappearance of itching following subtotal parathyroidectomy. *New England Journal of Medicine*, **279**, 697–700 (1968)

55 MASSRY, S. G., STEIN, R., GARTY, J., ARIEFF, A. I., COBURN, J. W., NORMAN, A. W. and FRIEDLER, R. M. Skeletal resistance to the calcemic action of parathyroid hormone in uremia: Role of $1,25(OH)_2D_3$. *Kidney International*, **9**, 467–474 (1976)

56 MATTHEWS, C., HEIMBERG, K. W., RITZ, E., AGOSTINI, B., FRITZSCHE, J. and HASSELBACK, W. Effect of 1,25-dihydroxycholecalciferol on impaired calcium transport by the sarcoplasmic reticulum in experimental uremia. *Kidney International*, **11**, 227–235 (1977)

57 MEEMA, H. E., OREOPOULOS, D. G., RABINOVICH, S., HUSDAN, H. and RAPAPORT, A. Periosteal new bone formation (periosteal neostasis) in renal osteodystrophy. *Radiology*, **110**, 513–522 (1974)

58 MEEMA, H. E., RABINOVICH, S., MEEMA, S., LLOYD, G. J. and OREOPOULOS, D. G. Improved radiological diagnosis of azotemic osteodystrophy. *Radiology*, **102**, 1–10 (1972)

59 MEEMA, H. E. and SCHATZ, D. L. Simple radiologic demonstration of cortical bone loss in thyrotoxicosis. *Radiology*, **97**, 9–15 (1970)

60 MEHLS, O., RITZ, E., BURKHARD, K., GILL, G., LINK, W., WILLICH, E. and SCHARER, K. Slipped epiphysis in renal osteodystrophy. *Archives of Diseases of Children*, **50**, 545–554 (1975)

61 MIRAHMADI, K. S., DUFFY, B. S., SHINABERGER, J. H. JOWSEY, J., MASSRY, S. G. and COBURN, J. W. A controlled evaluation of clinical and metabolic effects of dialysate calcium levels during regular dialysis. *Transactions of the American Society of Artificial Internal Organs*, **17**, 118–124 (1971)

62 MUSPRATT, S. Thoracic deformity and flail chest in renal osteodystrophy. *Journal of the American Medical Association*, **243**, 1458–1459 (1980)

63 OLGAARD, K., HEERFORDT, J. and MADSEN, S. Scintigraphic skeletal changes in uremic patients on regular hemodialysis. *Nephron*, **17**, 325–334 (1976)

64 PARKINSON, I. S., FEEST, T. G., WARD, M. K., FAWCETT, R. W. P. and KERR, D. N. S. Fracturing dialysis osteodystrophy and dialysis encephalopathy: and epidemiological survey. *Lancet*, **1**, 406–409 (1979)

65 PIERIDES, A. M., EDWARDS, W. G. Jr, CULLU, U. X., McCALL J. T. and ELLIS, H. A. Hemodialysis encephalopathy with osteomalacic fractures and muscle weakness. *Kidney International*, **18**, 115–124 (1980)

66 PIERIDES A. M., SKILLEN, A. W. and ELLIS, H. A. Serum alkaline phosphatase in azotemic and hemodialysis osteodystrophy: a study of isoenzyme patterns, their correlation with bone histology, and their changes in response to treatment with $1\alpha OHD_3$ and $1,25(OH)_2D_3$. *Journal of Laboratory Clinical Medicine*, **93**, 899–909 (1979)

67 PORTALE, A. A., BOOTH, B. E., TSAI, H. C. and MORRIS, R. C. Jr. Reduced plasma concentration of $1,25(OH)_2D$ in children with moderate renal insufficiency (MRI). *Kidney International*, **16**, (1979) (Abstract)

68 PRICE, P. A., PARTHEMORE, J. G. and DEFTOS, L. J. New biochemical marker for bone metabolism. Measurement by radioimmuoassay of bone GLA protein in the plasma of normal subjects and patients with bone disease. *Journal of Clinical Investigation*, **66**, 878–883 (1980)

69 RECKER, R. R., BLOTCKY, A. J., LEFFLER, J. A. and RACK, E. P. Evidence for aluminum absorption from the gastrointestinal tract and bone deposition by aluminum carbonate ingestion with normal renal function. *Journal of Laboratory Clinical Medicine*, **80**, 810–815 (1977)

70 REISS, E. and CANTERBURY, J. M. Genesis of hyperparathyroidism. *American Journal of Medicine*, **50**, 679–685 (1971)

71 RITZ, E., MALLUCHE, H. H., KREMPIEN B. and MEHLS, O. Bone histology in renal insufficiency. In *Calcium Metabolism in Renal Failure and Nephrolithesis,* edited by D. S. David, pp. 197–233. New York: John Wiley and Sons (1977)

72 RITZ, E., MEHLS, O., BOMMER, J., SCHMIDT-GAYK, H., FIEGEL, P. and REITINGER, H. Vascular calcifications under maintenance hemodialysis. *Klinische Wochenschrift,* **55,** 375–378 (1977)

73 RITZ, E., PRAGER, P., KREMPIEN, B., BOMMER, J., MALLUCHE, H. H. and SCHMIDT-GAYK, H. Skeletal X-ray findings and bone histology in patients on hemodialysis. *Kidney International,* **13,** 316–323 (1978)

74 RUTHERFORD, W. E., BORDIER, P., MARIE, P., HRUSKA, K., HARTER, H., GREENWALT, A., BLONDIN, J., HADDAD, J., BRICKER, N. and SLATOPOLSKY, E. Phosphate control and 25-hydroxycholecalciferol administration in preventing experimental renal osteodystrophy in the dog. *Journal of Clinical Investigation,* **60,** 332–341 (1977)

75 SCHWARTZ, K. V. Heart block in renal failure and hypercalcemia. *Journal of the American Medical Association Letters,* **235,** 1550 (1976)

76 SHERRARD, D. J., COBURN, J. W., BRICKMAN, A. S., SINGER, F. R. and MALONEY, N. Skeletal response to treatment with 1,25-dihydroxy-vitamin D in renal failure. *Contributions to Nephrology,* **18,** 92–97 (1980)

77 SIMMONS, J. M., WILSON, C. J., POTTER, D. E. and HOLLIDAY, M. A. Relation of calorie deficiency to growth failure in children on hemodialysis and the growth response to calorie supplementation. *New England Journal of Medicine,* **285,** 653–656 (1971)

78 SIMPSON, W., ELLIS, H. A., KERR, D. N. S., McELROY, M., McNARY, R. A. and PEART, K. N. Bone disease in long-term haemodialysis: the association of radiological with histologic abnormalities. *British Journal of Radiology,* **49,** 105–110 (1976)

79 SLATOPOLSKY, E., CAGLAR, S., GRADOWSKA, L., CANTERBURY, J., REISS, E. and BRICKER, N. S. On the prevention of secondary hyperparathyroidism in experimental chronic renal disease using 'proportional reduction' of dietary phosphorus intake. *Kidney International,* **2,** 147–151 (1972)

80 SLATOPOLSKY, E., GRAY, R., ADAMS, N. D., LEWIS, J., HRUSKA, K., MARTIN, K., KLAHR, S., DeLUCA, H. and LEMANN, J. Low serum levels of $1,25(OH)_2D_3$ are not responsible for the development of secondary hyperparathyroidism in early renal failure. *Kidney International,* **14,** 733 (1978) (Abstract)

81 SMITH, R. and STERN, G. Myopathy, osteomalacia and hyperparathyroidism. *Brain,* **90,** 593–602 (1967)

82 SMITH, F. W. and JUNOR, J. R. Xeroradiography of the hand in patients with renal ostcodystrophy. *British Journal of Radiology,* **50,** 261–263 (1977)

83 SOMERVILLE, P. J. and KAYE, M. Resistance to parathyroid hormone in renal failure: Role of vitamin D metabolites. *Kidney International,* **14,** 245–254 (1978)

84 SOMERVILLE, P. J. and KAYE, M. Evidence that resistance to the calcemic action of parathyroid hormone in rats with acure uremia is caused by phosphate retention. *Kidney International,* **16,** 552–560 (1979)

85 SUNDARAM, M., JOYCE, P. F., SHIELDS, J. B., RIAZ, M. A. and SAGAR, S. Terminal phalangeal tufts: earliest site of renal osteodystrophy findings in hemodialysis patients. *American Journal of Roentgenology,* **133,** 25–29 (1979)

86 SWENSON, R. S., WEISINGER, J. R., RUGGERI, J. L., *et al.* Evidence that parathyroid hormone is not required for phosphate homeostasis in renal failure. *Metabolism*, **24**, 199–209 (1975)

87 TANAKA, Y. and DE LUCA, H. F. Biological activity of 24,24-difluoro-25-hydroxy-vitamin D₃. *Journal of Biological Chemistry*, **254**, 7163–7167 (1979)

88 TAYLOR, C. M., MAWER, E. B., WALLACE, J. E., St JOHN, J., COCHRAN, M., RUSSELL, R. G. G. and KANIS, J. A. The absence of 24,25-dihydroxycholecalciferol in anephric patients. *Clinical Science and Molecular Medicine*, **55**, 541–547 (1978)

89 TEITELBAUM, S. L., BERGFELD, M. A., FREITAG, J., HRUSKA, K. A. and SLATOPOLSKY, E. Do parathyroid hormone and 1,25-dihydroxyvitamin D modulate bone formation n uremia? *Journal of Clinical Endocrinology and Metabolism*, **51**, 247–251 (1980)

90 VERBERCKMOES, R., BOUILLON, R. and KREMPIEN, B. Disappearance of vascular calcifications during treatment of renal osteodystrophy. *Annals of Internal Medicine*, **82**, 529–533 (1975)

91 WARD, M. K., FEEST, T. G., ELLIS, H. A., PARKINSON, I. S. and KERR, D. N. S. Osteomalacic dialysis osteodystrophy: Evidence for a water-borne aetiological agent, probably aluminum. *Lancet*, **1**, 841–845 (1978)

92 WILLS, M. R. and JENKINS, M. V. The effect of uraemic metabolites on parathyroid extract induced bone resorption *in vitro*. *Clinica Chimica Acta*, **73**, 121–125 (1976)

93 ZIMMERMAN, H. B. Osteosclerosis in chronic renal disease. Report of 4 cases associated with secondary hyperparathyroidism. *American Journal of Roentgenology*, **88**, 1152–1169 (1962)

8
Asymptomatic hypercalcemia and primary hyperparathyroidism

Hunter Heath III and Don C. Purnell

STATEMENT OF THE PROBLEM

It is obvious from the nature of hyperparathyroidism that there will be cases ranging from a marked degree of the disease all the way down to the normal state. The less the degree of hyperparathyroidism, the less the chemical findings will deviate from normal and the more difficult the diagnosis will be.

Albright and Reifenstein[2]

Hypercalcemia has been recognized as a metabolic abnormality only within our century, and for many years was seldom recognized outside medical centers. After discovery that the parathyroid glands are essential for maintenance of the plasma calcium concentration, however, hyperparathyroidism was soon postulated, found, and treated surgically[19, 36]. Nonetheless, primary hyperparathyroidism was considered an uncommon disease and one generally accompanied by symptomatic hypercalcemia, plus varying combinations of urolithiasis, renal failure and bone disease[36]. The occasional serendipitous discovery of hypercalcemia in people having few or no symptoms, however, raised the possibility that hypercalcemia – and primary hyperparathyroidism – could exist in a mild form. Several important screening studies published in the 1960s suggested that the prevalence of primary hyperparathyroidism in the adult US population might range from 0.1–0.15%[9, 37].

Just as new technology creates opportunities, it sometimes carries trouble in its wake. This homily is certainly true of the automated, multiphasic serum chemistry machines which became available in the late 1960s. In center after center, the relatively inexpensive, accurate, routine determination of serum calcium resulted in startling increases in case-ascertainment of calcium metabolic disorders, particularly primary hyperparathyroidism[1, 24, 32, 34]. The advance in clinical chemistry exemplified by such machines as the SMA–12/60 has revolutionized our concepts about the prevalence of hypercalcemia in many diseases. Furthermore, routine clinical testing for hypercalcemia has enormously altered the perceived clinical spectrum of primary hyperparathyroidism.

In the 1980s hypercalcemia is often an incidental finding in patients having no symptoms or ones not clearly connected to the metabolic abnormality. The discovery of hypercalcemia immediately raises a host of diagnostic possibilities, and can lead to an expensive, uncomfortable and complex diagnostic effort; nonetheless, the story of hypercalcemia today is largely that of primary hyperparathyroidism. The purposes of this chapter are to place in perspective the problem of incidental hypercalcemia; to examine critically the factors pertinent to treatment decisions; to propose an effective diagnostic strategy; and to pose some questions much in need of answers.

DEFINITIONS

Because terminology and misunderstanding of it can lead to inappropriate diagnosis and treatment, a few words should be clearly defined.

Hypercalcemia

Few biological variables are normally distributed (statistically) in healthy populations, but fortunately the serum calcium concentration is nearly so[38]. Therefore, the mean plus and minus two standard deviations defines a range within which 95% of normal serum calcium values will fall. By such criteria, then, the adult normal range for total serum calcium in the Mayo Clinic laboratories is 8.9–10.1 mg/dl (2.22–2.52 mmol/l)[37,38]. Laboratories using automated analyzers generally report normal values as 8.5–10.5 mg/dl (2.12–2.62 mmol/l). Thus, we define hypercalcemia operationally as persistent elevation of serum total (or ionized) calcium concentration to levels above the 95% confidence limits for normal values *in that laboratory*. By 'persistent' hypercalcemia we mean that at least three serum calcium values drawn on separate occasions are elevated. Two *caveats* are in order: firstly, mild primary hyperparathyroidism can exist in persons whose serum total calcium levels are occasionally or often within normal limits. Secondly, implicit in the use of 95% confidence limits to define normality is the fact that, by definition, a few healthy people will have serum calcium persistently 'above normal'. The higher the value, of course, the less the likelihood that it *is* a normal variant. Thus, it is not possible to achieve 100% separation of 'hypercalcemia' from 'normocalcemia'.

Asymptomatic

The published literature on primary hyperparathyroidism does not always clearly distinguish between *symptoms* apparent to the affected people, and *signs* knowable only by medical evaluation. A hypercalcemic patient may have no symptoms or complaints, yet on examination have clearcut signs of adverse consequences of his disease, such as radiographically apparent renal stones, osteopenia, or reduced renal function. On the other hand, patients may have many symptoms which are difficult to relate to the hypercalcemia. For this discussion, a patient is considered asymptomatic if he presents no complaints which could reasonably be linked to the hypercalcemia. We shall make a distinction between asymptomatic, uncomplicated hypercalcemia and asymptomatic hypercalcemia which is complicated by deleterious effects of the disease.

Primary hyperparathyroidism

The diagnosis of primary hyperparathyroidism requires, at a minimum, persistent elevation of serum ionized calcium, with or without elevation of total calcium; lack of evidence for other causes of the hypercalcemia; and measurements of circulating immunoreactive parathyroid hormone (iPTH) consistent with the disease. Serum ionized calcium measurements will not however be available in many centers. Primary hyperparathyroidism cannot be diagnosed solely on the basis of elevated serum iPTH levels in normocalcemic people.

THE PROBLEM OF CALCIUM MEASUREMENT

One reason for the late emergence of hypercalcemic disorders in physicians' consciousness is that, until fairly recently, calcium measurement was tedious, expensive and often inaccurate. Despite improved methods, calcium measurement is still subject to error from a number of sources, and physicians interpreting calcium assays must be aware of these problems. Techniques for measurement of serum total and ionized calcium have been reviewed critically by Robertson and Marshall[55].

Total serum calcium

Circulating calcium consists of three phases: that non-covalently bound to plasma proteins (approximately 45%); that complexed with various anions (approximately 10%); and the so-called free, ionic or ionized calcium (approximately 45%). All three phases are measured in most total serum calcium assays. Calcium may be measured in plasma or serum, but for technical reasons results are more reliable using serum if the specimen must be frozen prior to assay.

Literally dozens of variant methods are available for serum calcium measurement[55], but for practical purposes only three need to be remembered. The reference method is atomic absorption spectrophotometry (AAS); it has a number of advantages, including accuracy, precision, high specificity for calcium, and relative simplicity. However, various colorimetric methods are most popular because of their use in automated serum chemistry systems, such as the Technicon Autoanalyzer. In the latter system, one detects a color reaction product of calcium with O-cresolphthalein. With careful technique, serum calcium values obtained by AAS and the automated chemistry methods are comparable[30, 55]. Calcium may also be measured by titration of a fluorescing calcium–calcein complex with a calcium-chelator such as EGTA. Commercially available semiautomated microfluorometric titrators are especially useful when available sample volume is small.

A variety of reports show that in the United States most clinical laboratories are using appropriate techniques for measurement of calcium in serum, and collaborative studies indicate good interlaboratory precision. However, as late as the 1970s, the stated normal ranges for serum calcium varied to an extent clearly incompatible with uniform clinical detection of hypercalcemic or hypocalcemic states[61] (*Table 8.1*). In fact, the ranges for lower (6.0–9.6 mg/dl, 1.5–2.4 mmol/l) and upper (10.0–12.0 mg/dl, 2.5–3.0 mmol/l) limits of normal far exceeded the entire normal range (10.1 − 8.9 = 1.2 mg/dl, 2.5 − 2.2 = 0.3 mmol/l) in a laboratory using

Table 8.1   Normal ranges for adult serum total calcium concentration reported by laboratories participating in a collaborative study of calcium measurement by atomic absorption spectroscopy. (Modified from Sideman *et al.*[61], courtesy of the Editor, © (1970) *Clinical Chemistry*)

| Normal range, mg calcium/dl* | | Normal range, mg calcium/dl* | |
lower limit	upper limit	lower limit	upper limit
9.0	11.5	9.0	11.0
9.0	11.0	6.0	12.0
8.9	10.2	8.2	10.2
7.9	10.0	8.8	10.2
9.0	11.0	8.8	10.8
9.0	11.0	8.7	10.0
8.5	11.0	8.7	10.3
9.0	11.0	9.0	11.0
8.6	10.4	9.0	11.0
9.0	11.0	8.6	10.3
9.0	11.0	8.8	10.6

* 1 mg calcium/dl = 0.25 mmol/l

meticulous techniques and careful selection of healthy people as normal volunteers[38]. It is plainly evident that a laboratory using 6.0–12.0 mg/dl (1.5–3.0 mmol/l) as the normal range for serum calcium would be unable to detect the majority of cases of primary hyperparathyroidism[34]. Ideally, each clinical laboratory should determine its own normal range for serum calcium; given practical constraints, however, the laboratory can at least participate in a quality control program, and use a normal range known to have been carefully derived with the same method. The lesson for the clinician is, 'know your laboratory'. An excessively wide normal range should be distrusted. In almost all modern laboratories, serum total calcium values of 10.5 mg/dl (2.62 mmol/l) and above strongly suggest hypercalcemia, and primary hyperparathyroidism has often been definitively diagnosed in patients having mean serum calcium values of 10.2–10.4 mg/dl (2.55–2.6 mmol/l)[34].

Serum ionized calcium

Because the total serum calcium concentration can be highly misleading when pH or protein levels are altered[35, 40], one would prefer to measure ionized calcium routinely. Several companies now offer devices for serum ionized calcium measurement based on so-called 'ion-specific electrode' technology, which have found some use in reasearch and in large clinical laboratories[11, 41]. The devices are fairly expensive, and are limited in their utility and rate of analysis. Furthermore, they are technically demanding in comparison to total calcium methods[35]. In our opinion fresh serum is best for ionized calcium measurement; we are skeptical of values determined with frozen specimens. Until ionized calcium assay technology advances considerably, total serum calcium values will remain the standard for clinical use. Fortunately, one can generally avoid being misled by maintaining awareness of potential artifacts in measurement of serum total calcium[35]. Where careful ionized calcium measurements are available, they may be of considerable help in cases of minimal or intermittent elevation of serum total calcium[11, 40-42, 46].

Single versus multiple values of serum calcium

A single, unexpectedly elevated value for serum calcium is often ignored by the physician[29]. Alternatively, a second value may be obtained, and if it is normal, the first may be discounted. This course is illogical: how does one know whether the normal or the high value is correct? In our view, a single elevated serum calcium result demands at least two subsequent determinations. If both are normal, then the first value was likely in error. Otherwise, hypercalcemia is verified. If one has multiple serum calcium values from an extended period of observation, the surety of hypercalcemia is obviously increased.

THE DIFFERENTIAL DIAGNOSIS OF HYPERCALCEMIA

All textbooks of medicine and endocrinology present lists of the possible causes of hypercalcemia. Such lists, however, often obscure more than they clarify, because of failure to deal with the enormous differences in the likelihood of various diagnoses. *Table 8.2* represents an effort to show, in a semiquantitative sense, relative probabilities of the underlying pathogeneses of hypercalcemia. The table must be interpreted carefully, because there are simply no adequate data available to rank-order the possibilities precisely. Several general points are worth remembering. Firstly, not all hypercalcemic patient populations have the same probability of a given underlying cause. Children and young adults, for example, have a much greater chance of immobilization hypercalcemia than do the middle-aged and elderly. Seemingly well, ambulatory patients are vastly less likely to have the hypercalcemia of cancer than are sick, hospitalized people.

Burt and Brennan[12] found a 5% prevalence of hypercalcemia among 17 706 admissions to the Clinical Center, National Institutes of Health. Of the 890

Table 8.2   Underlying causes of persistent hypercalcemia in adults, arranged by groups, approximately in descending order of probability

Probability	Cause
Asymptomatic, ambulatory patients	
Most common	Primary hyperparathyroidism (sporadic) (more than 85%)
	Drugs (such as thiazides, lithium, calcium-containing antacids, vitamin D)
Less common	Occult malignancies
	Granulomatous diseases
Uncommon	Familial benign hypercalcemia (familial hypocalciuric hypercalcemia)
	Multiple endocrine neoplasia syndromes (types 1, 2a and 2b)
Symptomatic and/or hospitalized patients	
Most common	Overt malignancies (38–58%)
	Primary hyperparathyroidism (13–33%*)
	Acute and chronic renal failure (secondary hyperparathyroidism, vitamin D therapy)
Less common	Drugs
	Thyrotoxicosis
	Granulomatous diseases
	Immobilization
Uncommon	Pheochromocytoma (sporadic)
	Multiple endocrine neoplasia syndromes
	Adrenal insufficiency
	Milk-alkali syndrome
	Myxedema
	Everything else

* In some studies[12, 25, 26], this figure may be elevated by specific referral of hyperparathyroid persons to interested physicians in the reporting center.

hypercalcemic patients, 338 (38%) had cancer-associated hypercalcemia, 174 (19.6%) had primary hyperparathyroidism, 95 (10.7%) had non-neoplastic causes, and, remarkably, in 283 (31.8%) no cause was determined. Two recent papers by Fisken *et al.*[25, 26] support and extend Burt and Brennan's[12] findings. In a major English hospital, a retrospective study of 469 hypercalcemic patients showed 47% to have cancer, and 13% to have primary hyperparathyroidism; however, 22% were undiagnosed[25]. In their prospective study[26], Fisken *et al.* found 58% of 153 hypercalcemic hospital patients to have cancer, but this time 33% had primary hyperparathyroidism with the undiagnosed group virtually disappearing. It is noteworthy that in both of the English papers, the 'miscellaneous' category of hypercalcemic etiologies was very small. Another major point made in both reports is that the cancer associated with hypercalcemia is almost always plainly evident, and most such patients (approximately 75%) have obvious metastases[25, 26].

In sharp contrast to data from hospital patients, Christensson *et al.*[15–17], detected 95 persistently hypercalcemic individuals in 15 903 ambulatory employed people screened. Of the 95, 82 (86%) appeared to have primary hyperparathyroidism, and only two (2.1%) had verified cancer (one breast, one hypernephroma). It is interesting that of the 20 hypercalcemic persons who were being treated with thiazide diuretics when hypercalcemia was found, at least 14 (70%) suffered from primary hyperparathyroidism[17]. Therefore, one must not assume that thiazides are solely responsible for hypercalcemia in a given case; the odds are rather strongly against it. Data from Fisken *et al.*[25, 26] and Christensson's studies are reanalyzed in *Figure 8.1*.

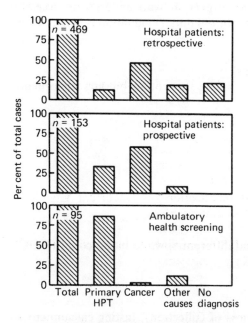

Figure 8.1 Distribution of etiologic diagnoses for hypercalcemic persons seen in hospital settings (*top and middle panels*) versus those in seemingly healthy persons (*bottom panels*). Bars represent per cent of total cases investigated. Primary HPT, primary hyperparathyroidism. (Data derived from Fisken *et al.*[25, 26] and Christensson *et al.*[15–17]

Our experience and the published work cited above support the contention that asymptomatic hypercalcemia which has no other obvious cause is very likely to represent mild primary hyperparathyroidism. If this belief is true, then one's diagnostic approach to such patients must be influenced by it. For instance, it would be folly to require that asymptomatic hypercalcemic patients all have sputum cytology, mammograms, barium enemas, and tests for adrenal insufficiency. The cost:benefit ratio would be astronomical. Asymptomatic persons with slightly elevated serum calcium and no apparent adverse effects of the disease surely should not be subjected to arteriography or other invasive diagnostic procedures.

DIAGNOSTIC TESTING IN ASYMPTOMATIC HYPERCALCEMIA

The goals of diagnostic testing must be to achieve diagnostic accuracy sufficient to guide action, at a cost in money and morbidity commensurate with the seriousness of the disease at hand. By these criteria, many hypercalcemic patients are subjected to inappropriate diagnostic evaluations. The approach we shall outline here is one which in our practice yields more than 90% accuracy in confirming parathyroid disease at surgery. We believe that the cost is reasonable, and that this scheme also will effectively differentiate non-parathyroidal causes for hypercalcemia from hyperparathyroidism.

The testing protocol is useful in differential diagnosis, but will simultaneously help learn the effects on the patient of hypercalcemia. The procedures may also be classified into those which we believe are always indicated during the first evaluation of hypercalcemia, those indicated only in some cases, and tests useful in followup of patients who either have no surgery or who undergo unsuccessful parathyroid exploration. A testing scheme for the initial evaluation is listed below.

(1) *Blood*
   Serum total calcium (3 determinations)
   Ionized calcium (if total calcium borderline or protein binding abnormality suspected)
   Inorganic phosphate
   Protein electrophoresis
   Creatinine
   Alkaline phosphatase
   Immunoreactive parathyroid hormone (iPTH)
   25-Hydroxyvitamin D (if vitamin D intoxication or concurrent vitamin D malnutrition suspected)
   Thyroxine
   Hemogram including blood smear and differential white blood count (WBC)
   Erythrocyte sedimentation rate (ESR)

(2) *Urine*
   Calcium content, 24-hour
   Creatinine (for clearance, completeness of collection), fasting calcium:creatinine ratio (if familial benign hypercalcemia/hypocalciuric hypercalcemia suspected)

(3) *Radiographs*
   Chest
   Kidneys (excretory urography with tomograms preferred)
   Bones (hand films with industrial technique *only* if alkaline phosphatase elevated)

Blood

Multiple serum calcium measurements are required to verify persistence of hypercalcemia, and to document its extent. Serum ionized calcium determination, even if readily available, need not be done routinely, but should be reserved for cases in which the total calcium abnormality is borderline or intermittent; a protein binding anomaly is suspected; or there are symptoms possibly attributable to hypercalcemia disproportionate to the serum total calcium values. Serum inorganic phosphorus levels are generally within normal limits in mild primary hyperparathyroidism[26], but seldom above the middle of the normal range. A high-normal or elevated serum phosphate concentration suggests non-parathyroidal hypercalcemia[26]. Serum protein electrophoresis is essential to detect monoclonal gammopathies and occult multiple myeloma, rare causes of asymptomatic hypercalcemia. Assessment of renal functional state indicates any adverse effects of hypercalcemia on the kidneys, and helps in interpreting serum phosphate, iPTH, etc. If the patient has serious parathyroid hormone (PTH)-induced bone disease, the serum alkaline phosphatase activity will be high. The value of isoenzyme fractionations in detecting increased serum alkaline phosphatase of skeletal origin is still debated. Serum thyroxine assay generally excludes the remote possibility that clinically unrecognized thyroid disease causes or modifies the hypercalcemia. Hematological indices may point toward unsuspected systemic ailments (such as multiple myeloma).

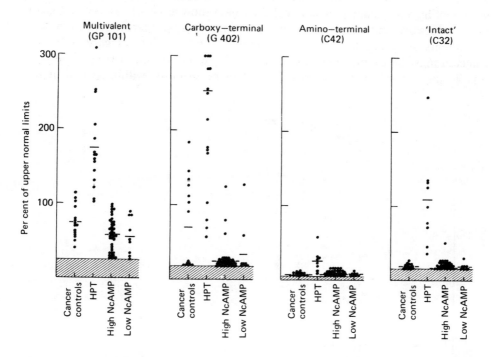

Figure 8.2   Results of parathyroid hormone radioimmunoassays (four different antisera, *top legend*) of serum from four groups of patients: cancer controls (normocalcemic), primary hyperparathyroid (HPT), hypercalcemic cancer patients with elevated nephrogenous cyclic AMP excretion (NcAMP), and hypercalcemic cancer patients with low NcAMP. Serum iPTH values are expressed as percentages of the upper limits of normal. Hatched areas represent lower limits of detectability. In all four PTH assays, patients with both types of cancer-associated hypercalcemia had lower values than did hyperparathyroid patients. (From Stewart *et al.*[63], reprinted, by permission of the *New England Journal of Medicine*, **303**, 1377, 1980)

Because it is so important, and because it may take weeks to get an answer, one should submit a specimen for serum iPTH measurement early in the diagnostic evaluation. PTH radioimmunoassays are difficult, tedious, and of variable characteristics and quality. For these and other reasons, PTH assays have received bad publicity lately[54, 65]. We think this pessimism is unwarranted. A large body of literature[10, 14, 21, 31, 33, 34], and 12 years' clinical experience at the Mayo Clinic[4, 8, 34, 37, 52, 53] sturdily support the utility of serum PTH assays in etiological diagnosis of hypercalcemia. It is beyond the scope of our chapter to discuss these issues in detail, but we offer the following observations. The majority of hyperparathyroid patients will have absolute elevations of serum iPTH, when the antiserum used has major immunochemical specificity which permits it to detect carboxyl-terminal fragments of the PTH molecule[10, 14, 21, 31, 33, 34]. For reasons yet unknown, so-called amino-terminal PTH assays are rather ineffectual in discriminating hyperparathyroid sera from normal[5, 44, 63]. There is great dispute over the prevalence of authentic 'ectopic secretion of PTH', but recent evidence suggests it is uncommon[51, 60, 63]. Stewart *et al.*[63] applied four different PTH radioimmunoassays to sera from a variety of hypercalcemic patients, and their data show as clearly as any that serum iPTH values are, in fact, powerful in separating hyperparathyroid sera from those of patients suffering from cancer-associated hypercalcemia (*Figure 8.2*). The clinician must be aware, however, that a variable proportion of truly hyperparathyroid patients will have serum iPTH values persistently 'within normal limits'.

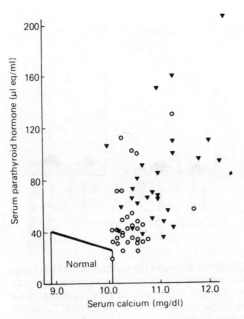

Figure 8.3   Serum immunoreactive parathyroid hormone (antiserum GP–1M) in unselected cases of primary hyperparathyroidism (HPT) occurring among residents of Rochester, Minnesota, USA, 1965–75. Even iPTH values 'within normal limits' may be judged inappropriately elevated for the level of serum calcium. (▼), Operated; (○) unoperated

Fortunately, when the PTH assay has been well-characterized, one may interpret the serum iPTH as a function of serum calcium (discriminant analysis), in which case an 'inappropriately elevated' (that is, within normal limits) iPTH level is consistent with, but not diagnostic of, primary hyperparathyroidism[4, 6, 33, 52, 53]. This point is illustrated for serum iPTH results in unselected cases of primary hyperparathyroidism in *Figure 8.3*. A working rule one might employ with any well-performed PTH assay is that values ranging from mid-normal range to the upper limit are consistent with hyperparathyroidism, but are best regarded as not diagnostic. One must then rely on the larger picture of historical, physical and biochemical evidence for a presumptive diagnosis. Serum iPTH values below the middle of the normal range, including 'undetectables', should be taken as warnings to look harder for non-parathyroidal causes of hypercalcemia.

Some authors suggest that serum 25-hydroxyvitamin D assay be done routinely, but we think its main role is to verify suspected hypervitaminosis D[47], or concurrent vitamin D deficiency[13].

Urine

The urinary excretion of calcium is a very useful but frequently neglected datum. Firstly, hypercalciuria is a risk factor, and might help in a decision for treatment. Secondly, the absolute amount of calcium in a 24-hour urine collection can be of limited diagnostic value. Extremely high values (for example more than 500 mg (12.5 mmol)/24 hour) characterize parathyroid-suppressed hypercalcemia (sarcoidosis, cancer, vitamin D intoxication, etc.). Extremely low values (less than 100 mg (2.5 mmol)/24 hour) raise the possibility of familial benign hypercalcemia/familial hypocalciuric hypercalcemia[28]. If the latter syndrome is suspected, then determination of the fasting urinary calcium:creatinine ratio may help distinguish the patient's condition from primary hyperparathyroidism[45].

Radiographs

Many physicians evaluating asymptomatic hypercalcemic patients carry out radiographic searches which are excessive, costly and unrewarding. Certainly, a chest film is in order, to detect hilar adenopathy, lung cancer and pulmonary metastases. If there are no symptoms or signs for guidance, routine metastic surveys, mammograms and gastrointestinal films are usually not indicated. A routine search for hyperparathyroid bone disease is futile; only about 8% of unselected cases will have specific signs[34]. We recommend that hand radiographs on industrial type film be obtained only if serum alkaline phosphatase activity is elevated. We have abandoned routine views of the skull (except when multiple endocrine neoplasia type 1 is suspected) and lamina dura. Non-specific findings of osteopenia are common in primary hyperparathyroidism[34], but are of no differential diagnostic value. We invariably recommend radiographic observation of the kidneys by intravenous pyelography (barring specific contraindications) when evaluating newly discovered hypercalcemia. The first goal is to exclude renal cell carcinoma, one of the tumors which can truly be occult and produce pseudohyperparathyroidism. Any masses found are next evaluated by ultrasonography or computed tomography (CT), which readily identifies simple renal cysts. The second goal is to learn whether the patient has suffered renal damage from hypercalcemia, either as nephrocalcinosis or (much more commonly) urinary tract stones[34]. Such calcifications are of prognostic and therapeutic, but not diagnostic, value.

Tests of dubious value

The procedures outlined above are highly effective, and we recommend abandonment of several procedures still occasionally used around the country, such as determination of tubular reabsorption of phosphate, chloride:phosphate ratios, and calcium infusion in attempts to discriminate adenomatous from hyperplastic parathyroid disease. For a time, it was believed that nephrogenous adenosine cyclic 3′, 5′-monophosphate (NcAMP) determinations would be even more effective than serum iPTH assay in the diagnosis of hyperparathyroidism. Regrettably, this optimistic view has weakened under the weight of recent evidence; a surprisingly large number of patients having cancer-caused hypercalcemia have low serum iPTH but elevated nephrogenous cyclic AMP excretion[8, 56, 63]. In fact, serum iPTH measurement emerges as superior to any variant of cyclic AMP determination in separating hyperparathyroidism from cancer-caused hypercalcemia[56, 63].

Procedures to localize hyperfunctioning parathyroid tissue

Space does not permit a detailed account, but it is generally agreed that invasive parathyroid localizing studies (arteriography, selective thyroid venous sampling) are not indicated before initial cervical exploration[23, 43]. Experienced surgeons have such high success rates in first operations for primary hyperparathyroidism that the cost and morbidity of invasive procedures are unacceptable[23]. However, recent evidence suggests that the relatively inexpensive non-invasive technique of grey-scale ultrasonography may often localize parathyroid adenomas as small as 500 mg[22]. Computed tomographic (CT) scanning also shows promise, particularly for mediastinal adenomas, but is considerably more expensive than ultrasonography. We reserve CT scanning for reoperative cases.

EPIDEMIOLOGY, AND THE BIOLOGICAL AND MEDICAL CONSEQUENCES OF PRIMARY HYPERPARATHYROIDISM

Epidemiology

Several approaches have been used to learn the frequency of primary hyperparathyroidism; these include serum calcium screening of seemingly healthy persons[15], of clinic outpatients[9, 37], and of hospital inpatients[25, 26, 62]; retrospective notations of hospital diagnoses[12]; and determination of population-based incidence rates in a community[34]. Each method yields a different kind of information, but there is a remarkable convergence of the data in recent years.

Screening of healthy persons

Christensson *et al.*[15–17] reported a prevalence of primary hyperparathyroidism of 0.36% in Swedish adult government employees. Our reanalysis of the data suggests that the prevalence in their study was actually higher still, 0.52% (82 of 95 hypercalcemic cases in 15 903 screened)[15–17].

Clinic outpatients

Two large US referral centers found prevalence rates of primary hyperparathyroidism to be 0.1%[9] and 0.15%[37] in rather large groups of patients (2005 and 50 330, respectively).

Hospital inpatients

Stenstrom and Heedman[62] reviewed the cases of primary hyperparathyroidism found in a large urban hospital over an 8-month period, and extrapolated these results to an incidence rate of 28 per 100 000 population/year. Mundy *et al.*[48] performed a similar review of mixed hospital and outpatients over a 5-month interval; once again, these results were used to estimate an incidence rate for primary hyperparathyroidism of 25 per 100 000/year.

Population-based incidence rates

A recent study from the Mayo Clinic shows that apparent incidence rates for primary hyperparathyroidism will vary markedly with several factors, but especially the availability and routine use of accurate serum calcium measurements[34]. Among residents of Rochester, Minnesota, the case-ascertainment rate for primary hyperparathyroidism averaged 7.8 per 100 000/year before routine serum calcium measurement (1 January 1965 to 30 June 1974). After addition of calcium assay to the serum chemistry panel performed in the Mayo Clinic laboratories, the incidence rate for primary hyperparathyroidism rose immediately to 51.1 per 100 000/year for the ensuing year. Subsequently, the rate stabilized at 27.7 cases per 100 000/year[34].

Thus, three recent studies done in three widely separated nations, by different methods, all suggest that a minimal incidence rate for primary hyperparathyroidism is 25–28 cases per 100 000 population annually. More importantly, the incidence rates are highest in women[34, 48] and rise linearly with age (*Table 8.3*). We can then

Table 8.3 Age-specific and sex-specific average annual incidence rates for primary hyperparathyroidism in Rochester, Minnesota*. (From Heath *et al.*[34], reprinted, by permission of *The New England Journal of Medicine*, **302**, 189, 1980)

Age group (Year)	Male Cases	Male Rate†	Female Cases	Female Rate†	Total Cases	Total Rate
			1 January 1965 to 30 June 1974			
39	4	2.5	3	1.6	7	2.0
40–59	5	12.0	10	20.4	15	16.5
60+	4	16.7	13	30.7	17	25.6
Total	13	5.7	26	9.5	39	7.8
Age-adjusted	—	6.7	—	10.2	—	8.8
			1 July 1974 to 31 December 1976			
39	2	4.5	4	8.0	6	6.4
40–59	3	25.9	14	103.6	17	67.7
60+	6	92.2	22	188.5	28	154.1
Total	11	17.6	40	53.2	51	37.1
Age-adjusted	—	22.3	—	56.3	—	42.1

* The ratio of the age-adjusted female rate to that in males was 1.5 in the first period and 2.5 in the second. The ratio increased in each age–sex group after calcium was included in the serum chemistry panel. In females, the age-adjusted rate increased to 5.5 times its level in the first period, and in males the increase was 3.3 times the first period level.
† New diagnoses per 100 000 population/year adjusted to US white population, 1970.

Table 8.4 Distribution of mean serum calcium concentration among Rochester, Minnesota residents having primary hyperparathyroidism, 1965–76. (From Heath *et al.*[34], reprinted, by permission of *The New England Journal of Medicine*, **302**, 189, 1980)

Serum calcium* (mg/dl)	1 January 1965 to 30 June 1974 n†	(%)	1 July 1974 to 31 December 1976 n†	(%)
10.1	2	(6)	3	(6)
10.2–10.5	17	(50)	18	(36)
10.6–11.0	8	(23.5)	18	(36)
11.1–11.5	6	(17.6)	4	(8)
11.6–12.0	0	(0)	4	(8)
12.1–13.0	1	(2.9)	3	(6)
≥ 13.1	0	(0)	0	(0)

* Mean of three determinations just prior to diagnosis or surgery; 1 mg/dl = 0.25 mmol/l.
† Total equals 84 cases, because serum calcium values were not available for the six cases found at autopsy.

Table 8.5 Clinical characteristics of patients with primary hyperparathyroidism in Rochester, Minnesota, 1965–76. (From Heath *et al.*[34], reprinted, by permission of *The New England Journal of Medicine*, **302**, 189, 1980)

Characteristics[a]	1 January 1965 to 30 June 1974		1 July 1974 to 31 December 1976	
	n	(%)	n	(%)
Urolithiasis	20	(51)	2	(4)*
Hypercalciuria (>250 mg/dl)	14	(36)	11	(22)
Emotional disorder[b]	10	(26)	10	(20)
Osteoporosis	8	(21)	6	(12)
Diminished renal function	7	(18)	7	(14)
Hyperparathyroid bone disease	4	(10)	4	(8)
Peptic ulcer disease	2	(5)	4	(8)
Pancreatitis	2	(5)	0	(0)
No problems related to primary hyperparathyroidism[c]	7	(18)	26	(51)†
Total	39	(100)	51	(100)

* $P > 0.001$
† $P > 0.005$
[a] Listed are problems generally accepted as potentially caused or aggravated by hypercalcemia and/or hyperparathyroidism.
[b] Depression, psychosis or severe neurosis.
[c] Only the problems in the table were considered; hypertension was not included.

define middle-aged and elderly women as the group most in need of routine search for primary hyperparathyroidism.

The recent epidemiological studies of primary hyperparathyroidism[34, 48] also emphasize an alteration in perceived clinical spectrum of the disease (*Tables 8.4* and *8.5*). Briefly, overt hyperparathyroid bone disease and symptomatic urolithiasis have become uncommon manifestations of primary hyperparathyroidism. In 57% of Mundy's cases[48], primary hyperparathyroidism was found unexpectedly by serum calcium screening. None of the 111 cases had radiographic evidence of bone disease, and only 7% had urolithiasis. In the Mayo Clinic series, 4% had renal calcifications, and 8% had signs of hyperparathyroid bone disease. In unexplained contrast, 48% of Mayo patients were hypertensive by strict criteria, but only 5% of the English cases were hypertensive[34, 48].

Biological and medical consequences of primary hyperparathyroidism

When one considers . . . the increased apparent and actual sense of wellbeing afforded the patient as a result of successful surgical treatment [of primary hyperparathyroidism], it seems reasonable to expand the indications as widely as possible.

Peskin *et al.*[50]

> On the basis of our experience . . . we consider parathyroid operation the
> treatment of choice for elderly hyperparathyroid patients, particularly those with
> . . . nonspecific symptoms . . . .
>
> Alveryd et al.[3]

> . . . little is to be gained by discovering and treating mild hyperparathyroidism.
>
> Williamson and Van Peenen[66]

The contrasting views of 'mild' primary hyperparathyroidism represented by the above quotations arise from our lack of definitive information about the extent to which the disease affects health and wellbeing. There is no dispute that many patients having primary hyperparathyroidism suffer serious complications of the disorder, and must be treated. Such cases will not be discussed further. What of the approximately 50% of cases in whom no classical indications for treatment are found? The possible biological consequences of primary hyperparathyroidism which are of greatest concern are on bone, kidney, and vasculature.

Bone

Most patients today have no radiographic signs of typical hyperparathyroid bone disease[34, 48], but some evidence suggests that the prevalence of osteoporosis may be increased in primary hyperparathyroidism[18, 20, 49, 59, 64]. This proposal would seem to be soundly based on the ability of PTH to stimulate osteoclasts.

Cohn et al.[18] found significant reduction of total body calcium by neutron activation analysis in nine hyperparathyroid patients. Dalen and Hjern[20] reported low bone mineral content in calcaneus, femoral shaft and forearm in 10 hyperparathyroid patients without X-ray evidence of skeletal alteration. Pak et al.[49] examined bone density by photon absorptiometry in 30 hyperparathyroid patients. Their results suggested that hyperparathyroid men and premenopausal women are not at great risk of bone loss, but that affected postmenopausal women are very likely to develop disproportionate osteopenia[49] (*Figure 8.4*). Tougaard et al.[64] found low forearm bone mineral content in six hyperparathyroid persons, and bone biopsy specimens had a subnormal phosphorus:hydroxyproline ratio (interpreted as evidence of decreased mineralization). Becker et al.[7] examined bone biopsies from 25 hyperparathyroid patients, 11 of whom had no skeletal symptoms or X-ray abnormalities, and normal serum alkaline phosphatase. Nine of the latter 11 were found to have evidence of increased PTH effect on bone, including increased osteoid and resorptive activity. Skeletal involvement in primary hyperparathyroidism, as assessed by retention of technetium 99m (^{99m}Tc) diphosphonate, was reported by Fogelman et al.[27] to occur even in patients with minimal hypercalcemia. Kaplan et al.[35] studied six 'asymptomatic' hyperparathyroid patients and seven with typical hyperparathyroid problems. In their view, both groups had evidence of adverse consequences of primary hyperparathyroidism, because both had varying combinations of hypercalciuria, low bone density, negative calcium balance, and decreased renal function.

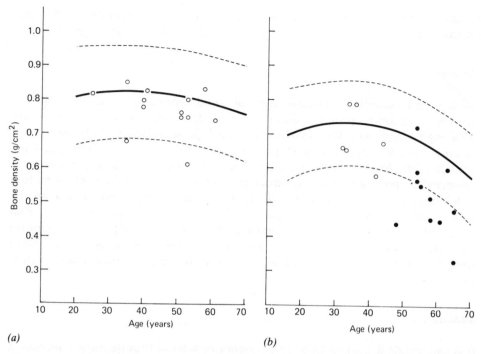

Figure 8.4a and b   Forearm bone density (single photon absorptiometry) in primary hyper-parathyroidism in males (*left*) and females (*right*). The solid and dashed lines represent normal means and 95% confidence limits. (From Pak *et al.*[49], courtesy of the Editor and Publishers, *Lancet*)

   The preceding studies have a number of limitations which suggest caution in generalizing from them. For example, the numbers of patients are small; perhaps more important, the cases were found several years ago, and may not be entirely representative of the 'mildest' hyperparathyroid cases seen today. A larger study initiated in 1968 at the Mayo Clinic partially clarifies the issues. Here 147 patients were recruited to followup; they all had serum calcium equal to or less than 11.0 mg/dl (2.75 mmol/l), and had no evident complications of the disease. Three papers describe the course of these patients[52, 53, 58]. At 30 months, 14% had gone on to surgery[53]; at 5 years, 20% of the original group had undergone parathyroid exploration[52]; and by 10 years, 26% had been treated surgically[58]. The Mayo study establishes that many patients with asymptomatic primary hyperparathyroidism can live at least a decade in peaceful coexistence with the disease. However, a number of patients died or were lost temporarily or permanently during the followup period. Furthermore, the study was not designed to pursue one of the most pressing questions: the effect of untreated primary hyperparathyroidism on skeletal mass, and the occurrence of osteoporosis.

   In summary, many patients who have primary hyperparathyroidism have some effects on bone metabolism, and often are subtly osteopenic. It is not known if *all* hyperparathyroid patients lose bone faster than they would otherwise. It is prudent to assume for now that all such persons are at risk of osteoporosis, but that postmenopausal women (who are the largest subgroup anyway) are at greatest risk.

Kidney

Most patients now diagnosed as hyperparathyroid have normal renal function[34, 48], and the Mayo followup study indicated no gross decreases of renal function in most surviving patients over 10 years of observation[58]. Some did show a decrease in renal function, and had parathyroid surgery because of this[52, 53]. The study could not exclude subtle losses of renal function which might be revealed by comparison to age-matched and sex-matched controls. In our view, available data permit no firm conclusions as to the long-term effects of chronic, mild hypercalcemia on the kidney, but we doubt that the result is positive. It may be important to note that renal function once lost in primary hyperparathyroidism usually does not improve after parathyroidectomy, and may worsen. The situation is, of course, often complicated by other factors such as atherosclerotic vascular disease or hypertension.

Vascular

It is conventional wisdom that the frequency of arterial hypertension is increased among hyperparathyroid patients[39]. Older reports of this association are suspect because of marked hypercalcemia and concurrent renal failure. Smaller series fail to account for the high prevalance of hypertension in the age-group at greatest risk of primary hyperparathyroidism[34]. One of us approached this problem with a case-control study of unselected hyperparathyroid patients, and found the relative risk of definite hypertension to be 1.98 (95% confidence limits, 1.27–3.1) in the cases[34]. Unfortunately, available data did not permit us to tell whether normalization of serum calcium favorably affected hypertension. We conclude provisionally that the risk of significant hypertension is increased in primary hyperparathyroidism, by still ill-defined mechanisms. Since there is no conclusive evidence that treatment of the hyperparathyroidism relieves hypertension, one cannot at present recommend parathyroid surgery solely to that end.

THERAPEUTIC DECISIONS IN ASYMPTOMATIC HYPERCALCEMIA

In some instances, decisions to treat a patient who has asymptomatic hypercalcemia come easily. 'Hypercalcemia' resulting from artifacts is merely ignored; that which results from drug ingestion simply indicates cessation or alteration of the treatment. Hypercalcemia accompanying malignant neoplasms, sarcoidosis, immobilization, etc., will be treated, *pari passu*, with the underlying disease. Parenthetically, one should resist the tendency to treat hypercalcemia itself aggressively – with measures such as saline infusion, furosemide (frusemide) or glucocorticoids – when the degree of calcemia is not threatening.

Primary hyperparathyroidism accompanied by symptoms of hypercalcemia, urolithiasis, hypercalciuria, hyperparathyroid bone disease, and excessive hypercalcemia (arbitrarily, more than 11.0 mg/dl, 2.75 mmol/l), clearly should have parathyroid exploration at the earliest opportunity (*Table 8.6*). Some hyperparathyroid patients have what one might term relative indications for surgical management. Such problems might include osteoporosis or concurrent disease likely to cause it, young age, solitary kidney, need to live far from modern medical help, and psychological distress over the uncertainties of the diagnosis. There will never be any substitute for a personal physician's well-reasoned advice in such cases.

Table 8.6   Indications for surgical treatment of primary hyperparathyroidism

Strong
    Serum calcium more than 11.0 mg/dl at all times
    Severe hypophosphatemia
    Decreased/decreasing renal function
    Metabolically active urolithiasis
    Symptoms of hypercalcemia, *per se*
    Soft tissue calcification
    Radiographic evidence of hyperparathyroid bone disease
    Prolonged observation impossible
    Intractable or recurrent peptic ulcer or pancreatitis
    Need for thiazide treatment of hypertension

Moderate
    Symptoms possibly resulting from hypercalcemia (such as fatigue, depression)
    Osteopenia
    Hypercalciuria without stones
    Elevated serum alkaline phosphatase in absence of liver disease, Paget's disease, etc.
    Sex hormone deficiency
    Young age

Weak or indeterminate
    Arterial hypertension
    Remote history of urolithiasis, peptic ulcer disease, pancreatitis
    Symptoms thought unlikely to result from hypercalcemia

We are left, then, with the central theme of this chapter: patients in whom one has no other likely explanation for hypercalcemia but primary hyperparathyroidism, and in whom symptoms and signs are absent or not clearly related to the parathyroid disease. There are simply not enough facts at hand to permit dogmatism, but we believe a rational approach is possible (*Figure 8.5*). Nonparathyroidal hypercalcemia falls away early in the schedule depicted, followed by hyperparathyroid patients having definite indications for treatment. As may be seen, our attitude toward the remaining cases is one of 'qualified aggressiveness'. The factors upon which we base this concept may be viewed in the context of cost–benefit ratios.

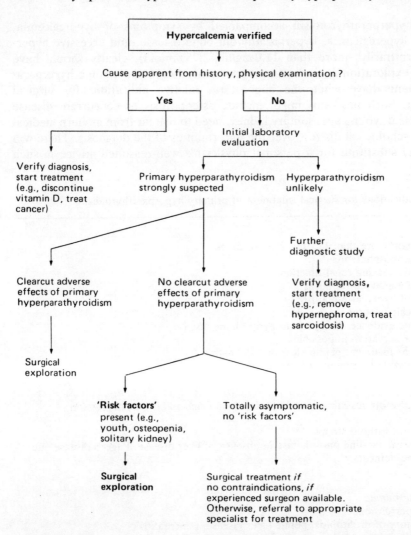

Figure 8.5 Branching decision tree in management of asymptomatic hypercalcemia

COST–BENEFIT CONSIDERATIONS IN DIAGNOSIS AND TREATMENT OF ASYMPTOMATIC PRIMARY HYPERPARATHYROIDISM

Diagnosis

The initial 'finding' of hypercalcemia is of very low cost, being made through serum chemistry surveys wherein the portion of the cost attributed to the calcium measurement is small. However, finding hypercalcemia necessitates a more costly general medical evaluation. We see this expense as unavoidable, because one simply cannot ignore a chemical abnormality which may point to serious, treatable disease. The only way to short-circuit these costs would be to reduce access to blood screening tests, a suggestion unlikely to be followed in the United States; or, to apply such screening procedures more selectively to the middle-aged and elderly, in whom the likelihood of hypercalcemia exceeds many-fold the probability in young people[34].

Treatment versus followup

While no reliable figures are available, an informal survey of US medical insurers and physicians shows that the costs of diagnosing as well as treating primary hyperparathyroidism vary enormously around the country. In some places, virtually any hypercalcemic person is hospitalized at once for a very expensive evaluation. Total costs are much lower when the diagnostic workup is conducted in an outpatient setting. Regional variations in hospital and surgical fees, and in length of hospital stay, also contribute to a wide range of costs for treating hyperparathyroidism. Therefore, one is forced in practice to assess the relative costs of treatment versus followup observation of primary hyperparathyroidism in one's own clinical environment.

In a previous study, we compared the cost of the outpatient diagnostic evaluation described above, and the hospital costs of surgery, with the costs of simple observation[34]. The costs are in 1977 dollars, and reflect only our own practice situation, but the relative figures may be of interest. The median total cost for definitive diagnosis and treatment was $1700. In contrast, the annual cost of followup evaluation for untreated primary hyperparathyroidism was approximately $300. The cost of followup is therefore not inconsequential: 5 years' followup costs would have, on the average, paid for definitive treatment[34]. Obviously, younger patients stand to incur substantial medical care costs if followed for decades. Some have argued that one may trim the followup studies to very few, and reduce costs of observation markedly; such a view presupposes that we know the risks of longstanding primary hyperparathyroidism, which we do not. If we undertake to merely observe asymptomatic hyperparathyroidism, we must be able to assure the patients year by year that all is well.

AN ARGUMENT FOR SURGICAL THERAPY IN MOST CASES OF WELL-DOCUMENTED PRIMARY HYPERPARATHYROIDISM

The rationale we shall describe fits our practice setting very well, and would do so in any highly specialized center[57]. We must emphasize that it is predicated on availability of excellent clinical laboratory support; internists and endocrinologists well-versed in diagnosis of hyperparathyroidism; and most importantly, surgeons specifically trained and experienced in parathyroid surgery. As we and others have emphasized repeatedly, parathyroid surgery is so difficult, and the consequences of failure are so serious, that inexperienced surgeons simply should not do parathyroid explorations. *To reiterate: the aggressive policy we recommend toward asymptomatic primary hyperparathyroidism is only feasible when expert parathyroid surgery is available.* If it is not, then careful medical observation is probably safer for the patient than is suboptimal surgery, with its risks of failure to find the diseased tissue, recurrent laryngeal nerve damage, inadvertent hypoparathyroidism, and scarring in the operative field which hinders subsequent exploration.

We propose that parathyroid surgery is generally indicated in well-documented primary hyperparathyroidism, for the reasons which follow.

(1) Removal of the diseased tissue is the ultimate diagnostic test; all diagnoses short of this are presumptive.
(2) Surgery may be cost-effective.
(3) Treatment relieves some patients of many years' anxiety about the disease.
(4) Patients do not stay in followup programs very well, and the dropouts can get into serious trouble.
(5) The patients never get any younger, and surgery seldom becomes safer for them.
(6) The definitive procedure simplifies present or future use of drugs such as thiazides and digitalis.
(7) We cannot predict who will develop problems from hyperparathyroidism.
(8) Particularly for perimenopausal and postmenopausal women (the largest single category in hyperparathyroidism), the possible skeletal consequences of untreated hyperparathyroidism are worrying.
(9) Because primary hyperparathyroidism will become more prevalent as our population ages, the disease might be less of a burden on the medical care system if treated at the outset, rather than managed by expensive and prolonged followup.

It is obvious that a policy such as the one proposed must be tempered with humane clinical judgement and common sense. One does not propose, for instance, cervical exploration for a 93-year-old demented nursing home resident with a serum calcium concentration of 10.4 mg/dl (2.6 mmol/l), no matter how certain the diagnosis of primary hyperparathyroidism! Nonetheless, there will remain a number of cases in which expert physicians of good intent will disagree.

QUESTIONS IN NEED OF ANSWERS

We shall continue to manage primary hyperparathyroidism amid controversy and uncertainty until a number of issues are resolved. For example:

(1) Is there a more secure way to diagnose PTH excess than by PTH radioimmunoassay? We seem to be near the limits of radioimmunoassay techniques, whether for technical or biological reasons is uncertain. New, highly sensitive assay procedures based upon specific cellular actions of PTH show great

promise, but for the moment the newer assays are costly, cumbersome and unproven in clinical circumstances. Is it possible that, just as there is no absolute demarcation between hypercalcemia and normocalcemia, there will be no final boundary between normal and excessive amounts of circulating PTH?

(2) Does asymptomatic primary hyperparathyroidism cause osteoporosis? In our view, available data are suggestive at best. There is great need for a large-scale, prospective clinical trial, using modern techniques for measurement of appendicular and axial bone mass[59], to resolve this question. If it were shown that most hyperparathyroid individuals lose bone at an excessive rate, then arguments about need for treatment would be greatly muted.

(3) What is the minimum one should do in followup observation of untreated hyperparathyroidism? Is an annual serum calcium really enough?

(4) Does untreated primary hyperparathyroidism affect longevity?

(5) Is the increasing case-ascertainment rate for hyperparathyroidism merely a result of serum calcium screening, or have environmental factors such as radiation actually increased the incidence?

(6) Does treatment of hyperparathyroidism benefit arterial hypertension?

SUMMARY

Primary hyperparathyroidism is a fairly common medical problem of the middle-aged and elderly in the western world; it is probably worthwhile to seek hypercalcemia in that population at periodic intervals. The precise consequences of very mild primary hyperparathyroidism for morbidity and longevity are still obscure. It may be worth noting in this context that within our professional lifetimes there was uncertainty as to the benefits of treating even moderately severe hypertension! The diagnosis of primary hyperparathyroidism can now be made with more than 90% certainty, and an experienced surgeon has more than a 90% chance of success at the first operation, with minimal risk of morbidity and mortality. Many patients who are 'asymptomatic' with primary hyperparathyroidism are suffering some possible or definite ill-effects of the disease, and in our view such patients deserve treatment by surgeons expert in parathyroid exploration. The smaller number of patients who have absolutely no detectable adverse consequences need personal physicians of wisdom and judgement to guide them in choice of management. Many imponderables must be taken into account in these decisions, especially the difficulty of keeping patients in long-term followup[58]. Until we have clearer information on the long-range consequences of untreated hyperparathyroidism, there will still remain many patients whose physicians choose watchful waiting. Fortunately, we can reassure such individuals that our current knowledge does not suggest great danger in untreated, mild primary hyperparathyroidism. In our practice setting, however, parathyroid exploration is safe, efficacious and cost-effective; therefore, we shall continue to recommend surgical therapy for most patients with securely diagnosed primary hyperparathyroidism.

Acknowledgements

Portions of the work described were supported by grants from the US Public Health Service, National Institutes of Health (GM-14231, AM-19607, AM-21101, AM-27440, and RR-585) and the Mayo Foundation.

References

1 AITKEN, R. E., BARTLEY, P. C., BRYANT, S. J. and LLOYD, H. M. The effect of multiphasic biochemical screening on the diagnosis of primary hyperparathyroidism. *Australian and New Zealand Journal of Medicine*, **5**, 224–226 (1975)

2 ALBRIGHT, F. and REIFENSTEIN, E. C., Jr. In *The Parathyroid Glands and Metabolic Bone Disease*, p. 73. Baltimore, Williams and Wilkins Co. (1948)

3 ALVERYD, A., BOSTROM, H., WENGLE, B. and WESTER, P. O. Indications for surgery in the elderly patient with primary hyperparathyroidism. *Acta Chirurgica Scandinavica*, **142**, 491–494 (1976)

4 ARNAUD, C. D., DI BELLA, F. P., BREWER, H. B., ZAWISTOWSKI, K. and VERHEYDEN, J. Human parathyroid hormone: biologic and immunologic activities of its synthetic (1–34) tetratriacontrapeptide and the utility of a carboxyl-terminal-specific radioimmunoassay in assessment of hyperparathyroid syndromes. In *Calcium Regulating Hormones* (Proceedings of the 5th Parathyroid Conference), edited by R. V. Talmage, M. Owen and J. A. Parsons, pp. 15–22. Oxford, Excerpta Medica ICS No. 346 (1975)

5 ARNAUD, C. D., GOLDSMITH, R. S., BORDIER, P. J., SIZEMORE, G. W., LARSEN, J. A. and GILKINSON, J. Influence of immunoheterogeneity of circulating parathyroid hormone on results of radioimmunoassays of serum in man. *American Journal of Medicine*, **56**, 785–793 (1974)

6 ARNAUD, C. D., TSAO, H. S. and LITTLEDIKE, T. Radioimmunoassay of human parathyroid hormone in serum. *Journal of Clinical Investigation*, **50**, 21–34 (1971)

7 BECKER, F. O., EISENSTEIN, R., SCHWARTZ, T. B. and ECONOMOU, S. G. Needle bone biopsy in primary hyperparathyroidism. *Archives of Internal Medicine*, **131**, 650–656 (1973)

8 BENSON, R. C., Jr, RIGGS, B. L., PICKARD, B. M. and ARNAUD, C. D. Radioimmunoassay of parathyroid hormone in hypercalcemic patients with malignant disease. *American Journal of Medicine*, **56**, 821–826 (1974)

9 BOONSTRA, C. E. and JACKSON, C. E. Serum calcium survey for hyperparathyroidism: Results in 50 000 clinic patients. *American Journal of Pathology*, **55**, 523–526 (1971)

10 BRADLEY, E. L., III, DI GIROLAMO, M., GOLDMAN, A. and McLARIN, C. Serum parathormone in the identification and surgical management of hyperparathyroidism. *Southern Medical Journal*, **71**, 1234–1237 (1978)

11 BURRITT, M. F., PIERIDES, A. M. and OFFORD, K. P. Comparative studies of total and ionized serum calcium values in normal subjects and patients with renal disorders. *Mayo Clinic Proceedings*, **55**, 606–613 (1980)

12 BURT, M. E. and BRENNAN, M. F. Incidence of hypercalcemia and malignant neoplasm. *Archives of Surgery*, **115**, 704–707 (1980)

13 Case records of the Massachusetts General Hospital, Case 4–1978. *New England Journal of Medicine*, **298**, 266–274 (1978)

14 CHRISTENSEN, M. S. Radioimmunoassay of human parathyroid hormone. *Danish Medical Bulletin*, **26**, 157–174 (1979)

15 CHRISTENSSON, T., HELLSTROM, K., WENGLE, B., ALVERYD, A. and WIKLAND, B. Prevalence of hypercalcaemia in a health screening in Stockholm. *Acta Medica Scandinavica*, **200**, 131–137 (1976)

16 CHRISTENSSON, T., HELLSTROM, K. and WENGLE, B. Clinical and laboratory findings in subjects with hypercalcaemia. *Acta Medica Scandinavica*, **200**, 355–360 (1976)

17 CHRISTENSSON, T., HELLSTROM, K. and WENGLE, B. Hypercalcemia and primary hyperparathyroidism. Prevalence in patients receiving thiazides as detected in a health screen. *Archives of Internal Medicine*, **137**, 1138–1142 (1977)

18 COHN, S. H., ROGINSKY, M. S., ALOIA, J. F., ELLIS, K. J. and SKUKLA, K. K. Alternations in skeletal calcium and phosphorus in dysfunction of the parathyroids. *Journal of Clinical Endocrinology and Metabolism*, **36**, 750–755 (1973)

19 COPE, O. The story of hyperparathyroidism at the Massachusetts General Hospital. *New England Journal of Medicine*, **274**, 1174–1182 (1966)

20 DALEN, N. and HJERN, B. Bone mineral content in patients with primary hyperparathyroidism without radiological evidence of skeletal changes. *Acta Endocrinologica*, **75**, 297–304 (1974)

21 DI BELLA, F. P., KEHRWALD, J. M., LAAKSO, K. and ZITZNER, L. Parathyrin radioimmunoassay: diagnostic utility of antisera produced against carboxyl-terminal fragments of the hormone from the human. *Clinical Chemistry*, **24**, 451–454 (1978)

22 EDIS, A. J. and EVANS, T. C. Jr. High-resolution, real-time ultrasonography in the preoperative location of parathyroid tumors. *New England Journal of Medicine*, **301**, 532–534 (1979)

23 EDIS, A. J., SHEEDY, P. F. II, BEAHRS, O. H. and van HEERDEN, J. A. Results of reoperation for hyperparathyroidism, with evaluation of preoperative localization studies. *Surgery*, **84**, 384–393 (1978)

24 ESSELSTYN, C. B., Jr and CRILE, G., Jr. Hyperparathyroidism–epidemic or endemic? Diagnosis and treatment. *Cleveland Clinic Quarterly*, **37**, 87–91 (1970)

25 FISKEN, R. A., HEATH, D. A. and BOLD, A. M. Hypercalcaemia – a hospital survey. *Quarterly Journal of Medicine*, **49**, 405–418 (1980)

26 FISKEN, R. A., HEATH, D. A., SOMERS, S. and BOLD, A. M. Hypercalcemia in hospital patients. Clinical and diagnostic aspects. *Lancet*, **1**, 202–207 (1981)

27 FOGELMAN, I., BESSENT, R. G., BEASTALL, G. and BOYLE, I. T. Estimation of skeletal involvement in primary hyperparathyroidism. *Annals of Internal Medicine*, **92**, 65–67 (1980)

28 FOLEY, T. P., Jr., HARRISON, H. C., ARNAUD, C. D. and HARRISON, H. E. Familial benign hypercalemia. *Journal of Pediatrics*, **81**, 1060–1071 (1972)

29 FRIEDMAN, G. D., GOLDBERG, M., AHUJA, J. N., SIEGELAUB, A. B., BASSIS, M. L. and COLLEN, M. I. Biochemical screening tests. Effect of panel size on medical care. *Archives of Internal Medicine*, **129**, 91–97 (1972)

30 GAMBINO, S. R. and FONSECA, I. Comparison of serum calcium measurements obtained with the SMA–12/60 and by atomic absorption spectrophotometry. *Clinical Chemistry*, **17**, 1047–1049 (1971)

31 HABENER, J. F. and SEGRE, G. V. Parathyroid hormone radioimmunoassay. *Annals of Internal Medicine*, **91**, 782–785 (1979)

32 HAFF, R. C., BLACK, W. C. and BALLINGER, W. F. Primary hyperparathyroidism: changing clinical, surgical and pathologic aspects. *Annals of Surgery*, **171**, 85–92 (1970)

33 HAWKER, C. D. and DI BELLA, F. P. Radioimmunoassay for intact and carboxyl-terminal parathyroid hormone: clinical interpretation and diagnostic significance. *Annals of Clinical and Laboratory Science*, **10**, 76–88 (1980)

34 HEATH, H. III, HODGSON, S. F. and KENNEDY, M. A. Primary hyperparathyroidism: incidence, morbidity, and potential economic impact in a community. *New England Journal of Medicine*, **302**, 189–193 (1980)

35 KAPLAN, R. A., SNYDER, W. H., STEWART, A. and PAK, C. Y. C. Metabolic effects of parathyroidectomy in asymptomatic primary hyperparathyroidism. *Journal of Clinical Endocrinology and Metabolism*, **42**, 415–426 (1976)

36 KEATING, F. R. and COOK, E. N. The recognition of primary hyperparathyroidism. An analysis of twenty-four cases. *Journal of the American Medical Association*, **129**, 994–1002 (1945)

37 KEATING, F. R., Jr., JONES, J. D. and ELVEBACK, L. R. Distribution of serum calcium and phosphorus values in unselected ambulatory patients. *Journal of Laboratory and Clinical Medicine*, **74**, 507–514 (1969)

38 KEATING, F. R., Jr., JONES, J. D., ELVEBACK, L. R. and RANDALL, R. V. The relation of age and sex to distribution of values in healthy adults of serum calcium, inorganic phosphorus, magnesium, alkaline phosphatase, total proteins, albumin, and blood urea. *Journal of Laboratory and Clinical Medicine*, **73**, 825–834 (1969)

39 KLEEREKOPER, M., RAO, D. S. and FRAME, B. Hypercalcemia, hyperparathyroidism, and hypertension. *Cardiovascular Medicine*, **3**, 1283–1295 (1978)

40 LADENSON, J. H., LEWIS, J. W. and BOYD, J. C. Failure of total calcium corrected for protein, albumin and pH to correctly assess free calcium status. *Journal of Clinical Endocrinology and Metabolism*, **46**, 986–993 (1978)

41 LADENSON, J. H., LEWIS, J. W., McDONALD, J. M., SLATOPOLSKY, E. and BOYD, J. C. Relationship of free and total calcium in hypercalcemic conditions. *Journal of Clinical Endocrinology and Metabolism*, **48**, 393–397 (1979)

42 LOW, J. C., SCHAAF, M., EARLL, J. M., PIECHOCKI, J. T. and LI, T. K. Ionic calcium determination in primary hyperparathyroidism. *Journal of the American Medical Association*, **223**, 152–155 (1973)

43 MALLETTE, L. E., GOMEZ, L. and FISHER, R. G. Parathyroid angiography: a review of current knowledge and guidelines for clinical application. *Endocrine Reviews*, **2**, 124–135 (1981)

44 MARTIN, K. J., HRUSKA, K., FREITAG, J., BELLORIN-FONT, E., KLAHR, S. and SLATOPOLSKY, E. Clinical utility of radioimmunoassays for parathyroid hormone. *Mineral and Electrolyte Metabolism*, **3**, 283–290 (1980)

45 MARX, S. J., SPIEGEL, A. M., BROWN, E. M., KOEHLER, J. O., GARDNER, D. G., BRENNAN, M. F. and AURBACH, G. D. Divalent cation metabolism. Familial hypocalciuric hypercalcemia versus typical primary hyperparathyroidism. *American Journal of Medicine*, **65**, 235–242 (1978)

46 MONCHIK, J. M. and MARTIN, H. F. Ionized calcium in the diagnosis of primary hyperparathyroidism. *Surgery*, **88**, 185–192 (1980)

47 MORITA, R., FUKUNAGA, M., DOKOH, S., YAMAMOTO, I. and TORIZUKA, K. Differential diagnosis of hypercalcemia by measurement of parathyroid hormone, calcitonin, and 25-hydroxyvitamin D. *Journal of Nuclear Medicine*, **19**, 1225–1263 (1978)

48 MUNDY, G. R., COVE, D. H. and FISKEN, R. Primary hyperparathyroidism: changes in the pattern of clinical presentation. *Lancet*, **1**, 1317–1320 (1980)

49 PAK, C. Y. C., STEWART, A., KAPLAN, R., BONE, H., NOTZ, C. and BROWNE, R. Photon absorptiometric analysis of bone density in primary hyperparathyroidism. *Lancet*, **2**, 7–8 (1975)

50 PESKIN, G. W., GREENBURG, A. G. and SALK, R. P. Expanding indications for early parathyroidectomy in the elderly female. *American Journal of Surgery*, **136**, 45–48 (1978)

51 POWELL, D., SINGER, F. R., MURRAY, T. M., MINKIN, C. and POTTS, J. T., Jr. Nonparathyroid humoral hypercalcemia in patients with neoplastic diseases. *New England Journal of Medicine*, **289**, 176–181 (1973)

52 PURNELL, D. C., SCHOLZ, D. A., SMITH, L. H., SIZEMORE, G. W., BLACK, B. M., GOLDSMITH, R. S. and ARNAUD, C. D. Treatment of primary hyperparathyroidism. *American Journal of Medicine*, **56**, 800–809 (1974)

53 PURNELL, D. C., SMITH, L. H., SCHOLZ, D. A., ELVEBACK, L. R. and ARNAUD, C. D. Primary hyperparathyroidism: a prospective clinical study. *American Journal of Medicine*, **50**, 670–678 (1971)

54 RAISZ, L. G., YAJNIK, C. H., BOCKMAN, R. S. and BOWER, B. F. Comparison of commercially available parathyroid hormone immunoassays in the differential diagnosis of hypercalcemia due to primary hyperparathyroidism or malignancy. *Annals of Internal Medicine*, **91**, 739–740 (1979)

55 ROBERTSON, W. G. and MARSHALL, R. W. Calcium measurements in serum and plasma – total and ionized. *CRC Critical Reviews in Clinical Laboratory Sciences*, 271–304 (1979)

56 RUDE, R. K., SHARP, C. F., Jr, FREDERICKS, R. S., OLDHAM, S. B., ELBAUM, N., LINK, J., IRWIN, L. and SINGER, F. R. Urinary and nephrogenous adenosine 3′, 5′-monophosphate in the hypercalcemia of malignancy. *Journal of Clinical Endocrinology and Metabolism*, **52**, 765–771 (1981)

57 RUSSELL, C. F. and EDIS, A. J. Surgery for primary hyperparathyroidism: experience with 500 consecutive cases and evaluation of the role of surgery in the asymptomatic patient. *British Journal of Surgery* (in press)

58 SCHOLZ, D. and PURNELL, D. C. Asymptomatic primary hyperparathyroidism: 10-year prospective study. *Mayo Clinic Proceedings*, **56**, 473–478 (1981)

59 SEEMAN, E., WAHNER, W. H., OFFORD, K. P., KUMAR, R., JOHNSON, W. J. and RIGGS, B. L. Differential effects of endocrine dysfunction on the axial and the appendicular skeleton. *Journal of Clinical Investigation* (in press)

60 SEYBERTH, H. W., SEGRE, G. V., MORGAN, J. L., SWEETMAN, B. J., POTTS, J. T., Jr and OATES, J. A. Prostaglandins as mediators of hypercalcemia associated with certain types of cancer. *New England Journal of Medicine*, **293**, 1278–1283 (1975)

61 SIDEMAN, L., MURPHY, J. J., Jr and WILSON, D. T. A collaborative study of the serum calcium determination by atomic absorption spectroscopy. *Clinical Chemistry*, **16**, 597–601 (1970)

62 STENSTROM, G. and HEEDMAN, P. Clinical findings in patients with hypercalcemia: a final investigation based on biochemical screening. *Acta Medica Scandinavica*, **195**, 473–477 (1974)

63 STEWART, A. F., HORST, R., DEFTOS, L. J., CODMAN, E. C., LANG, R. and BROADUS, A. E. Biochemical evaluation of patients with cancer-associated hypercalcemia. *New England Journal of Medicine*, **303**, 1377–1383 (1980)

64 TOUGAARD, L., HAU, C., RODBRO, P. and DITZEL, J. Bone mineralization and bone mineral content in primary hyperparathyroidism. *Acta Endocrinologica*, **84**, 314–319 (1977)

65 WATSON, L., MOXHAM, J. and FRASER, P. Hydrocortisone suppression test and discriminant analysis in differential diagnosis of hypercalcemia. *Lancet*, **1**, 1320–1325 (1980)

66 WILLIAMSON, E. and VAN PEENEN, H. J. Patient benefit in discovering occult hyperparathyroidism. *Archives of Internal Medicine*, **133**, 430–431 (1974)

9
Familial hypocalciuric hypercalcemia
Stephen J. Marx

INTRODUCTION

Familial hypocalciuric hypercalcemia (FHH) is a disorder that has been recognized with increasing frequency in the past decade. In the first full report, Foley et al.[6] described a kindred with 12 hypercalcemic members. No member experienced obvious disease-related morbidity so they described the disorder as familial benign hypercalcemia. In the past 8 years my colleagues and I have made this diagnosis in 15 apparently distinct kindreds with 2–23 affected members[12]. Relative hypocalciuria (hypercalcemia without hypercalciuria) has been a distinctive feature in these kindreds as well as in the first reported kindred; therefore we have used the descriptive term, familial hypocalciuric hypercalcemia. This review covers the clinical and biochemical features of the disorder as it has occurred in the 15 kindreds and in additional kindreds reported from other centers.

RECOGNITION AND CLINICAL FEATURES OF FAMILIAL HYPOCALCIURIC HYPERCALCEMIA

Recognition of hypercalcemia

Most commonly, hypercalcemic members of these kindreds exhibit no symptoms attributable to their metabolic disorder. Hypercalcemia is discovered most commonly in the course of family screening[6, 12, 15]. The second commonest reason for recognition of hypercalcemia has been use of multichannel blood analysis in routine health examination or during evaluation for conditions unrelated to familial hypocalciuric hypercalcemia. Recognition in this setting puts patients at high risk of being referred for parathyroid surgery which will not benefit them. The least common cause for recognition of hypercalcemia in these patients has been evaluation for complications directly attributable to the disease.

Symptoms

Approximately two-thirds of the affected patients exhibit one or more symptoms attributable to hypercalcemia (*Table 9.1*). The commonest symptoms are muscular fatigue, sleepiness, mental disturbances such as forgetfulness or difficulty concentrating, headaches, and arthralgias. These mild symptoms have been recognizable only by directly comparing large numbers of affected patients to their unaffected relatives (*Table 9.1*)[12]; they rarely cause the patients to seek medical attention.

Table 9.1 Symptoms in affected (hypercalcemic) versus unaffected members of 15 kindreds with familial hypocalciuric hypercalcemia (FHH)

Symptom	Hypercalcemic (%)	Normocalcemic (%)
Fatigue	31*	5
Weakness	20*	3
Mental problem	24*	7
Headache	24**	9
Arthralgia	30**	15
Polydipsia/polyuria	18**	7
Bone pain	10	3
Pruritis	7	4
Abdominal pain	8	5
Constipation	6	7

* Higher incidence in affected hypercalcemic members than in unaffected normocalcemic members, $P<0.005$.
** Higher incidence in affected hypercalcemic members than in unaffected normocalcemic members, $P<0.05$.

Signs

Only one form of morbidity has been directly linked to familial hypocalciuric hypercalcemia; in the 15 kindreds we have evaluated, there have been three cases of severe neonatal primary hyperparathyroidism[25, 27, 12a]. Severe neonatal primary hyperparathyroidism is a syndrome of severe hypercalcemia (often in the range of 5 mmol/l, 10 mEq/l), undermineralization of the skeleton, and respiratory distress (reflecting the metabolic disturbance and the softened, deformed thoracic cage). It is rare, and whether associated with familial hypocalciuric hypercalcemia or not the parathyroid glands have inevitably shown diffuse hyperplasia[16]. Subtotal parathyroidectomy has been followed by rapid recurrence of the full syndrome; thus, the appropriate treatment is total parathyroidectomy. Severe neonatal primary hyperparathyroidism is uncommon in the disease, and there has otherwise been no increased fetal or postpartum wastage among affected cases.

Pancreatitis has been a rare but dangerous complication[12]. Adult onset diabetes mellitus, hyperthyroidism and hypothyroidism, cardiovascular disease, and chronic pulmonary disease have all been more common in hypercalcemic than in normocalcemic kindred members, but the differences in prevalence have not been statistically significant[12]. More important than the possibility of subtle morbidity has been the lack of morbidity attributable to the common complications of typical primary hyperparathyroidism[11]. The incidence of nephrolithiasis, hypertension, osteopenia, or peptic ulcers has been low, probably similar to that in the general population. Affected females have generally had normal reproductive histories. However, both symptomatic and asymptomatic hypocalcemia have occurred in unaffected offspring of hypercalcemic mothers, and it is important to evaluate offspring for hypercalcemia or hypocalcemia.

RADIOGRAPHIC FEATURES

Growth and development have been normal in affected patients. The incidence of osteoporosis and fracture is not increased. In the light of the biochemical evidence for varying degrees of mild hyperparathyroidism (*see below*), there is a need for more detailed evaluation of skeletal composition in this disorder. Chondrocalcinosis occurs prematurely in these patients with a prevalence of 30% beyond age 45[12]. It does not generally cause arthritis, but one patient with chondrocalcinosis has had attacks that probably do represent pseudogout. Nephrocalcinosis has been absent in radiographs of 40 patients that we have evaluated.

COMPOSITION OF SERUM

Hypercalcemia is a lifelong trait in these families. Patients with familial hypocalciuric hypercalcemia exhibit a range of calcium concentrations in serum indistinguishable from that in patients with typical primary hyperparathyroidism[17]. Younger persons have exhibited serum calcium concentrations higher than those found in older persons[12]. Longitudinal studies have not yet been reported. Calcium concentration in serum of hypercalcemic members occupies a relatively narrow range that is characteristic for each kindred[12]. In four families, the elevation of total calcium concentration in serum was directly proportional to elevation in ionized calcium[6, 17]. Furthermore, fractionation by electrophoresis has indicated similar distribution of the principal serum components in patients with familial hypocalciuric hypercalcemia versus those with typical primary hyperparathyroidism. This does not exclude the hypothetical possibility that a similar disorder within some very unusual kindreds could reflect increased calcium binding in serum.

With regard to many serum components, average values for subjects with familial hypocalciuric hypercalcemia are intermediate between the values for normals and for subjects with typical primary hyperparathyroidism. This has been observed for bicarbonate, chloride, phosphate, and parathyroid hormone (PTH) and for alkaline phosphatase[6, 12, 17, 18]. Because of the wide and overlapping ranges of values for each of these components they have limited value in diagnosis.

Mild hypermagnesemia occurs in 50% of hypercalcemic subjects with familial hypocalciuric hypercalcemia. This is in distinct contrast to the variable depression of magnesium concentration in serum that characterizes typical primary hyperparathyroidism[12]. Furthermore serum calcium is positively correlated with serum magnesium concentration in familial hypocalciuric hypercalcemia but negatively in typical primary hyperparathyroidism. Thus, when present, mild hypermagnesemia in the absence of depressed glomerular filtration rate (GFR) or a high dietary load of magnesium is a useful diagnostic feature.

URINARY EXCRETION OF CALCIUM AND CREATININE

Creatinine clearance in a large number of subjects with familial hypocalciuric hypercalcemia has been randomly distributed about the normal age-dependent means[17]. This is noteworthy as it implies that lifelong hypercalcemia of moderately severe degree need not result in renal compromise.

Calcium excretion in 24-hour urine is similar to that in the normocalcemic normal population[12]. Since hypercalcemia is generally associated with hypercalciuria, this represents a relative (but not necessarily absolute) hypocalciuria, and it is one of the most striking features of this disorder. If it is true that urine calcium has a near normal distribution in the disease, it is perhaps not surprising that a few members of otherwise typical kindreds may actually exhibit hypercalciuria! This is not a paradox, but it serves to emphasize the difficulty of establishing this diagnosis without undertaking family evaluations. The 24-hour urine excretion of calcium is almost always below 6.25 mmol (12.5 mEq) with the subject taking a low calcium 10 mmol (20 mEq)/day diet (*Figure 9.1*). However, similar values of urine calcium are encountered in approximately one-third of patients with typical primary hyperparathyroidism. Much of this overlap is accounted for by the frequent

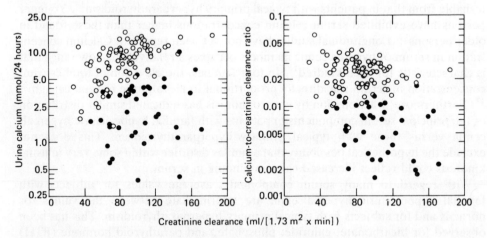

Figure 9.1 Indices of urinary calcium excretion in patients with familial hypocalciuric hypercalcemia (●) versus patients with typical primary hyperparathyroidism (○). All data were obtained from inpatients receiving a calcium-restricted diet (approximately 10 mmol(20 mEq)/day calcium). Calcium and creatinine in urine were means from multiple 24-hour specimens; total calcium and creatinine in serum were means from multiple preprandial morning specimens. *Left*: 24-hour urinary calcium; *right*: calcium-to-creatinine clearance ratio

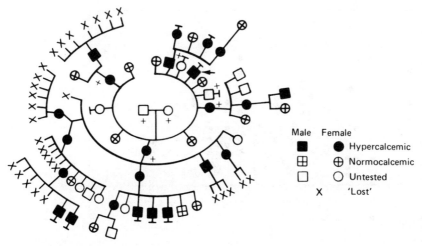

Figure 9.2 A large kindred with familial hypocalciuric hypercalcemia. Four members, including the proband (arrowed), underwent parathyroid explorations, and three remain hypercalcemic

impairment of creatinine clearance with a parallel depression of calcium clearance in typical primary hyperparathyroidism. Expression of urine calcium as a clearance ratio

calcium clearance/creatinine clearance $= (U_{ca} \times S_{cr})/(U_{cr} \times S_{ca})$

allows improved discrimination between the two hypercalcemic groups (*Figure 9.1*). We have employed total, not ultrafiltrable, calcium concentration serum to calculate this index.

PARATHYROID FUNCTION

Radiommunoassay of parathyroid hormone (PTH) in serum shows a normal value for most subjects with familial hypocalciuric hypercalcemia[6, 7, 18], and several workers believe this is a *sine qua non* for the diagnosis of familial benign hypercalcemia[6, 7]. In contrast we have found mild elevations of plasma PTH concentration in 20% of patients with the disease, though we believe that familial hypocalciuric hypercalcemia and familial benign hypercalcemia are alternate names for the same disorder. Other indices of circulating PTH bioactivity (urinary adenosine cyclic 3',5'-monophosphate (cAMP) and theoretical renal phosphate threshold) have also suggested values intermediate between those for normals and for persons with typical primary hyperparathyroidism[7, 18]. However, these indices are dependent on factors other than PTH (urinary cAMP is also dependent on renal responsivity to PTH, and this responsivity is greater in familial hypocalciuric hypercalcemia than in typical primary hyperparathyroidism[19]; renal transport of phosphate is also dependent on calcium concentration in serum).

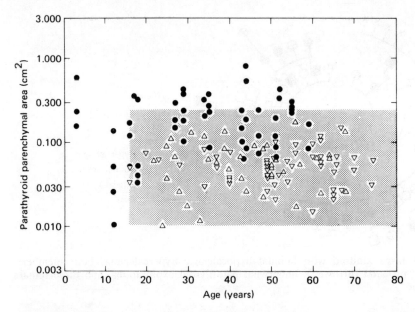

Figure 9.3 An index of parathyroid gland secretory mass as a function of age. Histological slides were used to derive the parenchymal cross-sectional area for each gland. Symbols represent 55 glands from 18 patients with familial hypocalciuric hypercalcemia (●), 42 glands from 32 operations not directed at the parathyroids (△), and 50 glands from post-mortem examinations of 30 cases without known parathyroid disease (▽)

Histological sections from parathyroid explorations have shown mild hyperplasia in 70% of familial hypocalciuric hypercalcemia patients undergoing surgery (*Figure 9.3*)[28]. The degree of hyperplasia was variable; at the upper extreme were 3.5 diffusely hyperplastic glands (weighing 2.5 g) that had been removed from a 54-year-old female. We believe that subtle grades of dysfunction are present in the parathyroids of all patients with familial hypocalciuric hypercalcemia.

RESPONSE TO PARATHYROID SURGERY

Hypercalcemia usually persists after attempted subtotal parathyroidectomy in familial hypocalciuric hypercalcemia[12, 15]. After 52 explorations in 27 members of the 15 kindreds we have followed, 21 remain hypercalcemic, one is normocalcemic, and five have developed chronic hypocalcemia requiring treatment with calcium and/or calciferol (*Table 9.2*). For most patients preoperative and postoperative concentrations of calcium in serum have been similar. It is because of this outcome of surgery that recognition of the disorder is particularly important. Efforts should be made to establish the diagnosis preoperatively so that management can be properly tailored to the underlying disorder.

Table 9.2 Results of parathyroid exploration among previously hypercalcemic members from 15 familial hypocalciuric hypercalcemia (FHH) kindreds

Total operations	Outcome of last operation		
(*n*)	Hypercalcemia (*n*)	Normocalcemia (*n*)	Hypocalcemia (*n*)
1	12	1	2
2	3	0	3
3	5	0	0
4	1	0	0

GENETICS

In all reported kindreds the pattern of hypercalcemia has been consistent with autosomal dominant transmission. The penetrance for expression of hypercalcemia has been near 100% at all ages in familial hypocalciuric hypercalcemia kindreds. And recognition of hypercalcemia before age 10 in relatives is an extremely useful component in diagnosis. Severe neonatal primary hyperparathyroidism is an unusual feature in these kindreds, and its occurrence is probably not a random event[12a, 16, 25, 27]. We believe that severe neonatal primary hyperparathyroidism in familial hypocalciuric hypercalcemia kindreds represents the interaction of the familial hypocalciuric hypercalcemia gene with genetic or other factors in the parents. In some cases it may represent a double dose of an allele for the disease, while in others it may result from a different form of synergism.

EPIDEMIOLOGY

The fraction of all hypercalcemia patients with familial hypocalciuric hypercalcemia is not known. Certain population surveys have accepted chronic asymptomatic hypercalcemia as sufficient evidence for the diagnosis of typical primary hyperparathyroidism; in the context of the present discussion, such an assumption would be misleading. The 15 probands of our familial hypocalciuric hypercalcemia kindreds include an employee of our medical center, an employee of a neighboring medical center, and a local patient attending the immunology clinic of our center. The disorder is undoubtedly commoner than its infrequent recognition would suggest. In a recent survey of 67 patients referred to our service for hypercalcemia after unsuccessful parathyroid exploration, six proved to be probands for kindreds with this condition[20]. This diagnosis had been suspected in none prior to referral. Assuming a 5% failure rate for parathyroidectomy and a 10% rate of familial hypocalciuric hypercalcemia among patients with failed parathyroidectomy, one can estimate that the prevalence of the disease is ½% ($0.05 \times 0.10 = 0.005$ or 1 in 200) in patients who were undergoing parathyroidectomy for hypercalcemia during the time of that study. Since familial hypocalciuric hypercalcemia is overrepresented among the young and among patients with asymptomatic hypercalcemia (two groups less likely to be referred for parathyroidectomy), its prevalence among all hypercalcemic patients is undoubtedly higher than 1/2%.

PATHOPHYSIOLOGY

The decreased renal clearance of calcium and magnesium imply a disturbance of renal tubular function (with the exception of the hypothetical possibility of abnormal serum binding of calcium and magnesium in a rare kindred). Parathyroid hormone is the principal known humoral regulator of the renal transport of filtered calcium and magnesium. Infusion of PTH causes a greater increase in urine and plasma cAMP in familial hypocalciuric hypercalcemia than in typical primary hyperparathyroidism[19]. Increased renal responsivity to endogenous PTH may contribute to the increased renal resorption of filtered calcium and magnesium. However, there are two reasons for believing that this is not the full explanation of the disorder. Firstly, hypercalcemia resulting from low renal clearance of calcium should lead to suppression of the parathyroid gland, but instead parathyroid hyperplasia is present in familial hypocalciuric hypercalcemia. Secondly, low renal clearance of calcium persists in the disease even after parathyroidectomy has induced a state that is otherwise identical to postsurgical hypoparathyroidism[1]; thus low renal clearance of calcium is expressed even after successful cure of hyperparathyroidism.

Explanations of pathophysiology of familial hypocalciuric hypercalcemia must account for both renal and parathyroid function in this disorder. Is it possible that renal function is not at all abnormal in this condition and that the difference between it and typical primary hyperparathyroidism represents the occurrence of an underlying or evoked renal leak of calcium in so-called 'typical' primary hyperparathyroidism? We consider this unlikely because renal transport of calcium in parathyroidectomized subjects with familial hypocalciuric hypercalcemia is different from that in other parathyroidectomized subjects[1]. If we return then to the concept that renal and parathyroid function are both disturbed in familial hypocalciuric hypercalcemia, we are left with a physiological disturbance with no obvious cause. There is an interesting pharmacological model that may ultimately shed some light on this issue. Lithium decreases the renal clearance of both calcium and magnesium under certain conditions[22]. In addition, chronic lithium therapy may also be associated with hyperparathyroidism[5]. Thus this drug which has been shown to affect many cellular processes may provide a clue to the process(es) disturbed in familial hypocalciuric hypercalcemia.

Detailed studies of renal function in this disease have been performed. Three interesting observations have been made, all consistent with the hypothesis that renal tubular cells in familial hypocalciuric hypercalcemia exhibit decreased sensitivity to extracellular calcium ion. We shall reveiw these observations and also indicate some alternate interpretations.

The observation that there is greater cAMP response to PTH in familial hypocalciuric hypercalcemia than in typical primary hyperparathyroidism has been cited above. When PTH is given acutely to rats, the magnitude of the urinary cAMP response correlates inversely with serum calcium concentration[3]. Thus a renal cell not sensitive to extracellular calcium ion might elaborate more cAMP into urine (and plasma) than a renal cell in typical primary hyperparathyroidism (with a response to PTH that is suppressed by high extracellular concentrations of calcium ion). An alternate explanation for this observation is that high circulating PTH 'downregulates' the renal cAMP response to PTH. Since PTH levels are lower in familial hypocalciuric hypercalcemia than in typical primary hyperparathyroidism, the renal response to PTH in this disorder may not be similarly downregulated.

Low renal clearance of calcium persists in familial hypocalciuric hypercalcemia patients rendered hypoparathyroid[1]. Hypoparathyroidism is unusual after parathyroid surgery in this disorder and has occurred in five of 27 members of the 15 kindreds we have followed (*see Table 9.2*). Renal clearance of calcium is generally high in hypoparathyroidism. However, even in hypoparathyroidism, there is a threshold value for calcium in serum below which fractional renal clearance of calcium reaches a minimum. Factors determining this threshold have not been explored. One possibility is that renal tubules autoregulate calcium transport in response to the concentration of calcium ion in extracellular fluid. And, as an extension of this reasoning, the renal tubular cells in familial hypocalciuric hypercalcemia may continue to transport calcium in the 'hypocalcemic' mode even when serum calcium concentration is elevated. An alternate explanation for the low renal clearance of calcium in hypoparathyroid familial hypocalciuric hypercalcemia patients is that the kidneys manifest an exquisite hyperresponse of the calcium transport mechanism to PTH, and that minimal amounts of residual PTH are sufficient to elicit this response.

Chronic hypercalcemia generally causes impaired urine-concentrating ability, but familial hypocalciuric hypercalcemia is the only known exception[13]. The model of lithium mimicry of familial hypocalciuric hypercalcemia breaks down here as lithium impairs urine-concentrating ability. The persistence of maximal urine-concentrating ability in familial hypocalciuric hypercalcemia could reflect insensitivity of the urine-concentrating mechanism to deleterious effects of high concentrations of extracellular calcium ion. An alternate explanation for this finding is that hypercalcemia *per se* is not deleterious to urine-concentrating mechanisms but that the associated hypercalciuria is nephrotoxic. Since fractional renal tubular resorption of calcium is increased in familial hypocalciuric hypercalcemia the urine-concentrating mechanism might be spared from this nephrotoxicity.

Impaired renal tubular sensitivity to extracellular calcium ion could account for the above three sets of observations. While plausible alternate explanations for each observation exist, the attractiveness of the unifying explanation is that it could also account for the observations concerning the parathyroid gland. Impaired response to extracellular calcium ion would result in persistent secretion of PTH or even hyperplasia in the face of hypercalcemia. The calcium-insensitivity hypothesis raises several important questions. What could cause impairment of parathyroid and renal responsiveness to extracellular calcium ion? Could it be an excess or deficiency of some humoral factor that has not yet been recognized? Could it be mutation(s) of intracellular pathway(s) involved in calcium recognition? Do tissues other than the parathyroid and kidney express the defect(s)? If hypercalcemia is an appropriate homeostatic response to the underlying defect(s), are efforts to treat the hypercalcemia inappropriate (see pages 228–229)?

DIAGNOSIS

Hypercalcemia occurring before age 10

This is an uncommon finding[16]. Many etiologies (such as vitamin D intoxication, malignancy, granulomatous disorders, and immobilization) should be immediately apparent. The one condition that is difficult to distinguish is typical primary hyperparathyroidism. A diagnosis of familial hypocalciuric hypercalcemia should become immediately apparent by analysis of serum calcium in each parent (and preferably also any siblings). The recognition of a hypercalcemic relative supports the diagnosis of familial hypocalciuric hypercalcemia, and confirmation of relative hypocalciuria in other hypercalcemic members of a family should be sought. Familial hypercalcemia with the expression of hypercalcemia before age 10 is uncommon in other disorders (*Table 9.3*). Only two kindreds with familial multiple endocrine neoplasia type 1 (FMEN1) have been reported to contain members expressing hypercalcemia before age 10[2,4]. Hypercalcemia has not been reported before age 10 in affected persons with familial multiple endocrine neoplasia type 2 (FMEN2). A syndrome resembling idiopathic hypercalcemia of infancy has been reported in one kindred[21]. As in the sporadic form of idiopathic hypercalcemia of infancy[23] there are distinguishing features, which include hypercalciuria, nephrocalcinosis, supravalvular aortic stenosis, and mental retardation.

Table 9.3 Distinct syndromes of familial primary hyperparathyroidism

	Familial hypocalciuric hypercalcemia (FHH)	Familial multiple endocrine neoplasia type 1 (FMEN1)	Familial multiple endocrine neoplasia type 2 (FMEN2)
Genetics	Autosomal dominant	Autosomal dominant	Autosomal dominant
Penetrance of hypercalcemia	Near 100% at all ages	Approx. 80% after age 35	Approx. 30% after age 35
Recurrence after subtotal parathyroidectomy	Rapid and near 100%	Late 25%	Late 25%
Endocrine outside parathyroid	None	Pancreatic islet and anterior pituitary	C-cell and adrenal medulla
Other	Severe, neonatal primary hyperparathyroidism	Lipoma(s)	

Hypercalcemia occurring after age 10

The difficulty of distinguishing familial hypocalciuric hypercalcemia from typical primary hyperparathyroidism increases in proportion to the patient's age. At present there is no test or battery of tests that unequivocally establishes the diagnosis of familial hypocalciuric hypercalcemia. However, a calcium-to-creatinine clearance ratio below 0.012 should raise the suspicion of this diagnosis, and a ratio below 0.005 is highly suggestive. This information is based, however, on data representing the mean of multiple 24-hour urine specimens collected from inpatients on a metabolic ward where they received a calcium-restricted diet (elimination of dairy products resulted in a daily calcium content of approximately 10 mmol, 20 mEq). Even more so than with young children, firm diagnosis of familial hypocalciuric hypercalcemia in adults depends on establishing a pattern of features in the family. The most useful features are hypercalcemia (often asymptomatic) in multiple members particularly before age 10, relative hypocalciuria in hypercalcemic members, and failure to establish normocalcemia after parathyroidectomy. We have, however, encountered exceptions to each of these features, and there is a clear need for a simple diagnostic criterion. Features that we have not found commonly useful in diagnosis include the mild hypermagnesemia and the exaggerated cAMP response to PTH infusion. The commonest and most difficult problem in diagnosis is the patient exhibiting hypocalciuric hypercalcemia but no family members with hypercalcemia. Depending on the degree of hypocalciuria, we have been increasingly inclined to manage these patients as if they have familial hypocalciuric hypercalcemia because of possible unsatisfactory response to parathyroid surgery.

RELATION TO THE FAMILIAL MULTIPLE ENDOCRINE NEOPLASIA SYNDROMES

The familial multiple endocrine neoplasia (FMEN) syndromes are characterized by proliferation and hormone hypersecretion in multiple endocrine tissues. Morbidity results from the metabolic disturbance or the malignant potential of the proliferative process.

In kindreds with familial multiple endocrine neoplasia type 1 the endocrine tissues most commonly affected are the parathyroids, the pancreatic islets, and the anterior pituitary[2]. Penetrance is highest for primary hyperparathyroidism, and 95% of persons exhibiting obvious endocrine features of this condition are hypercalcemic. The penetrance of hypercalcemia increases with age; the disorder is rare below age 10 but quite common after age 35[16]. Because of the high penetrance of hyperparathyroidism, familial multiple endocrine neoplasia type 1 can present as (isolated) familial primary hyperparathyroidism in small kindreds[14]. And four of the six largest kindreds (six or more affected members) reported as familial primary hyperparathyroidism have already been reclassified as familial multiple endocrine neoplasia (one) or familial multiple endocrine neoplasia (three)[12]. Approximately 30% of persons expressing type 1 will exhibit dysfunction of the pancreatic islets.

Gastrinoma is the commonest islet disturbance, and ulcer disease or malignant gastrinoma is a major form of morbidity. Other pancreatic islet manifestations include insulinoma and pancreatic cholera. Approximately 15% of affected persons exhibit morbidity from anterior pituitary involvement. This is divided among prolactin, adrenocorticotrophic hormone (ACTH), and growth hormone (GH) producing tumors; hypopituitarism from tumor growth is another complication. Approximately 15% of affected patients have single or multiple lipomas; this causes no morbidity but may be useful in diagnosis.

In kindreds with type 2 the endocrine tissues affected are the C-cells of the thyroid, chromaffin tissue in the adrenal medulla and para-aortic region, and the parathyroids[24, 26]. Primary hyperparathyroidism is the least common of the disturbances, being manifest in approximately 20% of affected patients. More commonly, mild and asymptomatic hyperplasia of the parathyroids is recognized as an incidental finding during thyroid surgery. C-cell hyperplasia and cancer (medullary carcinoma of the thyroid) are associated with hypersecretion of calcitonin, a hormone causing no definite morbidity. Less frequently, medullary carcinoma of the thyroid is associated with watery diarrhea of uncertain etiology or with ectopic hypersecretion of adrenocorticotrophic hormone. Since the cancer is occasionally aggressive, procedures have been developed to diagnose this disorder in premalignant and premetastatic stages. Though the degree of expression in the different endocrine organs varies from one kindred to another, in general adrenal medullary hyperfunction causes as much morbidity as C-cell dysfunction.

Familial multiple endocrine neoplasia type 3 (FMEN3) shares many features with type 2[9]. The C-cell and adrenal medullary involvement are indistinguishable. Most important for the present review is the fact that primary hyperparathyroidism is virtually non-existent in type 3[8]. The other feature that distinguishes type 3 from type 2 is the occurrence of multiple neuromatous lesions; these include cutaneous and mucosal neuromas lending a pathognomonic appearance to the face, mouth, or eyes, as well as ganglioneuromas causing motility disorders of the intestines. Patients with type 3 also frequently display diffuse myopathy and a marfanoid body habitus.

The etiologies of these three syndromes are not known. The hyperparathyroidism that occurs in both type 1 and type 2 is typical primary hyperparathyroidism in that it is accompanied by calcareous renal disease[10] and in so far as it is often improved by standard subtotal parathyroidectomy (though the postoperative recurrence rate of hyperparathyroidism is greater in the familial multiple endocrine neoplasia syndromes than in sporadic primary parathyroid hyperplasia). To date patients with familial hypocalciuric hypercalcemia have not been reported to have any of the disorders of the other endocrine organs seen in the familial hyperparathyroid syndromes.

MANAGEMENT

Decisions about management must be made in the face of our present uncertainty concerning pathophysiology. Hopefully, further information will remove some of this uncertainty in the near future. We have followed a policy of avoiding parathyroid surgery in familial hypocalciuric hypercalcemia. Hypercalcemic relatives should be informed about the favorable prognosis to prevent future surgical misadventures. This is not to imply that parathyroid surgery is always contraindicated. Just as increased affinity of hemoglobin for oxygen can result in degrees of reactive erythremia that require intervention, insensitivity to calcium ion could result in manifestations of hypercalcemia or of PTH excess that are deleterious. Severe neonatal primary hyperparathyroidism is a clear indication for surgical treatment; however, asymptomatic neonatal hypercalcemia with calcium concentrations in the range of 6.0 mmol/l (12.0 mEq/l) is probably common in these kindreds and should not be considered as an indication for intervention.

Symptoms, signs, or biochemical disturbances will occasionally be sufficiently severe to warrant intervention. There is no published information concerning pharmacotherapy. Our unpublished experience suggests that 'loop' diuretics or calcitonin (two classes of calciuretic agent) will not be effective for management outside the hospital; a trial of phosphate orally should be considered. Two forms of surgical intervention have met with limited success. The first is total parathyroidectomy; this may, in fact, be difficult to accomplish, and several patients have remained hypercalcemic after attempted total parathyroidectomy. In some other patients, total parathyroidectomy has led to clinical hypoparathyroidism. Though the low renal clearance of calcium persists, these patients require calcium and/or calciferols to maintain normocalcemia. The second is total parathyroidectomy with autografting of parathyroid tissue to an accessible site such as the forearm (with or without an interval of tissue cryopreservation to ascertain the completeness of parathyroidectomy). Wells et al.[29] reported carrying this out in three siblings; each developed graft-dependent recurrent hypercalcemia, but after subtotal graft resection normocalcemia was achieved with a follow up period of approximately 1 year.

SUMMARY

Familial hypocalciuric hypercalcemia or familial benign hypercalcemia is an autosomal dominant trait with a high penetrance for expression of hypercalcemia at all ages. Commonly subjects are asymptomatic, and when symptoms or signs occur they are similar to those in typical primary hyperparathyroidism but milder. The renal clearance of filtered calcium and magnesium is lower than in patients with comparable hypercalcemia from typical primary hyperparathyroidism. This is notable because PTH itself decreases the renal clearance of calcium. The calcium-to-creatinine clearance ratio can be useful in diagnosis. PTH concentrations in blood are occasionally elevated, but in general they are lower than those found in patients with typical primary hyperparathyroidism and comparable degrees of hypercalcemia. Familial hypocalciuric hypercalcemia represents an atypical form of primary hyperparathyroidism in so far as the parathyroid glands are mildly hyperplastic, but standard subtotal parathyroidectomy rarely, if ever, produces stable normocalcemia.

Diagnosis is dependent upon recognition of characteristic features in multiple members of a kindred. Patients should be managed conservatively unless there are complications clearly attributable to the metabolic disturbance. Severe neonatal primary hyperparathyroidism is a rare event in these kindreds but one requiring urgent treatment by total parathyroidectomy; it may represent a double dose of the familial hypocalciuric hypercalcemia allele or synergism of this allele with other factors. The etiology of this disease is unknown, but renal tubular function and parathyroid function are both suggestive of insensitivity to ionized calcium in extracellular fluid. Though familial hypocalciuric hypercalcemia is uncommon (accounting for perhaps 1–2% of cases of asymptomatic hypercalcemia), recognition is important because of unresponsiveness to standard subtotal parathyroidectomy but a generally favorable prognosis.

References

1 ATTIE, M. F., GILL, J. R. Jr, STOCK, J. L., SPIEGEL, A. M., DOWNS, R. W. Jr, LEVINE, M. A. and MARX, S. J. Parathyroid hormone (PTH) independent abnormality of renal tubular transport of calcium in familial hypocalciuric hypercalcemia. *Clinical Research*, **28**, 384 (Abstract) (1980)

2 BALLARD, H. S., FRAME, B. and HARTSOCK, R. Familial multiple endocrine adenoma –peptic ulcer complex. *Medicine*, **43**, 481–516 (1964)

3 BECK, N., SINGH, H., REED, S. W. and DAVIS, B. B. Direct inhibitory effect of hypercalcemia on renal actions of parathyroid hormone. *Journal of Clinical Investigation*, **53**, 717–725 (1974)

4 BETTS, J. B., O'MALLEY, B. P. and ROSENTHAL, F. D. Hyperparathyroidism: a prerequisite for Zollinger–Ellison syndrome in multiple endocrine adenomatosis type 1 – report of a further family and review of the literature. *Quarterly Review of Medicine*, **73**, 69–76 (1980)

5 CHRISTIANSEN, C., BAASTRUP, P. C., LINDGREEN, P. and TRANSBØL, I. Endocrine effects of lithium: II. 'Primary' hyperparathyroidism. *Acta Endocrinologica*, **88**, 528–534 (1978)

6 FOLEY, T. P., Jr, HARRISON, H. C., ARNAUD, C. D. and HARRISON, H. E. Familial benign hypercalcemia. *Journal of Pediatrics*, **81**, 1060–1067 (1972)

7 HEATH, H. III and PURNELL, D. C. Urinary cyclic 3′,5′-adenosine monophosphate responses to exogenous and endogenous parathyroid hormone in familial benign hypercalcemia and primary hyperparathyroidism. *Journal of Laboratory and Clinical Medicine*, **96**, 974–984 (1980)

8 HEATH, H. III, SIZEMORE, G. W. and CARNEY, J. A. Preoperative diagnosis of occult parathyroid hyperplasia by calcium infusion in patients with multiple endocrine neoplasia, type 2a. *Journal of Clinical Endocrinology and Metabolism*, **43**, 428–435 (1976)

9 KHAIRI, M. R. A., DEXTER, R. N., BURZYNSKI, N. J. and JOHNSTON, C. C. Jr. Mucosal neuroma, pheochromocytoma and medullary thyroid carcinoma: multiple endocrine neoplasia type 3. *Medicine*, **54**, 89–112 (1975)

10 LAMERS, C. B. H. W. and FROELING, P. G. A. M. Clinical significance of hyperparathyroidism in familial multiple endocrine adenomatosis type I (MEAI). *American Journal of Medicine*, **66**, 422–424 (1979)

11 MALLETTE, L. E., BILEZEKIAN, J. P., HEATH, D. A. and AURBACH, G. D. Primary hyperparathyroidism: clinical and biochemical features. *Medicine*, **53**, 127–146 (1974)

12 MARX, S. J., ATTIE, M. F., LEVINE, M. A., SPIEGEL, A. M., DOWNS, R. W. Jr and LASKER, R. D. The hypocalciuric or benign variant of familial hypercalcemia: clinical and biochemical features in fifteen kindreds. *Medicine*, **60**, 397–412 (1981)

12a MARX, S. J., ATTIE, M. F., SPIEGEL, A. M., LEVINE, M. A., LASKER, R. D. and FOX, M. An association between neonatal severe primary hyperparathyroidism and familial hypocalciuric hypercalcaemia in three kindreds. *New England Journal of Medicine*, **306**, 257–264 (1982)

13 MARX, S. J., ATTIE, M. F., STOCK, J. L., SPIEGEL, A. M. and LEVINE, M. A. Maximal urine-concentrating ability: familial hypocalciuric hypercalcemia versus typical primary hyperparathyroidism. *Journal of Clinical Endocrinology and Metabolism*, **52**, 736–740 (1981)

14 MARX, S. J., POWELL, D., SHIMKIN, P. M., WELLS, S. A., KETCHAM, A. S., McGUIGAN, J. E., BILEZEKIAN, J. P. and AURBACH, G. D. Familial hyperparathyroidism: mild hypercalcemia in at least nine members of a kindred. *Annals of Internal Medicine*, **78**, 371–377 (1973)

15 MARX, S. J., SPIEGEL, A. M., BROWN, E. M. and AURBACH, G. D. Family studies in patients with primary parathyroid hyperplasia. *American Journal of Medicine*, **62**, 698–706 (1977)

16 MARX, S. J., SPIEGEL, A. M., BROWN, E. M., GARDNER, D. G., DOWNS, R. W. Jr, ATTIE, M. and AURBACH, G. D. Familial hypocalciuric hypercalcemia. In *Pediatric Diseases Related to Calcium*, edited by H. F. DeLuca and C. S. Anast, pp. 413–431. New York, Elsevier-North Holland Inc. (1980)

17 MARX, S. J., SPIEGEL, A. M., BROWN, E. M., KOEHLER, J. O., GARDNER, D. G., BRENNAN, M. F. and AURBACH, G. D. Divalent cation metabolism: familial hypocalciuric hypercalcemia versus typical primary hyperparathyroidism. *American Journal of Medicine*, **65**, 235–242 (1978)

18 MARX, S. J., SPIEGEL, A. M., BROWN, E. M., WINDECK, R., GARDNER, D. G., DOWNS, R. W. Jr, ATTIE, M. and AURBACH, G. D. Circulating parathyroid hormone activity: familial hypocalciuric hypercalcemia versus typical primary hyperparathyroidism. *Journal of Clinical Endocrinology and Metabolism*, **47**, 1190–1197 (1978)

19 MARX, S. J., SPIEGEL, A. M., SHARP, M. F., BROWN, E. M., GARDNER, D. G., DOWNS, R. W. Jr, ATTIE, M. F. and STOCK, J. L. Adenosine 3′,5′-monophosphate response to parathyroid hormone: familial hypocalciuric hypercalcemia versus typical primary hyperparathyroidism. *Journal of Clinical Endocrinology and Metabolism*, **50**, 546–549 (1980)

20 MARX, S. J., STOCK, J. L., ATTIE, M. F., DOWNS, R. W. Jr, GARDNER, D. G., BROWN, E. M., SPIEGEL, A. M., DOPPMAN, J. L. and BRENNAN, M. F Familial hypocalciuric hypercalcemia: recognition among patients referred after unsuccessful parathyroid exploration. *Annals of Internal Medicine*, **92**, 351–356 (1980)

21 MEHES, K., SZELID, Z. and TOTH, P. Possible dominant inheritance of the idiopathic hypercalcemia syndrome. *Human Heredity*, **25**, 30–34 (1975)

22 MILLER, P. D., DUBOVSKY, S. L., McDONALD, K. M., ARNAUD, C. and SCHRIER, R. W. Hypocalciuric effect of lithium in man. *Mineral and Electrolyte Metabolism*, **1**, 3–11 (1978)

23 SEELIG, M. S. Vitamin D and cardiovascular, renal and brain damage in childhood and infancy. *Annals of the New York Academy of Science*, **147**, 537–582 (1969)

24 SIZEMORE, G. W., CARNEY, J. A. and HEATH, H. III. Epidemiology of medullary carcinoma of the thyroid gland: a 5-year experience (1971–1976). *Surgical Clinics of North America*, **57**, 622–645 (1977)

25 SPIEGEL, A. M., HARRISON, H. E., MARX, S. J., BROWN, E. M. and AURBACH, G. D. Neonatal primary hyperparathyroidism with autosomal dominant inheritance. *Journal of Pediatrics*, **90**, 269–272 (1977)

26 STEINER, A. L., GOODMAN, A. D. and POWERS, S. R. Study of a kindred with pheochromocytoma, medullary thyroid carcinoma, hyperparathyroidism and Cushing's disease: multiple endocrine neoplasia type 2. *Medicine*, **47**, 371–409 (1968)

27 THOMPSON, N. W., CARPENTER, L. C., KESSLER, D. L. and NISHIYAMA, R. H. Hereditary neonatal hyperparathyroidism. *Archives of Surgery*, **113**, 100–103 (1978)

28 THORGEIRSSON, U., COSTA, J. and MARX, S. J. The parathyroid glands in familial hypocalciuric hypercalcemia. *Human Pathology*, **12**, 229 (1981)

29 WELLS, S. A. Jr, FARNDON, J. R., DALE, J. K., LEIGHT, G. S. and DILLEY, W. G. Long-term evaluation of patients with primary parathyroid hyperplasia managed by total parathyroidectomy and heterotopic autotransplantation. *Annals of Surgery*, **191**, 451–457 (1980)

10
Hypercalcaemia of malignancy

D. A. Heath

Malignancy is the commonest cause of hypercalcaemia in any general hospital. In a retrospective survey of 469 inpatients with hypercalcaemia seen in a general hospital, the cause was apparent in 367. Of these malignancy was responsible for the hypercalcaemia in 60%[15].

In a subsequent prospective survey of 166 patients in the same hospital the cause of the hypercalcaemia was found in 153 and 59% were associated with malignant conditions[16]. As less severely ill populations are considered so the percentage of cases of hypercalcaemia due to malignancy falls. The same group studying the causes of hypercalcaemia throughout the entire City of Birmingham, involving inpatients, outpatients and some general practitioner patients, found malignancy to be the cause in 38% of patients[33]. In 'fit-patient' screening malignancy is a rare cause of hypercalcaemia. In the performance of nearly 16 000 biochemical screens of employees in Sweden aged between 20 and 63 years, hypercalcaemia was found in 178 individuals of whom only two had malignancy[7].

MALIGNANT STATES ASSOCIATED WITH HYERCALCAEMIA

Hypercalcaemia has been associated with a wide range of malignant states and the prevalence of hypercalcaemia varies considerably depending whether patients are serially studied or, if looked at once, whether it is at presentation or at autopsy. The tumours most likely to be responsible for hypercalcaemia also vary considerably in the published series, depending probably in the main part on the particular interests or expertise of the reporting group. The early literature raised the hope that a significant number of patients with malignancy and hypercalcaemia had a treatable tumour. On successful treatment the hypercalcaemia was completely corrected, suggesting that the tumour produced a humoral agent responsible for the hypercalcaemia. For this situation the term pseudohyperparathyroidism was coined[26]. When evidence was subsequently presented that this humoral agent might be parathyroid hormone (PTH) the term ectopic PTH syndrome became widely used even when PTH estimations were not performed. As will be seen later, it now appears that in the vast majority of malignant states with hypercalcaemia the tumour is metastatic and rarely curable and that ectopic PTH secretion is extremely rare. For this reason the terms pseudohyperparathyroidism and particularly the ectopic PTH syndrome seem inappropriate and will not be used further in this chapter.

Table 10.1 Hypercalcaemia in patients with malignant disease. (From Fisken *et al.*[15], courtesy of the Editor and Publishers, *Lancet*)

Primary site	Total number of cases	Number (%) of case with obvious metastatic disease
Bronchus	54	33 (61)
Breast	44	43 (98)
Ear, nose or throat	15	10 (66)
Ureters, bladder or urethra	15	4 (27)
Myeloma	14	14 (100)
Female genital tract	14	12 (86)
Oesophagus	13	8 (62)
Unknown primary site	10	10 (100)
Lymphoma	9	8 (89)
Kidney	7	3 (43)
Large bowel	5	4 (80)
Thyroid	4	4 (100)
Two primary sites	4	2 (50)
Liver and biliary system	3	2
Prostate	3	1
Melanoma	2	2
Testis	1	1
Osteosarcoma	1	1
Pancreas	1	1
Total	219	163 (75)

Table 10.1 lists the primary sites of 219 cases of hypercalcaemic malignancy seen at the Queen Elizabeth Hospital over a 32-month period[15]. As in most reported series from non-specialized centres the commonest malignancies were carcinoma of the lung and breast which accounted for 45% of the total series. There then follows a long list of other tumours that were occasionally associated with hypercalcaemia. *Table 10.2* is derived from *Table 10.1* but has further grouped together tumours arising from a related system. Such a grouping is of importance when it comes to investigation of a patient for a possible malignant cause for hypercalcaemia and helps to place in order our various investigative procedures. Conspicuous by their near absence from this list are malignancies of the gastrointestinal tract (other than oesophagus) and haematological malignancies (other than myeloma). Of course the order in *Table 10.1* in part reflects the commonness of certain tumours in the general population. By relating the patients with hypercalcaemia due to a particular

Table 10.2 Hypercalcaemia in patients with malignant disease. (After Fisken *et al.*[15])

Primary site	% of cases
Lung	24
Breast	20
Renal tract	11
Ear, nose and throat	7
Female genital tract	6
Oesophagus	6
Myeloma	6
Others	20

Table 10.3 Prevalence of hypercalcaemia with different primary sites of tumour. (From Fisken *et al.*[15], courtesy of the Editor and Publishers, *Lancet*)

Primary site	%
Myeloma	33
Oesophagus	6.5
Bronchus	6.4
Thyroid	5.7
Breast	5.3
Ear, nose and throat	4.1
Lymphoma	2.4
Bladder, ureter and urethra	2.3
Female genital tract	1.8
Large bowel	1.1

Figures give the number of cases with hypercalcaemia as a percentage of the total number of cases of that type of tumour admitted to the hospital during the study period.

tumour to the total number of tumours of that type seen in hospital during the period of study, Fisken *et al.*[15] were able to derive figures for prevalence of hypercalcaemia with different primary sites (*Table 10.3*). When looked at in this manner the malignant state most likely to be complicated by hypercalcaemia was myeloma where a third of cases developed this complication. As mentioned earlier these figures probably seriously underestimate the likelihood of hypercalcaemia occurring during the total course of the disease.

Of further great importance is the recognition that the majority of patients with hypercalcaemia of malignancy have obvious widespread metastases at the time that they are recognized to be hypercalcaemic. This information is given in *Table 10.1* where the overall incidence of metastases was 75%. As the vast majority of patients in this study did not have radiological or isotopic surveys of their skeleton or isotopic liver scans, it is quite obvious that 75% is a serious underestimation of the incidence of metastases. To further emphasize the rarity of these patients having a tumour that is curable by primary resection is the fact that in the entire series only one patient had a removal of a tumour which led to the patient becoming normocalcaemic – this was a patient with bronchial carcinoma and he had developed obvious metastases 4 months after attempted curative surgery (Fisken and Heath, unpublished observations). As might be expected, if hypercalcaemia is usually a manifestation of advanced malignancy, it was rare for the hypercalcaemia to present before the malignancy. In the Birmingham series in only four of the 219 cases was the hypercalcaemia known about before a diagnosis of malignancy was made. In three of these four cases malignancy was rapidly found on initial investigation. The exception was a case of cholangiocarcinoma which did not become apparent until the patient had been known to be hypercalcaemic for 9 months. Undoubtedly hypercalcaemia can occur in malignancy at a time when the tumour is non-metastatic and amenable to treatment. Powell *et al.*[31] reported 10 cases where treatment of the primary tumour cured the hypercalcaemia and eradicated the malignant process. However, these cases were collected over a period of several years and involved referral from a wide area of the United States (Powell, personal communication). In a subsequent review of the world literature 64 cases were found where removal of a tumour corrected the hypercalcaemia[44]. The understanding of these facts must inevitably influence the way we approach a patient with asymptomatic hypercalcaemia as it would appear extremely unlikely that such a patient will be harbouring a treatable, occult malignancy responsible for the hypercalcaemia.

HYPERCALCAEMIA ASSOCIATED WITH SPECIFIC NEOPLASTIC CONDITIONS

Carcinoma of the lung

It has been well demonstrated that hypercalcaemia occurs most typically with squamous cell carcinoma of the lung despite the fact that adenocarcinoma and small cell carcinoma more frequently metastasize to bone[1]. The incidence of hypercalcaemia in bronchogenic carcinoma has varied a little but two recent series have produced figures of 6.4% and 6.8%[6, 15].

Carcinoma of the breast

As shown in *Table 10.1* hypercalcaemia is almost invariably associated with metastatic disease, usually including extensive skeletal deposits. Although oestrogen and antioestrogen therapy may control the hypercalcaemia they can also cause a rapid rise in serum calcium on initiation of therapy[45]. Claims that a hypercalcaemia response predicted a likely remission of the disease with continuation of drug therapy have been challenged[29]. Subsequent rechallenge with the drug after one hypercalcaemic episode does not always result in hypercalcaemia but readministration should be closely monitored.

Carcinoma of the kidney and urogenital tract

Fisken *et al.*[15] noted that whereas 75% of all their cases of malignant hypercalcaemia had overt metastases, only 32% of tumours arising from the upper and lower renal tract were thus affected. Also, of seven patients known to be alive 1 year after the onset of hypercalcaemia, three had carcinoma of the bladder, a tumour site which represented less than 5% of the total series. This much more favourable outcome in tumours arising from these sites raises the possibility that the hypercalcaemia is due to a different mechanism in these cases or, less likely, that the tumours are functionally more active and thus come to notice at an earlier stage. Somewhat similar findings are to be found in the review of cases where removal of the tumour corrected the hypercalcaemia. Skrabanek *et al.*[44] found 64 cases in the world literature, of which seven were phaeochromocytomas and probably non-malignant. Of the remaining 59 cases, 30 arose from the kidney or urogenital system – a surprisingly high proportion. Although at present this finding may be due to case selection, the differences are sufficiently striking to warrant further study.

Haematological malignancies

Hypercalcaemia has always been recognized as a common complication of myeloma but has been thought to be a rather rare late complication in the leukaemias. In both conditions osteoclast-activating factor (OAF) has been shown to be produced by the malignant cells and the involvement of this agent in the aetiology of the hypercalcaemia will be discussed later. The incidence of hypercalcaemia in myeloma was found to range between 21% and 33% in three published series[6, 15, 50]. Recent evidence suggests that hypercalcaemia is more common in leukaemia than was previously believed. Burt and Brennan[6] reporting on a large number of cases found that approximately 5% of cases of chronic myeloid or lymphocytic leukaemia had associated hypercalcaemia while 10% of acute myeloid and 18% of acute lymphocytic leukaemias were affected.

Lymphomas

The incidence of hypercalcaemia in the various lymphomas has been well documented by Burt and Brennan[6]. In Hodgkin's disease they report a figure of 5.4% while in non-Hodgkin's lymphoma the figure rose from 2.4% to 18% as the histological appearances became less differentiated.

THE MECHANISM OF HYPERCALCAEMIA IN MALIGNANCY

Due to metastases to bone

Many patients with hypercalcaemia of malignancy will have extensive skeletal metastases and this is almost invariably true of hypercalcaemia associated with carcinoma of the breast. However, skeletal metastases *per se* cannot be the explanation of all cases of malignant hypercalcaemia and there appears to be a poor correlation between the presence of skeletal metastases and the occurrence of hypercalcaemia in many cases. In carcinoma of the lung, small cell, squamous cell carcinomas as well as adenocarcinomas frequently have skeletal metastases yet hypercalcaemia is almost entirely restricted to cases of squamous cell carcinoma[1]. Carcinomas of the stomach and large bowel not infrequently metastasize to bone yet are rarely complicated by hypercalcaemia. It is known that some tumour cells are able to resorb bone directly *in vitro*. In experiments on five lines of cells derived from patients with breast carcinoma Eilon and Mundy[14] were able to demonstrate direct resorption of bone *in vitro* independently of osteoclast stimulation. Normal lymphocytes and malignant cells derived from patients with chronic lymphatic leukaemia, ovarian and lung carcinoma and chondroblastoma, none of whom had skeletal metastases or hypercalcaemia, lacked the ability to resorb bone directly. Other workers have found that 60% of human breast tumours are able to cause bone resorption in organ culture[38] but that this resorption is dependent upon the ability of the tumour cells to produce prostaglandins and other non-dialysable osteolytic agents[11]. Tumours with *in vitro* osteolytic activity were more likely to have metastasized and to have been complicated by hypercalcaemia[38]. These experiments would lend support to the concept that certain tumour deposits have the potential to cause more local bone resorption than others dependent on the production of locally acting humoral agents. Of interest in this area is the fact that products released during the process of bone resorption appear to be chemotactic to both tumour cells[35] and to monocytes which are probably precursors of the osteoclast[32]. This raises the possibility that once bone resorption is increased either by local or distant mechanisms factors are released from bone which will increase the possibility of further skeletal metastases.

Using nephrogenous cyclic AMP (NcAMP) as an indicator of parathyroid hormone-like material secreted by tumours it was found in 50 consecutive tumours with hypercalcaemia that 18% had reduced NcAMP production suggesting to the authors that in these patients the hypercalcaemia was due to local osteolysis[46]. The larger group with elevated NcAMP (82%) were thought to have hypercalcaemia due to the production by the tumour of a distant humoral factor. Supporting their concept was the fact that all patients in the low NcAMP had evidence of extensive skeletal metastases whereas only just over 50% of the other group had skeletal metastases and these were not extensive.

Production by the tumour of parathyroid hormone

With the advent of radioimmunoassay for PTH a number of isolated case reports of elevated PTH in the presence of malignant hypercalcaemia appeared, including examples of PTH arteriovenous gradients across the tumour and PTH being identified in tumour extracts (see Skrabanek *et al.*[44]). This initially appeared to be an occasional finding but two groups in particular reported series in which the vast majority of cases of hypercalcaemia of malignancy had elevated immunoreactive PTH (iPTH) concentrations[2, 40]. In these series the PTH was not as elevated as the values seen in hyperparathyroidism with a similar degree of hypercalcaemia and it was inferred that the tumours were producing a variant of the PTH molecule which was immunologically different from normal human PTH but with biological activity. More recent studies have failed to confirm these findings and most current PTH assays find low levels of the hormone in the majority of cases of malignancy. Reviewing the previous reports, current thinking would be that true PTH production by tumours has been either adequately documented in only a small number of cases[43] or may never have been properly proven[44]. It should be remembered that there are considerable variations between differing PTH assays and that the same sample in two different assays may give apparently discrepant results. Thus, when identical samples were assayed in four different centres the correlation between the assays was poor and in one case varied from undetectable to unequivocally elevated[39]. Although differences in antibody recognition may play a part in these discrepancies, it is my own view that the major part is due to non-specific effects in the assay. There does, however, remain the occasional patient with hypercalcaemia of malignancy who does have an elevated PTH concentration. In my own experience this amounts to around 5–8% of samples from known malignant cases. In part this is due to the occurrence of primary hyperparathyroidism in patients with malignancy (*see below*). Whether this is the explanation in most or all cases, or whether it reflects non-specific artifacts or true ectopic production of PTH by the tumour, is not yet known. The studies of Drezner and Lebowitz[12] indicate that hyperparathyroidism may explain some of the cases of malignancy with elevated PTH concentration though it is likely that they were dealing with a very atypical collection of cases.

Overall therefore it would appear that tumours rarely, if ever, produce PTH ectopically.

Production by the tumour of vitamin D-like sterols

Despite a lack of evidence in support of this theory it continues to be quoted as a proven explanation of some cases of hypercalcaemia of malignancy. The report by Gordan *et al.*[17] of an osteolytic sterol in human breast cancer has not been substantiated by any other group and the compound was probably a prostaglandin. It precedes the recent advance in vitamin D analytical methodology, and more recent work using these newer techniques has failed to find any support for the concept[18].

Production by the tumour of prostaglandins

The excessive production of prostaglandin E_2 by tumours and its likely involvement in the associated hypercalcaemia has been well documented by Tashjian and his workers for two animal models[49]. A number of different prostaglandins have been shown *in vitro* to be potent bone-resorbing agents[24] and a variety of tumour cells in culture have produced prostaglandins[38]. In some studies cells derived from tumours metastatic to bone or associated with hypercalcaemia have produced greater amounts of prostaglandins in culture[38]. Several studies have demonstrated either increased plasma PGE concentrations[9] or increased urinary excretion of a PGE metabolite[41] in patients with hypercalcaemic malignancies. The report of a case of hypercalcaemia associated with a renal-cell adenocarcinoma where indomethacin consistently corrected the hypercalcaemia[5] further raised the possibility that prostaglandins were a likely aetiological agent in hypercalcaemia of malignancy in man. Since that report occasional further cases have been shown to respond to indomethacin or aspirin[28, 41] but the experience of most workers is that a response to drugs which inhibit prostaglandin synthetase is unusual. In the hypercalcaemia of breast cancer indomethacin was singularly ineffective[8], and yet breast cancer cells in culture can readily be shown to produce prostaglandins. This raises considerable doubts about the involvement of prostaglandins in the aetiology of the hypercalcaemia of a significant proportion of human tumours.

Production of osteoclast-activating factors

Peripheral blood leucocytes when activated by non-specific mitogens or by antigens to which they have been previously exposed, produce a potent bone resorbing factor called osteoclast-activating factor (OAF)[21]. Gel filtration studies on osteoclast-activating factor show the presence of two compounds, one with a molecular weight of between 12 500 and 25 000 daltons and the other with a molecular weight of between 1330 and 3500 daltons. These two compounds have been called big and little OAF respectively and are interconvertible by simple physical means[31]. Osteoclast-activating factor is physicochemically and immunologically distinct from PTH, vitamin D compounds and prostaglandins. Compounds with similar characteristics to OAF are produced by cultured malignant cells from patients with myeloma and a number of other B-cell lymphoproliferative disorders[30]. In subsequent studies a correlation was found between the amount of OAF produced *in vitro* and the degree of skeletal involvement *in vivo* though not with the serum calcium concentration[13]. Production of osteoclast-activating factor by stimulated leucocytes is blocked by indomethacin and other compounds which interfere with prostaglandin production and these effects are overcome by the addition of prostaglandins of the E series[51].

It would appear that activated lymphocytes are the source of osteoclast-activating factor but this is dependent on the presence of E-series prostaglandins which are released by associated monocytes[52]. The action of osteoclast-activating factor in causing bone resorption is inhibited by cortisol at doses as low as 10^{-9} M whereas OAF production was only inhibited at doses in excess of 10^{-5} M[48]. This inhibition of the action of OAF could explain the fact that corticosteroids are usually effective in controlling the hypercalcaemia associated with myeloma and leukaemia.

Hence there appears to be reasonable laboratory evidence and some clinical evidence to incriminate osteoclast-activating factor in the aetiology of a proportion of cases with hypercalcaemia associated with haematological malignancies. There is, however, no evidence at present that osteoclast-activating factor is produced by other malignancies.

Other factors

That other factors may be involved in the aetiology of the hypercalcaemia of malignancy is obvious from our present inability to satisfactorily explain many of the cases currently being investigated. Uncharacterized non-dialysable osteolytic agents have been found in the culture medium in which human breast tumours have been growing. Such agents were distinct from prostaglandins[11]. Other workers have detected a material in the plasma of patients with hypercalcaemia without skeletal secondaries which has similar biological actions to PTH in a cytochemical bioassay. This material on gel filtration eluted as a major peak in the void volume of the column and was only partially inactivated by PTH antibodies[47]. In support of the view that tumours produce a substance with biological actions similar to PTH is the similarity of the biochemical changes in malignancy and hyperparathyroidism (*see below*), and the finding of histological evidence of osteitis fibrosa in patients dying with malignancy and hypercalcaemia, yet in whom no evidence of parathyroid overactivity could be found at post-mortem[42].

Associated hyperparathyroidism

Quite obviously any known cause of hypercalcaemia may by chance be associated with malignancy. The concurrence of malignancy and primary hyperparathyroidism (HPT) has been reported on numerous occasions. As both conditions are common this is not surprising. However, analysis of cases has shown that the malignancies are almost always of epithelial origin suggesting that such occurrences are more than a chance event[22]. At present this issue cannot be resolved. Certainly the finding of elevated PTH concentrations in a hypercalcaemic patient known to have had or to have malignancy should raise the possibility of associated primary hyperparathyroidism.

Hypercalcaemia associated with other endocrine tumours

Hypercalcaemia commonly occurs in the setting of the multiple endocrine neoplasia syndromes where it is usually due to parathyroid hyperplasia or occasionally to a single parathyroid adenoma. Hypercalcaemia may be due to a phaeochromocytoma *per se* and be completely corrected by removal of the adrenal tumour. Although catecholamine stimulation of PTH secretion has been suggested as the mechanism of the hypercalcaemia[25] serum PTH is usually normal or low[10, 20, 36]. Catecholamines cause hypercalcaemia in the parathyroidectomized rat[23] and may therefore be the direct aetiological cause of the elevated serum calcium. Similarly hypercalcaemia associated with a vasoactive intestinal peptide (VIP) secreting pancreatic tumour may be corrected by removal of the pancreatic tumour[4]. This is in contradistinction to hypercalcaemia associated with the other hormonally active pancreatic tumours where hypercalcaemia indicates a concurrent parathyroid disorder. Finally, in acromegaly hypercalcaemia may occasionally be completely corrected by successful treatment of the excessive growth hormone secretion[34].

BIOCHEMICAL CHANGES IN MALIGNANT HYPERCALCAEMIA

Despite many claims there are few, if any, biochemical investigations which reliably differentiate between hypercalcaemia of malignancy and other causes of hypercalcaemia. In a prospective study of 153 consecutive cases of hypercalcaemia the measurement of serum phosphate, chloride, chloride–phosphate ratio and hydrogen ion concentration were found to be of no value in separating cases of hyperparathyroidism from malignancy[16]. Urinary studies of phosphate and cyclic AMP (cAMP) excretion were similarly found to be unhelpful (Fisken *et al.*, unpublished observations). Despite the similarity between the biochemical tests in hyperparathyroidism and malignancy there is rarely great difficulty differentiating the two conditions due to the fact that the malignancy state is usually apparent and frequently of a disseminated nature. Serum PTH assays vary in their ability to differentiate between the two conditions. Most assays give good separation but some are of little value[39].

MANAGEMENT OF MALIGNANT HYPERCALCAEMIA

Except when hypercalcaemia is very severe initial management will be directed to the cause of the hypercalcaemia. As mentioned above the underlying malignant disorder is usually readily apparent. In addition to specific symptoms or signs of malignancy, unexpected weight loss, anaemia or a high erythrocyte sedimentation rate (ESR) make the possibility of an underlying malignancy more likely though all of these features can occur in hyperparathyroidism[27]. A low serum albumin or high globulin should always raise the suspicion of malignancy. Where malignancy is suspected but not clinically apparent careful examination of the breasts, and investigation of the respiratory, genitourinary and female reproductive tract are most likely to bring to light the underlying primary tumour. Routine barium studies of the upper and lower intestinal tract are rarely of value unless symptoms of oesophageal disease are present.

Although curative treatment of the underlying malignant condition is the ideal management of the hypercalcaemia this is rarely possible. Often scant attention is paid to the hypercalcaemia associated with known malignancy[15] possibly due to the fact that some of the symptoms of hypercalcaemia may mimic the symptoms of the underlying malignancy or side-effects of the treatment given for the tumour. When hypercalcaemia is severe and causing marked symptoms the initial treatment should always be intravenous fluids, up to 10 l of fluids during the first 24 hours. Careful monitoring of the patient is required and hypokalaemia readily develops unless potassium supplements are given. I tend not to give frequent injections of diuretics reserving them should any evidence of heart failure develop. Such treatment is usually successful in dropping the serum calcium significantly and improving the clinical state of the patient sufficiently to avoid other emergency treatments. If further emergency treatment is required there is considerable debate as to the safest and most effective regime. It is my own view that calcitonin is not often very effective although the combination of calcitonin and steroids has been claimed to the effective[3]. Steroids are effective in only about 50% of patients with hypercalcaemic malignancy and are relatively slow to work. Intravenous phosphate therapy is very effective but considered by many to be too dangerous though a review of the literature does not necessarily support this view[19].

For these various reasons I use mithramycin as an adjunct to fluids in those cases requiring urgent additional therapy. A dose of 25 µg/kg is given as a bolus intravenous injection which is repeated on the second day if necessary. Mithramycin does not work immediately and a significant fall in serum calcium is usually not apparent until at least 24 hours. This further emphasizes the need for vigorous intravenous therapy. This delay, although unfortunate, is offset by the very high percentage of cases that respond to the treatment. Used in the above doses serious toxic side-effects are rare. It cannot be stressed enough that the vast majority of cases do not require any emergency treatment other than intravenous fluids; that in the past various treatment regimes have been used too readily and that a number of patients have died as a result of their treatment rather than from hypercalcaemia.

With more moderate hypercalcaemia or following initial fluid replacement other safer therapy can be considered, particularly the use of oral therapy. Basically, two effective drugs can be considered – oral steroids and phosphate. Oral steroids are less frequently effective than phosphate but cause fewer initial side-effects. Overall around 50% of cases respond but this rate may be higher with haematological malignancies. Doses of 120 mg hydrocortisone or 60 mg prednisolone are often used initially reducing to the lowest possible maintenance dose if the hypercalcaemia is controlled. Oral phosphate is more frequently effective but has a high incidence of side-effects particularly abdominal discomfort and diarrhoea. A dose of 500 mg phosphate should initially be given 6-hourly, using if necessary drugs like codeine phosphate to minimize diarrhoea. Long-term outpatient therapy with either steroids or phosphate may sometimes be necessary if definitive treatment of the malignancy is not possible. Not all cases of hypercalcaemia need such treatment and it should be reserved for symptomatic patients or those with moderate to severe hypercalcaemia. All other patients should be advised to avoid dehydration and to present immediately if any symptoms of hypercalcaemia develop.

CONCLUSIONS

Hypercalcaemia is a common complication of many different malignant states. The exact mechanism of the hypercalcaemia is likely to vary in different malignancies and in many instances remains to be elucidated. The ectopic production of PTH is probably very rare. In most cases the malignant condition is far advanced and metastatic. Hypercalcaemia is often neglected and its treatment can often cause marked symptomatic improvement.

References

1 BENDER, R. A. and HANSEN, H. Hypercalcaemia in bronchogenic carcinoma: a prospective study of 200 patients. *Annals of Internal Medicine*, **80**, 205–208 (1974)

2 BENSON, R. C. Jr., RIGGS, B. L., PICKARD, B. M. and ARNAUD, C. D. Radiommunoassay of parathyroid hormone in hypercalcaemic patients with malignant disease. *American Journal of Medicine*, **56**, 821–826 (1974)

3 BINSTOCK, M. L. and MUNDY, G. R. Effect of calcitonin and glucocorticoids in combination on the hypercalcaemia of malignancy. *Annals of Internal Medicine*, **93**, 269–272 (1980)

4 BLOOM, S. R. and POLAK, J. M. Glucagonomas, vipomas and somatostatinomas. *Clinics in Endocrinology and Metabolism*, **9**, 285–297 (1980)

5 BRERETON, H. D., HALUSHKA, P. V., ALEXANDER, R. W., MASON, D. M., KEISER, H. R. and DE VITA, V. T. Jr. Indomethacin-responsive hypercalcaemia in a patient with renal cell adenocarcinoma. *New England Journal of Medicine*, **291**, 83–85 (1974)

6 BURT, M. E. and BRENNAN, M. F. Incidence of hypercalcaemia and malignant neoplasm. *Archives of Surgery*, **115**, 704–707 (1980)

7 CHRISTENSSON, T., HELLSTRÖM, K., WENGLE, B., ALVERYD, A. and WIKLAND, B. Prevalence of hypercalcaemia in a health screening in Stockholm. *Acta Medica Scandinavica*, **200**, 131–137 (1976)

8 COOMBES, R. C., NEVILLE, A. M., BONDY, P. K. and POWLES, T. J. Failure of indomethacin to reduce hydroxyproline excretion or hypercalcaemia in patients with breast cancer. *Prostaglandins*, **12**, 1027–1035 (1976)

9 DEMERS, L. M., ALLEGRA, J. C., HARVEY, H. A., LIPTON, A., LUDERER, J. R., MORTEL, R. and BRENNER, D. E. Plasma prostaglandins in hypercalcaemic patients with neoplastic disease. *Cancer*, **39**, 1559–1562 (1977)

10 DE PLAEN, J. F., BOERNER, F. and VAN YPERSELE DE STRIHOUS, C. Hypercalcaemic phaeochromocytoma. *British Medical Journal*, **2**, 734 (1976)

11 DOWSETT, M., EASTY, G. C., POWLES, T. J., EASTY, D. M. and NEVILLE, A. M. Human breast tumour-induced osteolysis and prostaglandins. *Prostaglandins*, **11**, 447–460 (1976)

12 DREZNER, M. K. and LEBOWITZ, H. E. Primary hyperparathyroidism in paraneoplastic hypercalcaemia. *Lancet*, **1**, 1004–1006 (1978)

13 DURIE, B. G. M., SALMON, S. E. and MUNDY, G. R. Relation of osteoclast activating factor production to extent of bone disease in multiple myeloma. *British Journal of Haematology*, **47**, 21–30 (1981)

14 EILON, G. and MUNDY, G. R. Direct resorption of bone by human breast cancer cells *in vitro*. *Nature*, **276**, 726–728 (1978)

15 FISKEN, R. A., HEATH, D. A. and BOLD, A. M. Hypercalcaemia – a hospital survey. *Quarterly Journal of Medicine*, **49,** 405–418 (1980)

16 FISKEN, R. A., HEATH, D. A., SOMERS, S. and BOLD, A. M. Hypercalcaemia in hospital patients. Clinical and diagnostic aspects. *Lancet*, **1,** 202–207 (1981)

17 GORDAN, G. S., CANTINO, T. J., ERHARDT, L., HANSEN, J. and LUBICH, W. Osteolytic sterol in human breast cancer. *Science*, **151,** 1226–1228 (1966)

18 HADDAD, J. G., COURANZ, S.J. and AVIOLI, L. V. Circulating phytosterols in normal females, lactating mothers and breast cancer patients. *Journal of Clinical Endocrinology and Metabolism*, **30,** 174–180 (1970)

19 HEATH, D. A. The use of inorganic phosphate in the management of hypercalcaemia. *Metabolic Bone Disease and Related Research*, **2,** 213–215 (1980)

20 HEATH, H. III and EDIS, A. J. Phaeochromocytoma associated with hypercalcaemia and ectopic secretion of calcitonin. *Annals of Internal Medicine*, **91,** 208–210 (1979)

21 HORTON, J. E., RAISZ, L. G. and SIMMONS, H. A. Bone resorbing activity in supernatant fluid from cultured human peripheral blood leucocytes. *Science*, **177,** 793–795 (1972)

22 KAPLAN, L., KATZ, A. D. and BEN-ISAAC, C. Malignant neoplasms and parathyroid adenoma. *Cancer*, **28,** 401–407 (1971)

23 KENNY, A. D. Effect of catecholamines on serum calcium and phosphorus levels in intact and parathyroidectomized rats. *Naunyn-Schmiedeberg's Archives of Pharmacology*, **248,** 144–152 (1964)

24 KLEIN, D. C. and RAISZ, L. G. Prostaglandins: stimulation of bone resorption in tissue culture. *Endocrinology*, **86,** 1436–1440 (1970)

25 KUKREJA, S. C., HARGIS, G. K., ROSENTHAL, I. M. and WILLIAMS, G. A. Phaeochromocytoma causing excessive parathyroid hormone production and hypercalcaemia. *Annals of Internal Medicine*, **79,** 838–840 (1973)

26 LAFFERTY, F. W. Pseudohyperparathyroidism. *Medicine (Baltimore)*, **45,** 247–260 (1966)

27 MALLETTE, L. E., BILEZIKIAN, J. P., HEATH, D. A. and AURBACH, G. D. Primary hyperparathyroidism: Clinical and biochemical features. *Medicine*, **53,** 127–146 (1974)

28 McKAY, H. A., GAVRELL, G. J., MEEHAN, W. L., KAPLAN, R. A. and LE BLANC, G. A. Prostaglandin-mediated hypercalcaemia in transitional cell carcinoma of the bladder. *Journal of Urology*, **119,** 689–692 (1978)

29 MINTON, M. J., SPARROW, G., RUBEN, R. D. and HAYWARD, J. L. Tamoxifen induced hypercalcaemia and response to treatment. *British Medical Journal*, **280,** 186–187 (1980)

30 MUNDY, G. R., COOPER, L. G., SCHECTER, R. A. and SALMON, S. E. Evidence for the secretion of an osteoclast stimulating factor in myeloma. *New England Journal of Medicine*, **291,** 1041–1046 (1974)

31 MUNDY, G. R., RAISZ, L. G., SHAPIRO, J. L., BANDELIN, I. G. and TURCOTTE, R. J. Big and little forms of osteoclast activating factor. *Journal of Clinical Investigation*, **60,** 122–128 (1977)

32 MUNDY, G. R., VARANI, J., ORR, W., GONDEK, M. D. and WARD, P. A. Resorbing bone is chemotactic for monocytes. *Nature*, **275,** 132–135 (1978)

33 MUNDY, G. R., COVE, D. H., FISKEN, R. A., HEATH, D. A. and SOMERS, S.   Primary hyperparathyroidism: changes in the pattern of clinical presentation. *Lancet*, **1**, 1317–1320 (1980)

34 NADARAJAH, A. M., HARTOG, M., REDFERN, B., THALASSINOS, N., WRIGHT, A. D., JOPLIN, G. F. and FRASER, T. R. Calcium metabolism in acromegaly. *British Medical Journal*, **4**, 797–801 (1968)

35 ORR, F. W., VARANI, J., GONDEK, M. D., WARD, P. A. and MUNDY, G. R. Partial characterization of a bone-derived chemotactic factor for tumour cells. *American Journal of Pathology*, **99**, 43–52 (1980)

36 PASSWELL, J., BOICHIS, H., LOTAN, D., DAVID, R., THEODOR, R., COHEN, B. E. and MANY, M. The metabolic effects of excess noradrenaline secretion from a phaeochromocytoma. *American Journal of Diseases of Children*, **131**, 1011–1014 (1977)

37 POWELL, D., SINGER, F. R., MURRAY, T. M., MINKIN, C. and POTTS, J. T. Jr. Non-parathyroid humoral hypercalcaemia in patients with neoplastic diseases. *New England Journal of Medicine*, **289**, 176–181 (1973)

38 POWLES, T. J., DOWSETT, M., EASTY, D. M., EASTY, G. C. and NEVILLE, A. M. Breast cancer osteolysis, bone metastasis and anti-osteolytic effect of aspirin. *Lancet*, **1**, 608–610 (1976)

39 RAISZ, L. G., YAJNIK, C. H., BOCKMAN, R. S. and BOWER, B. B. Comparison of commercially available parathyroid hormone immunoassays in the differential diagnosis of hypercalcaemia due to primary hyperparathyroidism or malignancy. *Annals of Internal Medicine*, **91**, 739–740 (1979)

40 ROOF, B. S., CARPENTER, B., FINK, D. J. and GORDAN, G. S. Some thoughts on the nature of ectopic parathyroid hormones. *American Journal of Medicine*, **50**, 686–691 (1971)

41 SEYBERTH, H. W., SEGRE, G. V., MORGAN, J. L., SWEETMAN, B. J., POTTS, J. T. Jr and OATES, J. A. Prostaglandins as mediators of hypercalcaemia associated with certain types of cancer. *New England Journal of Medicine*, **293**, 1278–1283 (1975)

42 SHARP, C. F. Jr, RUDE, R. K., OLDHAM, S. B., TERRY, R. and SINGER, R. R. Abnormal bone and parathyroid histology in pseudohyperparathyroidism. *Sixth International Congress of Endocrinology*, **190A** (1980)

43 SHERWOOD, L. M. The multiple causes of hypercalcaemia in malignant disease. *New England Journal of Medicine*, **303**, 1412–1413 (1980)

44 SKRABANEK, P., McPARTLIN, J. and POWELL, D. Tumour hypercalcaemia and 'ectopic hyperparathyroidism'. *Medicine*, **59**, 262–282 (1980)

45 SPOONER, D. and EVANS, B. D. Tamoxifen and life-threatening hypercalcaemia. *Lancet*, **2**, 413–414 (1979)

46 STEWART, A. F., HORST, R., DEFTOS, L. J., CADMAN, E. C., LANG, R. and BROADUS, A. E. Biochemical evaluation of patients with cancer associated hypercalcaemia: evidence for humoral and non-humoral groups. *New England Journal of Medicine*, **303**, 1377–1383 (1980)

47 STEWART, A., GOLTZMAN, D., DEFTOS, L., VIGNERY, A., HORST, A., KIRKWOOD, J. and BROADUS, A. Humoral hypercalcaemia. Further study of the mediator *in vivo* and *in vitro*. *Clinical Research*, **28**, 407A (1980)

48 STRUMPF, M., KOWALSKI, M. A. and MUNDY, G. R. Effects of glucocorticoids on osteoclast activating factor. *Journal of Laboratory and Clinical Medicine*, **92**, 772–778 (1978)

49 TASHJIAN, A. H. Jr. Role of prostaglandins in the production of hypercalcaemia by tumours. *Cancer Research*, **38,** 4138–4141 (1978)

50 WOODARD, H. Q. Changes in blood chemistry associated with carcinoma metastatic to bone. *Cancer*, **6,** 1219–1227 (1953)

51 YONEDA, T. and MUNDY, G. R. Prostaglandins are necessary for osteoclast activating factor production by activated peripheral blood leucocytes. *Journal of Experimental Medicine*, **149,** 279–283 (1979)

52 YONEDA, T. and MUNDY, G. R. Monocytes regulate osteoclast activating factor production by releasing prostaglandins. *Journal of Experimental Medicine*, **150,** 338–350 (1979)

11
Hypocalcemia and other abnormalities of mineral homeostasis during the neonatal period
Laura S. Hillman and John G. Haddad

INTRODUCTION AND *IN UTERO* CONDITIONS

We have elected to present neonatal hypocalcemia from the viewpoint of its occurrence as an 'early' (first 4 days of life), 'late' (5–10 days of life) or 'late-late' (2–12 weeks of life) phenomenon of the postnatal period. Maintenance of the calcium concentration in extracellular fluid is a multifactorial process, and the newborn period follows a rapid change from dependence on placental transfer of calcium to independent assimilation of calcium from the diet. Compounding the issue is the remarkable skeletal accretion of mineral which occurs during the first weeks of life. This latter process is an extension of the skeletal mineralization which occurs exclusively in the last trimester of pregnancy. Since intrauterine factors influence the course of subsequent events, a brief review of these factors is presented.

Placental transfer of calcium from mother to fetus sustains a calcium content of 20–30 g in the full-term infant. In many species, including humans, calcium (total and ionized), magnesium and inorganic phosphorus concentrations are higher in fetal than in maternal blood[26]. However, severe nutritional deficiency in the mother results in a decreased bone density in the neonate, and calcium supplementation of the malnourished mother during pregnancy increases the bone density of all fetal bones[55,69].

The stability of fetal calcemia may simply reflect the saturation of the active placental transport mechanism, or fetal calciotropic hormones may play a role. Intrauterine secretion of calcitonin has been demonstrated in ovine, porcine and bovine fetuses, and in human fetuses and neonates the calcitonin concentration of the thyroid is increased[60]. However, a direct effect of calcitonin on the placental pump seems unlikely since removal of the fetus did not influence calcium transfer by the perfused guinea pig placenta[95]. In contrast to the high calcitonin levels observed[1,39,76] cord parathyroid hormone levels are low[19,39,78] or similar to maternal levels[18]. In species other than man, the fetal parathyroids may play a more active role in mineral homeostasis[4]. Neither parathyroid hormone (PTH) nor calcitonin is appreciably transferred to the fetus from the maternal circulation.

A close correlation exists between maternal and cord plasma 25-hydroxyvitamin D levels, consistent with a passive or facilitated transfer of this sterol by the placenta (*Figure 11.1*)[36]. Within the normal range, infant values are 75–80% of maternal values; however, at high maternal values infant values are considerably lower, and at very low maternal levels infant values may exceed maternal

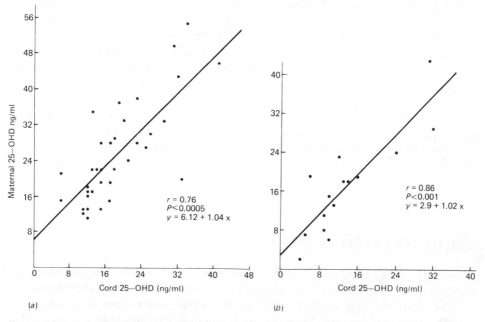

Figure 11.1 Correlation of maternal and cord serum 25-hydroxyvitamin D concentrations in term (a) and premature (b) pregnancy. (From Hillman and Haddad[36], courtesy of the Editor and Publishers, *Journal of Pediatrics*)

values[35, 36, 66]. This effect is not great enough to protect the infant from abnormally high or low serum 25-OHD in the mother[35, 36]. The major factor influencing maternal 25-OHD concentrations is season, with lower concentrations in winter[38]. This is modified only slightly by vitamin D intake[38]. There is no difference in serum 25-OHD concentrations of black and white women receiving adequate prenatal care and delivering at term[38]; however, among mothers delivering prematurely, blacks tend to have lower concentrations[37]. The potent sterol, 1,25-dihydroxyvitamin D has been reported to be absolutely low in cord plasma[88] or normal by adult standards but low for infants[11], consistent with the low fetal parathyroid activity. Concentration of the plasma transport protein for vitamin D and its metabolites (DBP) increases in maternal serum during pregnancy[33] and can be correlated with the 1,25-dihydroxyvitamin D concentration in maternal plasma[11]. In the last 5 weeks of pregnancy, however, the calculated 'free' concentration of 1,25-dihydroxyvitamin D increases in both the maternal and cord serum[11]. Since this is the most potent natural calciferol metabolite, the increase of its 'free' concentration could be responsible for changes in calcium movement at that period.

Quantitation of the placental transport of vitamin D metabolites is made complex by the demonstration of 25-OHD 1α-hydroxylase and 24-hydroxylase activity in placental tissue itself[98]. The ontogenesis, regulation and physiological role of this placental hydroxylase are totally unknown, and the destination(s) of its product is also not clear.

The possible role of 24,25-dihydroxyvitamin D in embryonic development and bone growth is controversial. Compared with adult normal values, $24,25(OH)_2D$ concentration is low in human maternal and cord serum[40, 97].

In fetal plasma, the interaction of high calcitonin, low parathyroid hormone (PTH), low-normal $1,25(OH)_2D$, and usually adequate 25-OHD may be ideal for the extensive bone mineralization which must take place during the last trimester of gestation.

Much remains to be learned about the ontogenesis of tissue responsiveness to calcitropic hormones. Considerable species variation exists in the maturity of the renal cortical adenylate cyclase system at birth[4]. The fetal rat intestine is unresponsive to $1,25(OH)_2D_3$ until birth, and the fetal renal 25-OHD 1α-hydroxylase activity is not maximal until hatching in chickens[9].

NORMAL POSTNATAL CHANGES

Postnatally, many changes in mineral homeostasis occur and it is important to understand these before one can understand disorders of mineral homeostasis.

After birth, the large supply of minerals from the mother is cut off and there is severely decreased mineral input to the circulation. To maintain serum levels, minerals may need to be mobilized from stores, primarily bone. This involves a reordering of hormonal balances. *Figures 11.2* and *11.3* present composites from many investigations of serum calcium and phosphorus during the first week of life in full-term infants[25].

Serum magnesium begins low, even though this is higher than maternal levels, and over the first 48 hours increases to normal adult levels, then transiently overshoots at 1 week[39, 90].

In full-term infants, 25-OHD concentrations remain stable during the first week[37, 39], $24,25(OH)_2D$ values remain low at 1 week[97] while $1,25(OH)_2D$ concentration increases over the first 24–48 hours, paralleling the increase in PTH (*see below*)[88].

Parathyroid hormone increases appropriately as serum calcium falls and by 48–72 hours in full-term infants has reached normal or elevated values[19, 39, 64]. This rise also parallels the rise in serum magnesium[19, 39, 64]. Calcitonin in serum increases after 1–2 hours of life, peaks at 12 hours and falls off rapidly[1, 20]. The stimulus for this surge is unknown. It is certainly not hypercalcemia and there is no correlation of calcitonin with catecholamines, glucagon or gastrin[20, 47]. The effect of the calcitonin surge is to further accentuate the fall in calcium and the

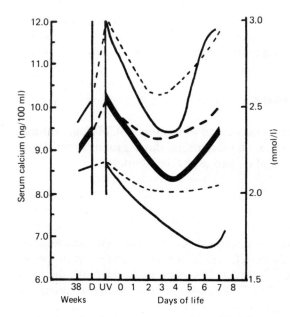

Figure 11.2 Calcium concentrations in plasma during late pregnancy, delivery (D) and first eight days of life (mean ± 2 SD). UV = umbilical venous; (---) breastfed, (——) bottle-fed. (From Forfar[25], courtesy of the Editor and Publishers, *Clinics of Endocrinology and Metabolism*)

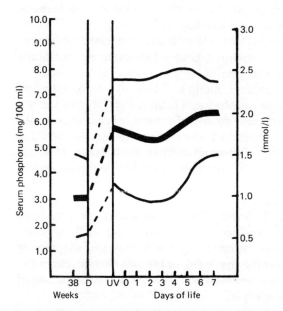

Figure 11.3 Phosphorus concentrations in plasma during late pregnancy, delivery (D) and the first 7 days of life (mean ± 2 SD). UV = Umbilical venous. (From Forfar[25], courtesy of the Editor and Publishers, *Clinics of Endocrinology and Metabolism*)

stimulation of PTH and $1,25(OH)_2D$. Growth hormone and cortisol also increase and may stimulate bone turnover or increase sensitivity to calcitonin[7], while estrogen rapidly falls, releasing its suppression of bone resorption.

EARLY NEONATAL HYPOCALCEMIA

Early neonatal hypocalcemia by definition occurs within the first 72 hours of life, usually at 24–48 hours. It most frequently occurs in three groups: premature infants, infants of diabetic mothers (IDM), and asphyxiated infants.

Premature infants

Premature infants have a greater fall in serum calcium than do full-term infants, with the nadir being both earlier, 24 hours, and lower; the decrease is inversely proportional to their gestational age[20, 91]. In 30–35% of premature infants, the total serum calcium will fall below 7.0 mg/dl (1.75 mmol/l). The fall in ionized calcium is not comparable to the fall in total calcium, and the ratio of ionized to total calcium is inversely related to total calcium[79, 80]. The disproportionate depression of protein-bound calcium is probably related to low serum protein concentrations and frequent acidosis, but cannot be totally explained by these factors[79, 80]. Sparing of ionized calcium may partly explain the lack of signs in most premature infants with early hypocalcemia. The lack of signs or good pathophysiological markers of 'significant' hypocalcemia make the decision to intervene very difficult and results in a general overtreatment of the condition. Occasionally hypomagnesemia occurs in premature infants with hypocalcemia, but this is usually transient and spontaneously corrects. Serum phosphorus is slightly higher in hypocalcemic premature infants than normocalcemic premature infants[91].

Conflicting data exist on the premature infant's ability to respond to the hypocalcemic challenge of an exchange transfusion. Further, some studies show a delay in the rise in serum PTH in premature infants[78, 92], while other studies would suggest that most premature infants can produce a normal or elevated serum PTH in response to their hypocalcemia[19, 39, 62]. In a small study shown in *Figure 11.4*, the authors found serum PTH in the majority of premature infants to be higher than in full-term infants, although a few infants with a delayed response were identified[39]. The variation in results probably reflects the difference in antibodies used. In general, there have been elevated PTH levels when C-terminal assays have been used, though high values have been reported in one study using an N-terminal assay[62]. Since C-terminal fragments are excreted by the kidney and glomerular filtration rate (GFR) is increasing over the first week of life and may be less in the premature, the possibility that elevated levels could represent an accumulation of C-terminal fragments must be acknowledged.

A second question is the ability of the premature infant's target organs to respond to PTH. Mallet *et al.*[62] gave 10 units PTH/kg to 16 premature infants and observed a low urinary cyclic AMP response on day 1, but a significant response on

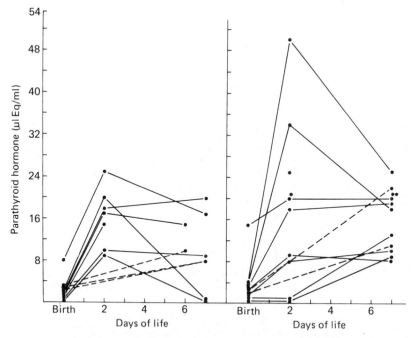

Figure 11.4 Serial parathyroid hormone serum concentrations in term (*left*) and premature (*right*) infants. (From Hillman *et al.*[39], courtesy of the Editor and Publishers, *Pediatric Research*)

day 3 with a much greater response on day 6. Similar results have been found in full-term infants with adult response levels reached at 2–4 months. Thus, the premature baby has at least the same postnatal delays in renal PTH responsiveness as the full-term infant, and although this may not represent an additional problem of prematurity, it may well interact with other factors to produce hypocalcemia with hyperphosphatemia.

The premature infant appears to have an exaggeration of the early serum calcitonin surge. Indeed, an inverse correlation between peak calcitonin and gestational age has been reported[20]. Infants with hypocalcemia have a higher mean calcitonin than normocalcemic infants[22], and an inverse correlation of calcitonin and calcium has been reported[74]. This suggests a role for calcitonin in the hypocalcemia seen at this period. *Figure 11.5* compares the calcitonin serum concentrations of premature and full-term infants.

In 80 premature infants there was no correlation between serum 25-OHD and serum calcium at 48 hours (Hillman, unpublished observations). In premature infants, $24,25(OH)_2D$ and $1,25(OH)_2D$ have not been extensively studied, mainly because of sampling limitations, and it has been speculated that premature infants may not be able to increase their $1,25(OH)_2D$ concentrations normally. However, Glorieux *et al.* have recently shown elevated $1,25(OH)_2D$ in premature infants given 2000 vitamin D and treatment trials with high doses of $1,25(OH)_2D$ (0.5 µg) have not prevented early neonatal hypocalcemia in premature infants[15, 28, 75].

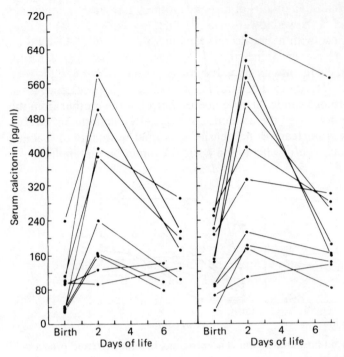

Figure 11.5 Serial calcitonin serum concentrations in term (*left*) and premature (*right*) infants. (From Hillman *et al.*[39], courtesy of the Editor and Publishers, *Pediatric Research*)

There are conflicting reports about whether 25-hydroxycholecalciferol will prevent early neonatal hypocalcemia[24, 75]. Treatment with 0.66 μg/kg 1α-OHD$_3$ has been reported to increase serum calcium[3].

Infants of diabetic mothers

In infants of diabetic mothers (IDM), the postnatal fall in serum calcium is exaggerated compared to that in neonates of similar gestational age. The same sparing of ionized calcium relative to total calcium seen in premature infants is also seen in infants of diabetic mothers[64]. Diabetics have a lower serum magnesium and lower PTH than normal women during pregnancy[18], and plasma magnesium is frequently low in infants of diabetic mothers. This is usually transient, but it is more frequent in those infants with more severe hypocalcemia[64]. Serum phosphorus also tends to be higher in the infant of a diabetic mother than in infants of normal mothers. These changes are consistent with a delayed increase in PTH secretion in the infant of a diabetic patient[64, 78]. Both magnesium and PTH are reported to be lower in the hypocalcemic infant of a diabetic mother than the normocalcemic infant of a diabetic mother and one may speculate that hypomagnesemia blunted the skeletal response to PTH and/or further delayed the release of PTH, which was already suppressed by the high maternal and cord ionized calcium. Calcitonin concentration is not increased in infants of diabetic mothers greater than in normal infants[7]. Fleischman *et al.*[24] showed lower serum 25-OHD in diabetic mothers and, thus, in their infants, those with hypocalcemia having lower serum 25-OHD than normocalcemic infants. However, Steichen *et al.*[89] have shown both normal serum 25-OHD and $1,25(OH)_2D$ in infants and diabetic mothers, with no difference between the serum $1,25(OH)_2D$ in those infants who became hypocalcemic from those who remained normocalcemic. Strict diabetic control of the mother from the first trimester markedly decreased the incidence of hypocalcemia in the infant, but the mechanism for this is unclear. Bone density is normal in infants of diabetic mothers at birth. Glorieux *et al.*[29] also found normal vitamin D_3 metabolism.

Asphyxiated infants

Asphyxiated infants, regardless of gestational age, have a hypocalcemia which is often early, within the first 24 hours, and severe[93]. Asphyxiated infants have a marked accentuation of the calcitonin surge and serum PTH is consistently elevated in full-term asphyxiated infants[78]. No vitamin D sterol estimations are available in this group. An increased phosphate release secondary to tissue hypoxia has also been postulated to play a role in this early hypocalcemia. Severe perinatal asphyxia may result in both neurological damage leading to seizures within the first day, and to hypocalcemia. The seizures, however, are not due to the low calcium and will not be corrected by calcium infusion.

Other infants at risk

Small-for-gestational age (SGA) infants as a group do not have hypocalcemia out of proportion to their gestational age[94]. However, pre-eclampsia and postmaturity with fetal growth retardation are associated with an increased incidence of hypocalcemia[53]. These infants have a much higher incidence of hypomagnesemia and a delay in the increase of their serum magnesium postnatally[46, 90].

Phototherapy has recently been reported to increase the incidence of hypocalcemia in premature infants but not in term or small-for-gestational-age infants[72]. The mechanism of this is unclear.

A frequently used procedure with profound effects on blood calcium is exchange transfusion with blood containing high concentrations of citrate and phosphate. During the course of an exchange, though total calcium may increase, ionized calcium falls often to less than 2.5 mg/dl (0.6 mmol/l) and the Q–T interval increases. Signs, especially seizures, are rarely seen[99]. Serum PTH initially shows a prompt increase[92, 99], and subsequent fall with return to normal by 48–72 hours postexchange[99]. PTH secretion may be further compromised by a fall in ionized magnesium during the exchange[99].

Thus, in summary, early neonatal hypocalcemia is an exaggeration of the normal physiological changes after birth. In all infants with early neonatal hypocalcemia, a number of factors play a role, though the predominant factor varies. In asphyxiated infants, an exaggeration of the normal calcitonin surge predominates, whereas in infants of diabetic mothers an exaggerated delay in the serum PTH rise may predominate. In premature infants, the calcitonin surge may be the primary factor, possibly compounded by a decreased compensatory PTH response. Vitamin D and its metabolites do not appear to play any clear role. Early neonatal hypocalcemia is self-limiting and without symptomatology or sequelae in the large majority of cases, and requires treatment only when very severe or clearly symptomatic.

Although pharmacological dosages of potent vitamin D metabolites may be able to prevent or mollify early neonatal hypocalcemia, this approach cannot be justified presently. We recommend expectant waiting, with treatment by intra-venous calcium infusion at serum calcium values of less than 5–6 mg/dl (1.25–1.5 mmol/l) in very small premature infants. A serum calcium of less than 6–7 mg/dl (1.5–1.75 mmol/l) may require treatment in a full-term infant, especially the infant of a diabetic mother. If oral treatment is possible, milder degrees may be treated.

LATE NEONATAL HYPOCALCEMIA

In contrast to early neonatal hypocalemia, infants with late neonatal hypocalcemia present between 5 and 10 days of age with signs, usually seizures, jitteriness or apnea. These infants have typical neurological abnormalities, including increased reflexes (52%), increased muscle tone (36%), jitteriness (36%), clonus (33%) and hyperactiveness (26%)[16]. They are usually full-term infants without antecedent neonatal problems. The entity is more common in the winter and in infants of mothers of greater parity and lower socioeconomic status[70]. The infants are usually receiving cow's milk or prepared formula and the syndrome is rare in breastfed infants. Total serum calcium is low, and serum phosphorus is increased in 85% of cases[16]. The phosphate load from the cow's milk had long been thought to explain the entity. Other studies have reported that 50% of these infants are also hypomagnesemic[16].

Association with vitamin D deficiency

Because of the winter predominance and enamel hypoplasia of the primary molars, which was felt to be consistent with *in utero* vitamin D deficiency, a theory of maternal vitamin D deficiency was put forth[68]. Cockburn *et al.*[17] recently published a very large study comparing women whose vitamin D intake during pregnancy was about 100 iu with a group supplemented to 500 iu (100 iu diet plus 400 iu supplement) and found significant differences in the infants' hypocalcemia at 6 days (6% versus 13% less than 7.4 mg/100 ml, 1.85 mmol/l), seizures (0.4% versus 0.9%), and enamel hypoplasia (48% of hypocalcemic controls and 7% of vitamin D treated). These differences were seen in both breastfed and bottle-fed infants. However, bottle-fed infants had a lower calcium and magnesium and higher phosphorus and more frequent seizures in spite of their supplementation. The infants' 6th-day serum calcium was predicted by type of feeding, vitamin D supplementation and sex, with other factors having little effect[17]. The incidence of late neonatal hypocalcemia is 0.03% in non-Asian Britons but is 2.3% in Asians who have very low maternal and cord 25-OHD[35]. A second double-blind study was performed by Brooke *et al.*[12] in Asian women residing in Britain where a placebo or 1000 iu/day vitamin D was used. Cord 25-OHD was 4 ng/ml in the control group and 56 ng/ml in the treated group. Weight gain was greater in the treated women and the incidence of small-for-gestational-age infants was lower (15% versus 29%). Fontanelle size was also smaller. Serum calciums at days 3 and 6 were higher and cord alkaline phosphatase was lower in infants of treated women. Five out of 67 control infants developed hypocalcemic seizures, whereas none of the treated infants developed seizures.

In the United States, maternal vitamin D levels were lower in winter than summer but were unrelated to any of the other epidemiological factors associated with neonatal tetany in Britain[38]. In seven characteristic, late neonatal hypocalcemic infants studied recently by Fakhraee *et al.*[23], five had normal serum 25-OHD concentrations. The other two had very low (both 1 ng/ml) levels consistent with negligible maternal intakes and very low maternal 25-OHD. Thus, 25-OHD deficiency was not the cause in the majority of cases seen in the United States.

In cases of very severe and longstanding maternal vitamin D deficiency which, if looked for, presents as osteomalacia in the mother, the infant will present with bone changes of fetal rickets in addition to hypocalcemia. Bone changes have not yet been evaluated in infants with classical late neonatal hypocalcemia.

Parathyroid hormone (PTH) deficiency and hypomagnesemia

The mineral derangements in late neonatal hypocalcemia are suggestive of a deficiency of parathyroid hormone and such cases had been called 'transient congenital hypoparathyroidism' prior to the availability of PTH measurements. In our seven cases, the mean serum PTH was less than 3 (nl 2–10) which was inappropriately low for their serum calcium[23]. On repeat after the hypocalcemia was no longer present, serum PTH was normal. In all seven cases, serum magnesium was low, and the high incidence of unexplained hypomagnesemia in our cases as well as the literature suggests that the delayed serum PTH rise could be secondary to hypomagnesemia. After treatment with 0.1–0.2 ml/kg of 50% magnesium sulfate, the serum calcium frequently corrects. Decreased gastrointestinal absorption of calcium and magnesium secondary to high phosphorus diet could also contribute to the syndrome.

Whether or not maternal vitamin D deficiency can be related to transient infant hypoparathyroidism is unclear. PTH does not cross the placenta, and in maternal vitamin D deficiency, both maternal and cord calcium concentrations are lower than normal, so that suppression of fetal parathyroid function is less likely[13]. A relationship through hypomagnesemia also seems unlikely, since cord serum magnesium was significantly higher in infants of vitamin D-deficient mothers than a vitamin D-supplemented treatment group[13]. It may be that both severe neonatal

25-OHD deficiency and infant functional hypoparathyroidism can lead to late neonatal hypocalcemia and that the chance occurrence of both can lead to an even more severe situation.

Sequelae and treatment

Late neonatal hypocalcemia has documented long-term effects. Since the infants are usually full-term, the teeth which are calcifying at that point are the primary molars. The enamel on these teeth is abnormal in over 50% of infants with a history of late neonatal hypocalcemia[68]. Similar changes were seen in the past in infants born to mothers with severe nutritional osteomalacia and infants with hypoparathyroidism. Long-term linear growth of these infants has not been reported. The seizures usually do not recur and are without neurological sequelae.

Late neonatal hypocalcemia requires immediate treatment. Seizure activity can be stopped by the intravenous bolus infusion of 200 mg/kg of calcium gluconate. Maintenance oral calcium supplementation can then be started. The serum magnesium must be checked immediately and if found to be low, 50% magnesium sulfate (0.2 ml/kg) should be given intramuscularly. If the infant is receiving cow's milk, this should be replaced with a commercial formula. If the serum phosphorus is below 9 mg/dl, a standard formula containing about 400 mg/l phosphorus will probably be tolerated. If the serum phosphorus is higher, a low phosphorus formula such as PM 60/40 should be used. Since such a formula also restricts calcium intake, continued calcium supplementation is necessary. After a few weeks, supplementation with calcium and restriction of phosphorus can be stopped. In the United States, unless the mother is known to have been on a vitamin D-deficient diet or to have had very little sun exposure, routine treatment with additional vitamin D is probably not warranted. If possible the infant's serum 25-OHD level can be checked to assure that it is normal. In high-risk British populations, limited supplementation with vitamin D would be appropriate and serum 25-OHD may be measured.

We have seen asymptomatic hypocalcemia in full-term infants undergoing surgery in the first week of life. These infants have not been fed and the only possible phosphate source is their tissue breakdown. In this group the total calcium is low, the phosphorus slightly elevated, and the magnesium low. Serum PTH values were within normal limits but inappropriately low for the degree of hypocalcemia. Correction of the hypomagnesemia corrected the hypocalcemia. The etiology of the hypomagnesemia is unclear but a decreased intake certainly contributes[23].

In summary, late neonatal hypocalcemia is a sporadic occurrence which is more frequent in vitamin D-deficient populations and prevented to a large degree by vitamin D supplementation of the mother. In vitamin D-sufficient populations, hypomagnesemia and an inappropriately low serum PTH are usually present, although unexplained. Late neonatal hypocalcemia is associated with seizures, neurological abnormalities, as well as potential long-term sequelae of enamel hypoplasia. It requires immediate treatment with intravenous calcium and often with intramuscular magnesium.

HYPOMINERALIZATION AND LATE-LATE HYPOCALCEMIA

The third group of infants developing hypocalcemia are premature infants who, during the first 3–4 months of life, have hypocalcemia associated with bone hypomineralization or frank rickets. Normal bone mineralization in the premature infant requires a continuous and substantial supply of calcium, phosphorus and vitamin D. Thus, premature infants are very susceptible to both vitamin D and/or phosphate deficiency rickets. It is, therefore, necessary to give detailed consideration to dietary intake of the premature infant.

Mineral and 25-OHD deficiency in premature infants fed standard formulae

The majority of premature infants in the United States, until very recently, received the same commercial formula as normal-term infants from birth to over 1 year of age. These formulae contain from 440–550 mg/l calcium and from 330–460 mg/l phosphorus and 400 iu/l vitamin D_2 or D_3. With normal absorption of calcium and phosphorus, the premature infant could not match normal *in utero* calcium or phosphorus accretion rates. When the infant reached 40 weeks postconceptual age, the premature infant's bones would be undermineralized relative to those of the infant born at term (40 weeks postconceptual age). This was indeed shown by bone densitometry[63, 86] and has also been demonstrated by performing serial radiographs of the hand and wrist[45, 46]. However, the variations seen in densitometric and radiological studies are quite large among infants of similar gestation and well-being. Thus, constitutional factors can modify changes which might be attributable to dietary content, assimilation, or retention of these minerals.

In addition to dietary mineral content, an effect of vitamin D was noted many years ago[96]. We followed serum 25-OHD concentrations in premature infants to see whether the low values seen at birth persisted[37, 45, 46]. Studies of premature infants fed formulae containing 400 iu/l vitamin D (without additional vitamin D supplementation) showed that infants born with low serum 25-OHD could not correct these low values over many weeks. Premature infants beginning life with normal serum 25-OHD could not maintain normal levels[37]. Because of this experience and sporadic reports of unsupplemented infants developing rickets[61], it was felt that a larger study of the significance of low serum 25-OHD needed to be carried out at the currently recommended daily dosage of 400 iu vitamin D in addition to that obtained from formula (usually approximately 100 iu). Eighty premature infants with a mean gestation 30.1 ± 2.6 weeks and mean birthweight of 1176 ± 266 g have been followed for the first 3 months of life[45]. The mean serum calcium at 3, 6 and 9 weeks was 9.0, 8.7 and 9.0 mg/dl (2.25, 2.2 and 2.25 mmol/l), with 41%, 51% and 45% less than 9 mg/dl (2.25 mmol/l). At 12 weeks of age the mean serum calcium increased to 9.8 mg/dl (2.45 mmol/l) with only 24% less than 9 mg/dl. These low values of serum calcium are physiologically important since they are accompanied by elevations of serum PTH and are correlated with the degree of demineralization at 12 weeks of age. In this population, serum phosphorus steadily falls between 3 and 9 weeks, with 3, 6 and 9 week mean values of 6.8, 6.3 and

5.6 mg/dl (2.2, 2.0 and 1.8 mmol/l) and 0%, 10% and 21% of values less than 4 mg/dl (1.3 mmol/l). At 12 weeks the average serum phosphorus rose to 7.0 ± 1.6 mg/dl (2.3 ± 0.5 mmol/l). However, 9% remained below 4 mg/dl (1.3 mmol/l) and 15% less than 5.5 mg/dl (1.8 mmol/l). Those infants with low serum phosphorus had more severe hypomineralization. Serum magnesium remained at normal adult levels after 48 hours (mean 1.8 mEq/l) and did not further increase at 12 weeks of age[45, 46].

When infants were supplemented with 400 iu vitamin D, four patterns emerged. The majority of infants who began life with a normal serum 25-OHD were able to maintain normal serum 25-OHD (25% of the total premature population). However, a smaller group (20% of the total prematures) still had falling serum 25-OHD concentrations; 54% of infants began life with low (less than 15 mg/ml) serum 25-OHD. Though 20% were now able to correct low serum 25-OHD before 9 weeks of age, 34% were still low at 9 weeks of age. At 12 weeks of age, an initial or subsequent increase in 25-OHD was seen in all groups except the falling group, which continued to fall. Thus, at 12 weeks of age 20% of premature infants had low serum 25-OHD. Those infants with low 25-OHD had significant hypomineralization and low serum calcium and phosphorus. At 12 weeks, serum 25-OHD was significantly correlated with serum calcium ($r = 0.47$, $P < 0.02$) and phosphorus ($r = 0.59$, $P = 0.01$) and was also correlated with the degree of hypomineralization. Three months is the age at which we[52] and others[14, 57] have observed vitamin D deficiency rickets in premature infants on other formula diets (*see below*). The finding of correlations of 25-OHD with serum calcium and phosphorus within the normal range consistent with a major function of 25-OHD was unexpected since so many other hormones interact in these systems.

To date, serial studies of the vitamin D metabolites have been limited to 25-OHD because of sample size requirements for both $1,25(OH)_2D$ and $24,25(OH)_2D$. Elevated serum $1,25(OH)_2D$ has been reported in premature infants with frank rickets secondary to prolonged total parenteral nutrition and in a group on standard formula[87].

It has been questioned whether the plasma vitamin D binding protein (DBP) plays a regulatory role in mineral homeostasis[11]. Cord vitamin D binding protein is normal in term infants (558 ± 78 μg/ml) but low in premature infants (359 ± 24 μg/ml)[33]. Serial data on 20 of our small premature infants showed that vitamin D binding protein remained low until 12 weeks of age when it increased significantly[50]. We have found that many other liver proteins follow a similar pattern: albumin, ceruloplasm[49], and somatomedin. This probably represents a maturation of liver function. The increase in 25-OHD at 12 weeks is possibly, at least in part, due to a maturation of the liver's ability to hydroxylate 25-OHD.

The other calcitrophic hormones have not been extensively studied past the first week of life. PTH certainly becomes elevated in the face of frank vitamin D deficiency rickets[52] and in severe hypomineralization with hypocalcemia[45, 46] so that the premature infant is able to respond to hypocalcemia with a PTH increase. Serum calcitonin measured serially in 28 premature infants has been found to remain elevated, falling slowly and not reaching normal levels until 12 weeks or later[41].

The end result of deficient mineral intake by *in utero* standards is poor mineralization of bone, or poor osteogenesis during the neonatal period of many premature infants. The percentage of premature infants with moderate osteopenia was 76% at 3 weeks, 59% at 6 weeks, 55% at 9 weeks, and 17% at 12 weeks[45]. Thus, as with most parameters related to vitamin D, the bones improved as postconceptual maturity was reached. The degree of hypomineralization still present at 12 weeks was correlated with the concurrent serum 25-OHD[45]. When frank rickets was seen, the serum 25-OHD was always less than 7 ng/ml. Severe osteopenia with fractures usually occurred between 8 and 12 ng/ml[44]. Abnormal wrist radiographs and impaired definition of metaphyseal lines in the radius and ulna are present in older infants at low serum 25-OHD concentrations (mean 8.4 ng/ml, all less than 12 ng/ml) prior to biochemical abnormalities of rickets[67]. Rib changes and craniotabes did not correlate with 25-OHD. The bone density slowly increased with postnatal age, but at a much lower rate than would have occurred *in utero* based on the bone density of infants of different gestation at birth[63]. Minton *et al.*'s[63] data suggest acceleration in bone accretion and length at 12 weeks in the less than 32-week group, a time similar to the increase in 25-OHD observed[45]. The few histological studies in bone of premature infants which we have done suggest that there is not an abundance of unmineralized osteoid as might be seen in a pure mineral or vitamin D deficiency state. Therefore, factors related to matrix production may also cause the marked paucity of bone present. Quantitative bone histomorphometry in three premature infants who died of bronchopulmonary dysplasia (BPD) showed changes more consistent with phosphate deficiency than classical vitamin D deficiency rickets[65]. The percentage of osteoid was only slightly increased, and the percentage of total osseous tissue was markedly decreased[65]. However, two of our cases with classical rickets on X-ray and very low serum 25-OHD had classical vitamin D deficiency rickets at post-mortem evaluation of bone with evidence of PTH elevation[52]. The association between bronchopulmonary dysplasia and rickets seems more than random and has been reported in several countries[10, 27]. In our experience, infants with bronchopulmonary dysplasia, especially those with growth problems, frequently had low serum 25-OHD concentrations. Indeed, myopathy and thoracic undermineralization could certainly aggravate bronchopulmonary dysplasia.

Assuming that the spontaneous resolution of neonatal osteopenia occurs, are there any long-term effects? Nutritional vitamin D deficiency rickets and experimentally produced rickets in animals are associated with a linear growth retardation. We have followed 36 infants with known postnatal vitamin D status to evaluate growth. At 1 year, the height percentile corrected for gestational age was significantly correlated with the 12-week serum 25-OHD (r = 0.45, *P* <0.01). Further analysis in the four groups of prematures by serum 25-OHD values showed that infants whose serum 25-OHD was normal at birth and remained normal at 9 weeks of age had a height percentile of 60 ± 32%, whereas the infants who were born with low serum 25-OHD which remained low at 9 weeks had a height percentile of 13.5 ± 15.9%[42]. This suggested that an early low serum 25-OHD, even if normalized prior to the infant's developing frank rickets, was associated with growth retardation. In 20% of prematures, enamel hypoplasia of the upper anterior incisors, which are the teeth calcifying at 28–30 weeks gestation, has been observed[30]. In our study, infants with enamel hypoplasia were infants with calcium and vitamin D problems[42].

Treatment and prevention possibilities

Infants who have developed frank rickets[52] or severe osteopenia and fractures with biochemical rickets[44] have been successfully treated with vitamin D 4000 iu daily p.o. for 2 weeks. Since many commercial laboratories now perform 25-OHD measurement, this can be obtained before and after treatment. One would, however, like to detect vitamin D deficiency in infants before fractures and rickets occur. At minimum, very small premature infants should have their serum calcium and phosphorus measured every 2 weeks. There is not a good correlation of the serum alkaline phosphatase with other biochemical and X-ray findings, and it cannot be used as a sole measurement. Alkaline phosphatase was also found to be an inadequate screen for subclinical rickets in older infants[67]. Evaluation of bone mineralization is necessary when biochemical abnormalities are noted, and routine X-ray screening at 6–9 weeks can be justified to identify severe osteopenia. A complete evaluation requires a serum PTH measurement. However, a urinary amino acid screen looking for a generalized aminoaciduria will often identify infants with an elevated PTH. In the face of a severe vitamin D deficiency, osteopenia, low normal calcium, low phosphorus, high alkaline phosphatase, and an elevated PTH or generalized aminoaciduria are seen.

Of course, prevention is preferable to treatment. Since it is agreed upon by most but not all investigators that nutritional supplies comparable to those *in utero* should be the goal, methods to increase the amount of calcium and phosphorus absorbed have been studied. Multiple factors play a role: calcium and phosphorus are absorbed independently and the calcium: phosphorus ratio of the diet has little effect; the amount of fat in the diet and the amount lost in the stool also does not appear to alter the calcium absorption; the type of fat appears to make a difference with diets high in medium-chain triglycerides increasing absorption of calcium; a low linoleate: stearate ratio similar to breast milk improves calcium absorption but endogenous calcium excretion into the gut, as shown with[46]Ca, is very large and very variable[6, 81, 83].

However, the major factor determining calcium absorption is postnatal age. Even in full-term infants, better absorption is observed at 4–6 weeks of age than at 5–7 days, regardless of the type of feeding. In premature infants, this is even more impressive with increases in absorption not occurring until 50–60 days of age[83]. The pattern of increased calcium absorption was independent of fat absorption, which remained low[83]. The time-course is reminiscent of what we have seen for serum 25-OHD concentrations in premature infants with sharp increases at 9–12 weeks postnatal age.

In spite of these limitations, the potential benefit of further calcium supplementation for low birthweight infants has been pursued. Several investigators have reported improved calcium retention[5, 21, 84] and improved mineralization[86]. Our experience with a similar formula giving 1200 mg/l calcium and 600 mg/l phosphorus is that mineralization (X-ray) is improved, but it is not completely corrected in most of the very small premature infants[46]. On this formula, we found an impressive urinary retention of phosphorus and a temporary lowering of serum phosphorus, and Shenai *et al.*[84] found phosphorus retention to be poorer than calcium retention. These data suggest that in a high calcium–phosphorus formula, the 2:1 ratio seen in low calcium–phosphorus breast milk may not be appropriate. Improved mineralization might be seen on a high calcium–high phosphorus formula with a calcium–phosphorus ratio below 2:1.

A major function of many of the vitamin D metabolites, the most potent of which is 1,25-dihydroxyvitamin D, is to increase gastrointestinal absorption of calcium and phosphorus. A deficiency in 25-OHD, $1,25(OH)_2D$, or both, can adversely affect calcium and phosphorus absorption. The lowest reported calcium absorption rates have come from studies in Britain and France where vitamin D supplementation of foods is rare and sun exposure frequently limited and where vitamin D supplementation of the infant was not part of the study design[5, 6, 81]. The highest absorption rates have been in the United States where vitamin D supplementation abounds and sun exposure is less limited so that the population in general has higher 25-OHD serum concentration, and where also by study design the infants had vitamin D intakes of about 800 iu[84, 86]. Our studies of a uniformly treated population of premature infants with total daily vitamin D intakes of about 500 iu indicate that most infants who are born with normal serum 25-OHD concentrations are able to maintain these normal concentrations and have fewer problems with hypomineralization or hypocalcemia than infants born with low 25-OHD concentrations. Further feeding of a high calcium–high phosphorus formula alone did not alter serum 25-OHD concentrations[48], and infants who had persistently low serum 25-OHD often did not normalize X-ray mineralization[46].

Thus, an alternative prophylaxis was to try to normalize 25-OHD levels in all infants. The production of 25-OHD requires two processes: first, the absorption of the parent compound, vitamin D, from the gastrointestinal tract; and second, the hydroxylation of the vitamin D in the liver to 25-OHD. Problems in performing either or, most likely, both of these steps would result in low 25-OHD, and feeding 25-hydroxycholecalciferol (25-HCC) would bypass either problem. We performed 25-hydroxycholecalciferol absorption tests on eight 2-week-old premature infants to define their abilities to absorb 25-hydroxycholecalciferol and to define dosage[43]. The premature infants had peak blood levels of 25-OHD at 4 or 8 hours after dosage similar to adults[34]. However, the increase over baseline was only half of what would be predicted from the adult data for dosage based on micrograms per kilogram (μg/kg)[43]. The absorption, however, was adequate for use of the preparation of 25-hydroxycholecalciferol and it was felt that 1 μg/kg daily should result in normal blood levels. Twenty-one infants were fed at that dosage for 3–4 weeks without vitamin D supplementation above that contained in the formula. Infants with normal baseline 25-OHD maintained normal values and infants with moderately low levels increased their serum 25-OHD concentration and then maintained normal levels. Infants with very low levels, less than 8, required many weeks to correct levels. Thus, as with the parent vitamin, it appears that one dosage will not be ideal for all infants. On 25-hydroxycholecalciferol supplements, both serum calcium and phosphorus improved and, except for the very small premature infants (less than 1000 g) in whom calcium and phosphorus intake may be limiting, mineralization on X-ray was improved but not normalized in all cases. 25-hydroxycholecalciferol is available in both Europe and the United States.

Senterre et al.[82] fed preterm infants 0.5 µg of $1,25(OH)_2D_3$ for a week and did balance studies which showed an increased calcium absorption of 47 ± 10 versus 25 ± 18% and an increased retention of 29 ± 10 versus 16 ± 10 mg/kg per day. Magnesium absorption was increased. Phosphorus absorption was 94% in both control and experimental groups. However, phosphorus retention increased from 29 ± 7 to 34 ± 9%, a slight but not significant difference[82]. In the normal adult, $1,25(OH)_2D$ production is tightly regulated and is independent of 25-OHD serum concentration, except in extreme deficiency. However, Glorieux et al.[28] found that in the first week of life, premature infants of birthweights of 1820–2460 g, fed vitamin D 2000 iu daily, were able to increase serum 25-OHD and serum 1,25-OHD, and surprisingly at 1 week of age serum 25-OHD and serum $1,25(OH)_2D$ were correlated. If this correlation persists in the premature infant, then the low levels of 25-OHD which we have defined in 34% of our population could also be associated with low $1,25(OH)_2D$. Long-term feeding of $1,25(OH)_2D$ to premature infants has not been tested. Indeed, given our lack of knowledge about their ability to autoregulate serum $1,25(OH)_2D$ and the lack of available microassays to measure serum $1,25(OH)_2D$, the feeding of $1,25(OH)_2D$, which is now available in most countries, to premature infants must be considered extremely dangerous.

Europeans have been routinely supplementing the diet of premature infants with 1000 iu daily for many years. Recent measurements of serum 25-OHD in infants fed daily 1000 iu[100] showed that although infants of 36–39 weeks readily increased serum 25-OHD levels to high levels, three premature infants of 32–34 weeks only slowly increased levels into the normal range in 4 weeks[100]. Robinson et al.[71] compared 400 iu and 1000 iu in infants of mean birthweight 1500 g and mean gestation of 30.5 weeks and showed that between 32.5 weeks of age and 36 or 39 weeks postconceptual age, there was a significant mean increase in both groups. However, if the data are carefully examined, only four out of nine infants had a significant increase at 400 iu and six out of nine increased at 1000 iu. This is consistent with our findings that with 400 iu supplementation, about 40% of infants with low levels can correct[45], and with preliminary data on 800 iu showing that a large number of infants still fail to correct low serum 25-OHD concentrations. Vitamin D intakes up to 1200 iu per day had no effects on calcium absorption in premature infants during the first month of life[81]. Increases in serum 25-OHD and $1,25(OH)_2D$ were seen on feeding 1200 and 2000 iu to more mature premature infants[28]. Thus, if absorption and hydroxylation limitations are to be reliably overcome, supplementation even exceeding the daily 1000 iu frequently used in Europe may be needed. Infants born with normal serum 25-OHD levels did not reach excessive levels on 800 iu supplements; however, higher doses have not been studied over several weeks.

In summary, the problems of hypomineralization and hypocalcemia seen in very premature infants are usually a combination of inadequate calcium and phosphorus intake and inadequate vitamin D metabolites. Some improvement has been documented with both calcium and phosphorus supplementation and with use of 25-hydroxycholecalciferol to normalize 25-OHD; however, neither treatment has been uniformly completely successful. Optimal mineralization and growth probably require both adequate substrate and adequate vitamins to assure maximal gastro-intestinal absorption and deposition in bone. Combination trials of increased calcium–phosphorus substrate and increased vitamin D or 25-hydroxy-cholecalciferol are in progress. At present we would recommend one of the newer commercially available formulae with increased calcium and phosphorus content intended for premature infants less than 1500 g plus daily vitamin D intake of between 400 and 1000 iu.

Phosphate deficiency in premature infants fed breast milk

Premature infants are more and more frequently being fed their mother's (and occasionally bank) breast milk. Recent studies have shown that the protein and sodium content of the breast milk of a woman delivering prematurely is higher than that of a woman delivering at term[77] and, thus, more adequate to meet the needs of the premature infant. Unfortunately, this is not the case with calcium and phosphorus, which are both deficient in breast milk (calcium 300 mg/dl, 75 mmol/l; phosphorus 150 mg/dl, 49 mmol/l). The 2:1 calcium phosphorus ratio at these low levels may increase calcium absorption and the fat content of breast milk also is ideal for optimal calcium absorption so that the actual amount of calcium absorbed may approach the amount of calcium absorbed from standard formula. Phosphorus absorption is almost complete (90%) from either standard formula or breast milk so that the low phosphorus content is the limiting factor. Term breastfed infants maximally conserve phosphorus at the kidneys and bone mineralization is usually adequate. Phosphate supplementation of full-term infants increases calcium and magnesium retention. What is marginal for the full-term infant who has completed the mineralization that occurs in the third trimester, appears to be inadequate for the premature infant attempting that mineralization *extra utero*. Senterre[81] did balance studies on 10 premature infants of 1500–2020 g birthweight and 32–36 weeks gestation and found that, although calcium absorption was 49 ± 11%, calcium retention was poor with urinary excretion of calcium reaching 10 ± 5 mg/kg per day, about 40% of the calcium absorbed. Almost all of the phosphorus ingested was absorbed (89 ± 5%) and retained (87 ± 8%); however, the amount of phosphorus available from human milk was limited. In the face of a limited total phosphorus supply, phosphorus will preferentially go to tissues and not bone, so that the absorbed calcium cannot be used for bone accretion and is excreted in the urine. In our experience, as urine phosphorus falls to undetectable levels, urine calcium begins to rise and sharply increases at about 7–8 weeks in the 1100 g premature infant. At this point, serum phosphorus often falls below 4 mg/dl (1.3 mmol/l) resulting in suboptimal mineralization. In a study of growth of premature infants fed breast milk, serum phosphorus fell below 3 mg/dl (1.0 mmol/l) frequently. Very small infants can exhibit rickets attributable to phosphate deficiency[73]. Here serum phosphorus is low and serum PTH is normal or low, aminoaciduria is not seen and serum alkaline phosphatase is again elevated. It is desirable to follow the serum and urine calcium and phosphorus of all small premature infants exclusively fed breast milk. If the serum phosphorus falls below 4.0 and the urine calcium increases, phosphorus supplementation might reasonably be given.

A major variable in these infants is their serum 25-OHD concentration, since in our experience, infants with low serum 25-OHD levels almost always require phosphorus supplementation. Given 400 iu vitamin D supplement, breastfed premature infants have serum 25-OHD concentrations similar to the formula-fed premature infants, with serum 25-OHD remaining low in many cases. The infants studied by Senterre[81] were not supplemented with any vitamin D and, thus, probably had low 25-OHD concentration superimposed on their dietary restrictions of phosphorus.

Recent studies have been unable to confirm large amounts of vitamin D metabolites in breast milk[51] or show substantial biological activity[59]. Nevertheless, full-term infants have had a much lower incidence of rickets if fed human milk than cow's milk. Two recent studies measuring serum 25-OHD in breastfed infants have shown normal serum 25-OHD in this group; however, one showed improved serum 25-OHD levels with vitamin D supplementation[31] and one did not[15]. There is a high incidence of vitamin D deficiency rickets in breastfed infants of mothers who are on unusual, vitamin D-deficient diets and who have limited sun exposure[2].

The deformity, growth retardation, and dental abnormalities of vitamin D-resistant rickets (X-linked phosphate diabetes) are well known. However, the long-term effects of dietary phosphate deficiency rickets are unknown, and long-term follow up studies of these breastfed premature infants are needed. A recent study of full-term infants showed that the demineralization defined by bone densitometry[32] at 6 months of age had resolved by 1 year of age. Part of this probably reflects an increased phosphorus content of a mixed diet.

Treatment of phosphorus deficiency involves either the introduction of a phosphate supplement or a cow's milk based formula. Rowe *et al.*[73] recommended 20–25 mg/kg phosphate as potassium phosphate and we have used that dosage with much success. Serum and urine abnormalities usually correct after a week and improved mineralization is seen by 2–3 weeks. Some have prevented problems by supplementing all breast milk fed to premature infants with phosphorus to a calcium–phosphorus ratio of about 1.2:1[28, 81]. This regimen appears to be successful in a large number of infants in Europe but has not gained popularity in the United States.

Combination vitamin D deficiency and phosphate deficiency in premature infants fed special formulae

A high incidence of severe hypomineralization, fractures or frank rickets is seen in small premature infants fed a diet which results in both vitamin D and phosphorus deficiency. This was beautifully demonstrated in a large group of very small premature infants divided into four groups: (1) human milk without additional vitamin D; (2) human milk plus vitamin D; (3) cow's milk without vitamin D; and (4) cow's milk plus vitamin D. It was clear that increasing the dietary minerals markedly reduced the incidence of rickets. However, in the cow's milk group without vitamin D, the biochemical changes of vitamin D deficiency rickets could be seen[96].

Table 11.1 Clinical and laboratory findings of nine infants who developed rickets. Summary of data presented by Hoff *et al.*[52]. The table appeared in L. Hillman. Problems of bone mineralization in low birthweight infants fed soy fomula. In *Ross Clinical Research Conference on Low Birthweight Infants fed Isomil*. Columbus, Ohio, Ross Laboratories (1979)

Birthweight	948 ± 153 g
Gestational age	27.7 ± 1.1 weeks
Age at diagnosis	12.6 ± 2.8 weeks
Mean vitamin D since birth	300 ± 181 iu
Mean vitamin D at diagnosis	587 ± 313 iu
Calcium	8.1 ± 0.7 mg/dl
Phosphorus ($n = 3$)	4.0 ± 0.5 mg/dl
Alkaline phosphatase	1010 ± 426 iu/dl
Parathyroid hormone ($n = 5$)	40 ± 15 µl Eq/ml
25-Hydroxyvitamin D	< 3.6 ± 2.1 ng/ml
Formula	4 PM 60/40, 5 soy
Other diagnoses	5 bronchopulmonary dysplasia; 2 jaundice
X-ray	6 severe, 3 moderate rickets, 5 with fractures
Pathology	2/2 severe rickets

1 mg Ca/dl = 0.25 mmol/; 1 mg P/dl = 0.32 mmol/l.

In our nursery over a 1-year period of time, nine infants were identified with frank rickets. Their 25-OHD serum concentrations were less than 7 ng/ml and the PTH and alkaline phosphatase were markedly elevated, all consistent with classical vitamin D deficiency rickets (*Table 11.1*)[52] and they responded to vitamin D therapy. Another group of 10 infants were observed to have severe osteopenia with fractures, but no rachitic changes by X-ray. Their average serum 25-OHD was 8–12 ng/ml and they had low serum calcium, phosphorus and elevations of serum PTH[44] (*Table 11.2*). These were all very small premature infants (less than 1000 g) and they were all on non-standard formulae: either PM 60/40 where the calcium and phosphorus content was the same as breast milk, or a soy formula which was lactose-free and high in phytate concentration, or Pregestimil, which is also lactose-free. In these infants we speculated that there was vitamin D-deficiency rickets and that a low calcium or, more important, low phosphorus intake and/or absorption was further contributing to the problem. When soy formula was fed as the standard formula in another nursery, rickets was diagnosed by X-ray in 22 infants, about one-third of the susceptible small prematures[57]. No measurements of 25-OHD or PTH were available on these infants. In a prospective study of soy formula versus cow's milk formula in matched infants[56] 50% of infants on soy

Table 11.2 Clinical and laboratory findings of seven infants who developed osteopenia and fractures. Patients reported in abstract by Hillman *et al.*[43]. The table appeared in L. Hillman. Problems of bone mineralization in low birthweight infants fed soy formula. In *Ross Clinical Research Conference on Low Birthweight Infants fed Isomil*. Columbus, Ohio, Ross Laboratories (1979)

Birthweight	1032	± 223	g
Gestational age	28.4 ±	1.9	weeks
Age at diagnosis	11.4 ±	2.7	weeks
Vitamin D at diagnosis	> 500		iu
Calcium	8.1 ±	0.88	mg/dl
Phosphorus ($n = 3$)	4.8 ±	0.99	mg/dl
Alkaline phosphatase	888	± 266	iu/dl
Parathyroid hormone ($n = 5$)	25	± 13	μl Eq/ml
25-Hydroxyvitamin D	9.4 ±	2.8	ng/ml
Formula	5 Isomil, 2 Pregestimil		
Other diagnoses	3 bronchopulmonary dysplasia,		
	2 jaundice		
X-ray	7 severe osteopenia,		
	5 with fractures		

1 mg Ca/dl = 0.25 mmol/; 1 mg P/dl = 0.32 mmol/l.

formula developed rickets, whereas none did on standard formula, clearly identifying the formula as contributory. Studies of the formula would suggest that poor phosphorus absorption is universally present with calcium absorption very variable[85], and poor absorption of vitamin D is also a possibility[44]. When comparing infants who developed rickets on soy formula with those who did not, there were no differences in calcium, phosphorus and vitamin D intakes; biochemical differences, low phosphorus and high alkaline phosphatase commenced very early[14]. The infants with rickets were more frequently black and born in the spring when maternal 25-OHD and, thus, infant 25-OHD serum concentrations are low, and when any 25-OHD stores would be minimal. Thus, 25-OHD deficiency may be an underlying problem which is accentuated by the phosphorus deficiency of the formula producing frank rickets where only moderate to severe osteopenia is usually seen on a standard formula. Other lactose-free formulae may cause problems but require further study.

Thus, phosphate deficiency, whether secondary to breast milk feedings or feeding of a formula with poor phosphorus absorption, can lead to undermineralization. Although in the extremely premature infant fed exclusively breast milk a pure phosphorus deficiency rickets has been reported, in most infants severe hypomineralization results from a combined deficiency of phosphorus and 25-OHD. The hypomineralization can usually be corrected by supplementation with either phosphate or vitamin D, and each situation needs to be individually evaluated with serum and urine calcium and phosphorus, PTH, and 25-OHD measurements.

Finally, infants who are not fed orally at all, and who are fed by hyperalimentation also have a high incidence of rickets[58]. It is not clear if this results from the selected population given hyperalimentation, limitation of calcium and phosphorus intake, limitations of vitamin D intake, and/or further deficits in liver hydroxylation secondary to cholestatic liver disease[54]. Binstadt and L'Heuseux[8] reported 15 newborns, mostly premature infants, who developed radiographic rickets after a mean of 46 days of hyperalimentation early in life. The intravenous phosphorus supplied was 100–150 mg/kg per day. Vitamin D intake was at least 400 iu in most infants. However, only 100 iu a day was given intravenously. The rickets rapidly responded to treatment with higher dosages of vitamin D.

SUMMARY

We have characterized three types of neonatal hypocalcemia based on their time of occurrence in life: early neonatal hypocalcemia, late neonatal hypocalcemia, and demineralization and 'late-late' hypocalcemia.

Early neonatal hypocalcemia is prevalent in premature infants, infants of diabetic mothers, and asphyxiated infants. An exaggeration of the calcitonin surge probably plays a major role in premature and asphyxiated infants, while infants of diabetic mothers and premature infants may have a prolonged functional hypoparathyroidism. Early neonatal hypocalcemia is very frequent. It is rarely symptomatic, and the need for treatment is often unclear. Late sequelae are not described.

Late neonatal hypocalcemia occurs in full-term, otherwise healthy infants and is most common in vitamin D-deficient populations. The major pathological problem appears to be transient decreased parathyroid function, and a phosphate load may exaggerate the problem. There is a high association with unexplained hypomagnesemia especially in vitamin D-sufficient populations, and decreased secretion of PTH secondary to hypomagnesemia may be one cause of abnormal parathyroid function. Late neonatal hypocalcemia is much less frequent than early neonatal hypocalcemia; however, the infants are usually symptomatic often with seizures and the entity always requires treatment with additional calcium and often magnesium supplementation and/or phosphate restriction. Abnormal calcification of infant teeth is a frequent long-term sequela; however, other development is apparently normal.

Late-late neonatal hypocalcemia is seen in very premature infants and is associated with severe osteopenia or rickets. Its etiology appears to be a combination of calcium and phosphorus deficiency and an effective vitamin D metabolite deficiency. Both high calcium–high phosphorus formulae and 25-hydroxycholecalciferol to normalize serum 25-OHD have improved mineralization and decreased hypocalcemia. Severe demineralization occurs most frequently when a phosphorus deficiency is superimposed on 25-OHD deficiency as was seen with soy formulae and formulae designed to mimic human milk. Human milk *per se*, when fed to the very small premature infant, often produces a classical phosphate-deficiency rickets.

References

1 ANAST, C. and DIRKSEN, H. Neonatal hypocalcemia. In *Vitamin D: Biochemical, Chemical and Clinical Aspects Related to Calcium Metabolism*, edited by A. W. Norman, K. Schaefer, J. W. Coburn, H. F. DeLuca, D. Fraser, H. G. Grigoleit and D. V. Herrath, p. 727. New York, Walter De Gruyter and Co. (1977)

2 BACHRACH, S., FISHER, J. and PARKS, J. S. An outbreak of vitamin D deficiency rickets in a susceptible population. *Pediatrics*, **64**, 871–877 (1979)

3 BARAK, Y., MILBAUER, B., WEISMAN, Y., EDELSTEIN, E. and SPIRER, Z. Response of neonatal hypocalcemia to 1α-hydroxyvitamin D_3. *Archives of Disease in Childhood*, **54**, 642–643 (1979)

4 BARLET, J. P. and GAREL, J. M. Hormonal regulation of calcium metabolism in the newborn. *Annales de Biologie Animale, Biochemie, Biophysique*, **18**, 69–80 (1978)

5 BARLTROP, D. and OPPÉ, T. Calcium and fat absorption by low birthweight infants from a calcium-supplemented milk formula. *Archives of Disease in Childhood*, **48**, 580–582 (1973)

6 BARLTROP, D., MOLE, R. and SUTTON, A. Absorption and endogenous faecal excretion of calcium by low birthweight infants on feeds with varying contents of calcium and phosphate. *Archives of Disease in Childhood*, **52**, 41–49 (1977)

7 BERGMAN, L., WESTERBERG, B., LINDSTEDT, G. and LUNDBERG, P.-A. Possible involvement of growth hormone in the pathogenesis of early neonatal hypocalcemia in infants of diabetic mothers. *Biology of the Neonate*, **34**, 72–79 (1978)

8 BINSTADT, D. H. and L'HEUREUX, P. R. Rickets as a complication of intravenous hyperalimentation in infants. *Pediatric Radiology*, **7**, 211–214 (1978)

9 BISHOP, J. E. and NORMAN, A. W. Studies on calciferol metabolism: metabolism of 25-hydroxyvitamin D_3 by the chicken embryo. *Archives of Biochemistry and Biophysics*, **167**, 769–773 (1975)

10 BOISSIERE, H., CAGNAT, R., POISSONNIER, M. and d'ANGELY, S. Dystrophie ostéomalacique du prématuré. *Annual de Pédiatrié*, **June/July**, 367 (1964)

11 BOUILLON, R., VAN ASSCHE, F. A., VAN BAELEN, H., HEYNS, W. and De MOOR, P. Influence of the vitamin D-binding protein on the serum concentration of 1,25-dihydroxyvitamin D_3: significance of the free 1,25-dihydroxyvitamin D_3 concentration. *Journal of Clinical Investigation*, **67**, 589–596 (1981)

12 BROOKE, O. G., BROWN, I. R. F., BONE, C. D. M., CARTER, N. D., CLEEVE, H. J. N., MAXWELL, J., ROBINSON V. P. and WINDES, S. M. Vitamin D supplements in pregnant Asian women: effects on calcium status and fetal growth. *British Medical Journal*, **280**, 751–754 (1980)

13 BROWN, I. R. F., BROOKE, O. G. and HASWELL, D. J. Vitamin D and plasma magnesium in pregnancy. *Clinica Chimica Acta*, **111,** 109–111 (1981)

14 CALLENBAC, J. C., SHEEHAN, M. B., ABRAMSON, S. J. and HALL, R. T. Etiologic factors in rickets of very low-birthweight infants. *Journal of Pediatrics*, **98,** 800–805 (1981)

15 CHAN, G. M., TSANG, R. C., CHEN, I.-W., DeLUCA, H. F. and STEICHEN, J. J. The effect of 1,25(OH)$_2$ vitamin D$_3$ supplementation in premature infants. *Journal of Pediatrics*, **93,** 91–96 (1978)

16 COCKBURN, F., BROWN, J. K., BELTON, N. R. and FORFAR, J. O. Neonatal convulsions associated with primary disturbance of calcium phosphorus, and magnesium metabolism. *Archives of Diseases in Childhood*, **48,** 99–107 (1973)

17 COCKBURN, F., BELTON, N. R., PURVIS, R. J., GILES, M. M., BROWN, J. K. and TURNER, T. L. *et al.* Maternal vitamin D intake and mineral metabolism in mothers and their newborn infants. *British Medical Journal*, **281,** 11–14 (1980)

18 CRUIKSHANK, D. P., PITKIN, R. M., REYNOLDS, W. A., WILLIAMS, G. A. and HARGIS, G. K. Altered maternal calcium homeostasis in diabetic pregnancy. *Journal of Clinical Endocrinology and Metabolism*, **50,** 264–267 (1980)

19 DAVID, L. and ANAST, C. S. Calcium metabolism in newborn infants: the interrelationship of parathyroid function and calcium, magnesium, and phosphorus metabolism in normal, 'sick', and hypocalcemic newborns. *Journal of Clinical Investigation*, **54,** 287–296 (1974)

20 DAVID, L., SALLE, B. L., PUTET, G. and GRAFMEYER, D. Serum immunoreactive calcitonin in low birthweight infants. Description of early changes; effect of intravenous calcium infusion; relationships with early changes in serum calcium, phosphorus, magnesium, parathyroid hormone and gastrin levels. *Pediatric Research*, **15,** 803–808 (1981)

21 DAY, G., CHANCE, G., RADDE, I., REILLY, B., PARK, E. and SHEEPERS, J. Growth mineral metabolism in very low birthweight infants. II. Effect of calcium supplementation on growth and divalent cations *Pediatric Research*, **9,** 568 (1975)

22 DIRKSEN, H. C. and ANAST, C. S. Hypercalcitonemia and neonatal hypocalcemia. *Pediatric Research*, **11,** 424 (1977)

23 FAKHRAEE, S. H., HILLMAN, L. S., SLATOPOLSKY, E. and BELL, M. J. Hypomagnesemia and parathyroid hormone (PTH). Deficiency in classical late neonatal hypocalcemia (CLNH) and surgically related late neonatal hypocalcemia (SLNH). *Pediatric Research*, **14,** 571 (1980)

24 FLEISCHMAN, A. R., ROSEN, J. F. and NATHENSON, G. 25-hydroxyvitamin D: serum levels and oral administration of calcifediol in neonates. *Archives of Internal Medicine*, **138,** 869–873 (1978)

25 FORFAR, J. O. Normal and abnormal calcium, phosphorus and magnesium metabolism in the perinatal period. *Clinics in Endocrinology and Metabolism*, **5,** 123–134 (1976)

26 GAREL, J. M. and BARLET, J. P. Calcitonin in mother, fetus and newborn. *Annales de Biologie Animale, Biochimie, Biophysique*, **18,** 53–68 (1978)

27 GLASGOW, J. F. T. and THOMAS, P. S. Rachitic respiratory distress in small preterm infants. *Archives of Disease in Childhood*, **52,** 268–273 (1977)

28 GLORIEUX, F., SALLE, B. L., DELVIN, E. E. and DAVID, L. Vitamin D metabolism in preterm infants: serum calcitriol levels during the first five days of life. *Journal of Pediatrics*, **99,** 640–643 (1981)

29 GLORIEUX, F. H., SALLE, B., DELVIN, E. E. and DAVID, L. Vitamin D metabolism in preterm infants (PI) and infants born from diabetic mothers (DM). *Pediatric Research*, **14,** 572 (1980)

30 GRAHNEN, H., SJOLIN, S. and STENSTROM, A. Mineralization defects of primary teeth in children born pre-term. *Scandanavian Journal of Dental Research*, **82,** 396–400 (1974)

31 GREER, F. R., SEARCY, J. E., LEVIN, R. S., STEICHEN, J. J., STEICHEN-ASCH, P. and TSANG, R. C. Bone mineral content and serum 25-hydroxyvitamin D concentration in breast-fed infants with and without supplemental vitamin D. *Journal of Pediatrics*, **98,** 696–701 (1981)

32 GREER, F. R., SEARCY, J. E., LEVIN, R. S., STEICHEN, J. J. and TSANG, R. C. Decreased bone mineral content (BMC) in breastfed infants without supplemental vitamin D (D): 'catch up' mineralization at 6 months and one year; possible effects on length. *Pediatric Research*, **15,** 533 (1981)

33 HADDAD, J. G., HILLMAN, L. and ROJANASATHIT, S. Human serum binding capacity and affinity for 25-hydroxyergocalciferol and 25-hydroxycholecalciferol. *Journal of Clinical Endocrinology and Metabolism*, **43,** 86–91 (1976)

34 HADDAD, J. G., Jr and ROJANASATHIT, S. Acute administration of 25-hydroxy-cholecalciferol in man. *Journal of Clinical Endocrinology and Metabolism*, **42,** 284–290 (1976)

35 HECKMATT, J. Z., DAVIES, A. E. J., PEACOCK, M., McMURRAY, J. and ISHERWOOD, D. M. Plasma 25-hydroxyvitamin D in pregnant Asian women and their babies. *Lancet*, **2,** 546–549 (1979)

36 HILLMAN, L. S. and HADDAD, J. G. Human perinatal vitamin D metabolism. I: 25-hydroxyvitamin D in maternal and cord blood. *Journal of Pediatrics*, **84,** 742–749 (1974)

37 HILLMAN, L. S. and HADDAD, J. G. Perinatal vitamin D metabolism. II: Serial concentrations in sera of term and premature infant. *Journal of Pediatrics*, **86,** 928–935 (1975)

38 HILLMAN, L. S. and HADDAD, J. G. Perinatal vitamin D metabolism. III: Factors influencing late gestational human serum 25-hydroxyvitamin D. *American Journal of Obstetrics and Gynecology*, **125,** 196–200 (1976)

39 HILLMAN, L., ROJANASATHIT, S., SLATOPOLSKY, E. and HADDAD, J. G. Serial measure-ments of serum calcium, magnesium, parathyroid hormone, calcitonin, and 25-hydroxyvitamin D in premature and term infants during the first week of life. *Pediatric Research*, **11,** 739 (1977)

40 HILLMAN, L., SLATOPOLSKY, E. and HADDAD, J. G. Perinatal vitamin D metabolism. IV: Maternal and cord serum 24,25-dihydroxyvitamin D concentrations. *Journal of Clinical Endocrinology and Metabolism*, **47,** 1073–1077 (1978)

41 HILLMAN, L. S., HOFF, N., SLATOPOLSKY, E. and HADDAD, J. G. Serial calcitonin serum concentrations in premature infants during the first 12 weeks of life. *Calcified Tissue International* (in press)

42 HILLMAN, L., HADDAD, J. G. and HUEBENER, D. Long-term effects of low 25-hydroxyvitamin D (25-OHD) serum concentrations in premature infants: a preliminary report. *4th Workshop in Vitamin D*, edited by A. W. Norman *et al.*, p. 81. New York, Walter de Gruyter and Co. (1979)

43 HILLMAN, L. S., MARTIN, L. A. and HADDAD, J. G. Absorption and maintenance dosage of 25-hydroxycholecalciferol (25-HCC) in premature infants. *Pediatric Research*, **13**, 400 (1979)

44 HILLMAN, L., HOFF, N., MARTIN, L. and HADDAD, J. G. Osteopenia, hypocalcemia, and low 25-hydroxyvitamin D (25-OHD) serum concentrations with use of soy formula. *Pediatric Research*, **13**, 400 (1979)

45 HILLMAN, L. S., HOFF, N., MARTIN, L. A. and HADDAD, J. G. Serum 25-hydroxyvitamin D (25-OHD) deficiency in premature infants. *Pediatric Research*, **13**, 475 (1979)

46 HILLMAN, L. S. and HADDAD, J. G. Vitamin D metabolism and bone mineralization in premature and small-for-gestational-age infants. In *Pediatric Diseases Related to Calcium*, edited by H. F. DeLuca and C. S. Anast, New York, Elsevier (1980)

47 HILLMAN, L., HADDAD, J. G., CRYER, P. and SCOTT, S. Failure to relate catecholamines and glucagon to the degree of calcitonin surge in normal newborn infants. *Pediatric Research*, **14**, 573 (1980)

48 HILLMAN, L., MARTIN, L., FIORI, B. and HADDAD, J. G. Failure of calcium (Ca) and phosphorus (P) supplementation to correct low serum 25-hydroxyvitamin D (25-OHD) concentrations in premature infants. *Pediatric Research*, **14**, 574 (1980)

49 HILLMAN, L., MARTIN, L. and FIORE, B. Effect of oral copper supplementation on serum copper and ceruloplasmin concentrations in premature infants. *Journal of Pediatrics*, **98**, 311–313 (1981)

50 HILLMAN, L. and HADDAD, J. G. Serum vitamin D binding protein (DBP) in preterm infants. *Pediatric Research*, **15**, 631 (1981)

51 HO, M., GREER, F. R., EVANS, D. D. and TSANG, R. C. Lack of 25-hydroxyvitamin D, 25-hydroxyvitamin D-like compound, or 1,25(OH)$_2$D in human milk. *Pediatric Research*, **14**, 501 (1980)

52 HOFF, N., HADDAD, J. G., TEITELBAUM, S., McALISTER, W. and HILLMAN, L. Serum concentrations of 25-hydroxyvitamin D in rickets of extremely premature infants. *Journal of Pediatrics*, **94**, 460–466 (1979)

53 KHATTAB, A. K. and FORFAR, J. O. The interrelationship between calcium, phosphorus and glucose levels in mother and infant in conditions commonly associated with placental insufficiency. *Biology of the Neonate*, **18**, 1–16 (1970)

54 KOBAYASHI, A., KAWAI, S., OHKUBO, M. and OHBE, Y. Serum 25-hydroxy-vitamin D in hepatobiliary disease in infancy. *Archives of Disease in Childhood*, **54**, 367–370 (1979)

55 KRISHNAMACHARI, K. A. V. R. and IYENGAR, L. Effect of maternal malnutrition on the bone density of the neonates. *American Journal of Clinical Nutrition*, **28**, 482–486 (1975)

56 KULKARNI, P. B. Prospective study of rickets in very-low-birth-weight infants fed by formula. In *Ross Clinical Research Conference, Low-birth-weight infants fed Isomil*. Columbus, Ohio, Ross Laboratories (1979)

57 KULKARNI, P. B., HALL, R. T., RHODES, P. G., SHEEHAN, M. B., CALLENDACH, J. C., GERMANN, D. D. and ABRAMSON, S. J. Rickets in low birthweight infants. *Journal of Pediatrics*, **96**, 249–252 (1980)

58 LEAPE, L. and VALAES, T. Rickets in low birthweight infants receiving total parenteral nutrition. *Journal of Pediatric Surgery*, **11**, 665–674 (1976)

59 LEERBECK, E. and SØNDERGAARD, H. The total content of vitamin D in human milk and cow's milk. *British Journal of Nutrition*, **44,** 7–12 (1980)

60 LEROYER-ALIZON, E., DAVID, L. and DUBOIS, P. M. Evidence for calcitonin in the thyroid gland of normal and anencephalic human fetuses: immunocytological localization, radioimmunoassay, and gel filtration of thyroid extracts. *Journal of Clinical Endocrinology and Metabolism*, **50,** 316–321 (1980)

61 LEWIN, P. K., REID, M., SWYER, P. R. and FRASER, D. Iatrogenic rickets in low-birthweight infants. *Journal of Pediatrics*, **78,** 207–210 (1971)

62 MALLET, E., BASUYAU, J.-P., BRUNELLE, P., DEVAUX, A.-M. and FESSARD, C. Neonatal parathyroid secretion and renal receptor maturation in premature infants. *Biology of the Neonate*, **33,** 304–308 (1978)

63 MINTON, S. D., STEICHEN, J. J. and TSANG, R. C. Bone mineral content in term and preterm appropriate-for-gestational-age infants. *Journal of Pediatrics*, **95,** 1037–1042 (1979)

64 NOGUCHI, A., EREN, M. and TSANG, R. C. Parathyroid hormone in hypocalcemic and normocalcemic infants of diabetic mothers. *Journal of Pediatrics*, **97,** 112–114 (1980)

65 OPPENHEIMER, S. J. and SNODGRASS, G. J. A. I. Neonatal rickets. *Archives of Disease in Childhood*, **55,** 945–949 (1980)

66 PAUNIER, L., LACOURT, G., PILLOUD, P., SCHLAEPPI, P. and SIZONENKO, P. 25-hydroxyvitamin D and calcium levels in maternal, cord and infant serum in relation to maternal vitamin D intake. *Helvetica Paediatrica Acta*, **33,** 95–103 (1978)

67 PETTIFOR, J. M., ISDALE, J. M., SAHAKIAN, J. and HANSEN, J. D. L. Diagnosis of subclinical rickets. *Archives of Disease in Childhood*, **55,** 155–157 (1980)

68 PURVIS, R. J., MacKAY, G. S., COCKBURN, F., BARRIE, W. J. H. WILKINSON, E. M., BELTON, N. R. and FORFAR, J. O. Enamel hypoplasia of the teeth associated and neonatal tetany: a manifestation of maternal vitamin D deficiency. *Lancet*, **2,** 811–814 (1973)

69 RAMAN, L., RAJALAKSHMI, K., KRISHNAMACHARI, K. A. V. R. and SASTRY, J. G. Effect of calcium supplementation to undernourished mothers during pregnancy on the bone density of the neonates. *American Journal of Clinical Nutrition*, **31,** 466–469 (1978)

70 ROBERTS, S. A., COHEN, M. D. and FORFAR, J. O. Antenatal factors associated with neonatal hypocalcemic convulsions. *Lancet*, **2,** 809–811 (1973)

71 ROBINSON, M. J., MERRETT, A. L., TETLOW, V. A. and COMPSTON, J. E. Plasma 25-hydroxyvitamin D concentrations in preterm infants receiving oral vitamin D supplements. *Archives of Disease in Childhood*, **56,** 144–155 (1981)

72 ROMAGNOLI, C., POLIDORI, G., CATALDI, L., TORTOROLO, G. and SEGNI, G. Phototherapy-induced hypocalcemia. *Journal of Pediatrics*, **94,** 815–816 (1979)

73 ROWE, J. C., WOOD, D. H., ROWE, D. W. and RAISZ, L. G. Nutritional hypophosphatemic rickets in a premature infant fed breast milk. *New England Journal of Medicine*, **300,** 293–296 (1979)

74 SALLE, B. L., DAVID, L., CHOPARD, J. P., GRAFMEYER, D. C. and RENAUD, H. Prevention of early neonatal hypocalcemia in low birthweight infants with continuous calcium infusion: effect on serum calcium, phosphorus, magnesium, and circulating immunoreactive parathyroid hormone and calcitonin. *Pediatric Research*, **11,** 1180–1185 (1977)

75 SALLE, B. L., DAVID, L., GLORIEUX, F. H., DELVIN, E., SENTERRE, J. and RENAUD, H. Early oral administration of vitamin D and its metabolites in premature neonates, effect on mineral homeostasis. *Pediatric Research*, **16**, 75–78 (1982)

76 SAMAAN, N. A., ANDERSON, G. D. and ADAM-MAYNE, M. Immunoreactive calcitonin in the mother, neonate, child and adult. *American Journal of Obstetrics and Gynecology*, **121**, 622–625 (1975)

77 SANN, L., BIENVENU, F., LAHET, C., BIENVENU, J. and BETHENOD, M. Comparison of the composition of breast milk from mothers of term and preterm infants. *Acta Paediatrica Scandinavica*, **70**, 115–116 (1981)

78 SCHEDEWIE, H. K., ODELL, W. D., FISHER, D. A., DRUTZIK, S. R., DODGE, M., COUSINS, L. and FISER, W. P. Parathormone and perinatal calcium homeostasis. *Pediatric Research*, **13**, 1–6 (1979)

79 SCOTT, S. M., LADENSON, J. H., AGUANNO, J. J. and HILLMAN, L. S. Ionized calcium in the sick neonate. *Pediatric Research*, **13**, 505 (1979)

80 SCOTT, S., LADENSON, J. H. and HILLMAN, L. S. Effect of treatment of early neonatal hypocalcemia (ENHC) on ionized calcium (Ca_i) and calcitonin (HCT). *Pediatric Research*, **14**, 581 (1980)

81 SENTERRE, J. Calcium and phosphorus retention in preterm infants. In *Intensive Care in the New Born, II*, edited by L. Stern, W. Oh and B. Friis-Hansen, pp. 205–215. New York, Masson Publishing USA, Inc. (1978)

82 SENTERRE, J., DAVID, L. and SALLE, B. Effect of 1,25–dihydroxycholecalciferol on calcium phosphorus and magnesium balance in preterm infants. *Annales d'Endocrinologie*, **40**, 163–164 (1979)

83 SHAW, J. C. L. Evidence for defective skeletal mineralization in low-birthweight infants: the absorption of calcium and fat. *Pediatrics*, **57**, 16–25 (1976)

84 SHENAI, J. P., REYNOLDS, J. W. and BABSON, S. G. Nutritional balance studies in very low-birthweight infants: enhanced nutrient retention rates by an experimental formula. *Pediatrics*, **66**, 233–238 (1980)

85 SHENAI, J. P., JHAVERI, D. M., REYNOLDS, J. W., HUSTON, R. K. and BABSON, S. G. Nutritional balance studies in very low-birthweight infants: role of soy formula. *Pediatrics*, **67**, 631–637 (1981)

86 STEICHEN, J. J. GRATTON, T. L. and TSANG, R. C. Osteopenia of prematurity: the cause and possible treatment. *Journal of Pediatrics*, **96**, 528–534 (1980)

87 STEICHEN, J. J., HO, M., HUG, G. and TSANG, R. C. Elevated serum 1,25(OH)$_2$ vitamin D (1,25(OH)$_2$D) concentrations in rickets of prematurity. *Pediatric Research*, **14**, 581 (1980)

88 STEICHEN, J. J., TSANG, R. C., GRATTON, T. L., HAMSTRA, A. and DeLUCA, H. F. Vitamin D homeostasis in the perinatal period. *New England Journal of Medicine*, **302**, 315–319 (1980)

89 STEICHEN, J. J., TSANG, R. C., HO, M., KNOWLES, H., LAVIN, J. and MIODOVNIK, M. 1,25(OH)$_2$ vitamin D (1,25(OH)$_2$D) and incidence of hypocalcemia in infants of diabetic mothers (IDM) in relation to prospective randomized treatment during pregnancy. *Pediatric Research*, **15**, 683 (1981)

90 TSANG, R. C. and OH, W. Serum magnesium levels in low birthweight infants. *American Journal of Diseases of Children*, **120**, 44–48 (1970)

91 TSANG, R. C., LIGHT, I. J., SUTHERLAND, J. M. and KLEINMAN, L. I. Possible pathogenetic factors in neonatal hypocalcemia of prematurity. *Journal of Pediatrics*, **82,** 423–429 (1973)

92 TSANG, R. C., CHEN, I.-W., FRIEDMAN, M. A. and CHEN, I. Neonatal parathyroid function: Role of gestation age and postnatal age. *Journal of Pediatrics*, **83,** 728–738 (1973)

93 TSANG, R. C. CHEN, I., HAYES, W., ATKINSON, W., ATHERTON, H. and EDWARDS, N. Neonatal hypocalcemia in infants with birth asphyxia. *Journal of Pediatrics*, **84,** 428–433 (1974)

94 TSANG, R. C., GIGGER, M., OH, W. and BROWN, D. R. Studies in calcium metabolism in infants with intrauterine growth retardation. *Journal of Pediatrics*, **86,** 936–941 (1975)

95 TWARDOCK, A. R. and AUSTIN, M. K. Calcium transfer in perfused guinea pig placenta. *American Journal of Physiology*, **219,** 540–545 (1970)

96 VON SUDOW, G. A study of the development of rickets in premature infants. *Acta Paediatrica Scandinavica*, **33,** Suppl 2, (1946)

97 WEISSMAN, Y., OCCHIPINTI, M., KNOX, G., REITER, E. and ROOT, A. Concentrations of 24,25-dihydroxyvitamin D and 25-hydroxyvitamin D in paired maternal-cord sera. *American Journal of Obstetrics and Gynecology*, **130,** 704–707 (1978)

98 WEISSMAN, Y., HARRELL, A., EDELSTEIN, S., DAVID, M., SPIRER, Z. and GOLANDER, A. 25-dihydroxy vitamin D_3 and 24,25-dihydroxy vitamin D_3 *in vitro* synthesis by human decidua and placenta. *Nature*, **281,** 317–319 (1979)

99 WIELAND, P., DUC, G., BINSWANGER, U. and FISCHER, J. Parathyroid hormone response in newborn infants during exchange transfusion with blood supplemented with citrate and phosphate: effect of IV calcium. *Pediatric Research*, **13,** 963–968 (1979)

100 WOLFE, H., GROFF, U. and OFFERMANS, G. The vitamin D_3 requirements for premature infants. *4th Workshop on Vitamin D*, edited by A. W. Norman *et al.* p. 87. New York, Walter de Gruyter and Co. (1979)

Index

Acromegaly, 242
Acro-osteolysis, 170
Adenoma, parathyroid, 181, 200, 241
Adenylate cyclase,
  calcitonin stimulation of, 13
  parathyroid hormone-sensitive, 2, 94, 95,
    99
    in *Hyp* mice, 21
Age,
  calcium absorption, 262
  extraskeletal calcification, 164
  osteoporosis, 47–50, 69
  primary hyperparathyroidism, 201
  rickets, osteomalacia, 128–133, 142
Alcohol, 56, 104
Alkaline phosphatase, serum,
  in infants, 262
  PTH-induced bone disease, 197
  in renal osteodystrophy, 168, 180
  in rickets, osteomalacia, 135, 139, 262
Alopecia, 28, 30, 35
Aluminium,
  dialysis osteomalacia, 157, 165, 176
  renal osteodystrophy treatment, 157, 176
Aluminium hydroxide, antacid,
  osteomalacia, 143
Aminoaciduria, 25, 26, 262
6-Aminohexane-1,1-bisphosphonate, 115
3-Amino 1-hydroxypropylidene-1,1-
  bisphosphonate (APD), 115, 121
Anabolic agents, 60, 73
Androgens, osteoporosis, 59, 60, 73, 82, 83
Androstenedione, 59, 60
Anticonvulsant drugs, 14, 128, 129, 144
APD, 115, 121
ARVDD, *see under* Rickets
Asphyxia, in infants, 99
Autosomal dominant hypophosphataemic
  rickets (ADHR), *see* Rickets

Autosomal recessive vitamin D-dependency
  rickets (ARVDD), *see* Rickets

Bed, oscillating, 52
Bendrofluazide, 52
Bisphosphonates, 114–121 (*see also*
    Diphosphonates)
  actions, 114
  bone scanning, 116
  medical uses, 116–120
  metabolism, 115
Bone,
  biopsy, mineralization, 117, 120
  disease,
    Fanconi's syndrome, 23
    hypophosphataemic, *see*
      Hypophosphataemic bone disease
  ectopic, 118
  formation, parathyroid hormone, 94
  hypomineralization, infants, 258–264
  loss, oophorectomy, 57–59, 61
  mass, 47, 48–50
    loss, *see* Osteoporosis
    measurements, 47, 54, 175
  metastases, 238
  mineralization, (*see also* Osteomalacia)
    bisphosphonates, 117, 118, 120
    defective, factors causing, 156–158
    in fetus, 247–249
    in osteoporosis treatment, *see*
      Osteoporosis
    in phosphopenic rickets, 17, 22
  osteoporotic, 47, 48
  pain, 160
  in primary hyperparathyroidism, 204–206
  resorption,
    bisphosphonates, reduction, 114, 117,
      120, 121

277